A City without Care

STUDIES IN SOCIAL MEDICINE

Allan M. Brandt, Larry R. Churchill, and Jonathan Oberlander, *editors*

This series publishes books at the intersection of medicine, health, and society that further our understanding of how medicine and society shape one another historically, politically, and ethically. The series is grounded in the convictions that medicine is a social science, that medicine is humanistic and cultural as well as biological, and that it should be studied as a social, political, ethical, and economic force.

A complete list of books published in Studies in Social Medicine is available at https://uncpress.org/series/studies-social-medicine.

KEVIN McQUEENEY

A City without Care

300 Years of Racism, Health Disparities, and Health Care Activism in New Orleans

The University of North Carolina Press *Chapel Hill*

This book was published with the assistance of the Authors Fund of the University of North Carolina Press.

© 2023 Kevin McQueeney
All rights reserved
Set in Arno Pro by Westchester Publishing Services
Manufactured in the United States of America

Library of Congress Cataloging-in-Publication Data
Names: McQueeney, Kevin, author.
Title: A city without care : 300 years of racism, health disparities, and health care activism in New Orleans / Kevin McQueeney.
Other titles: Studies in social medicine.
Description: Chapel Hill : University of North Carolina Press, [2023] | Series: Studies in social medicine | Includes bibliographical references and index.
Identifiers: LCCN 2022036485 | ISBN 9781469673912 (cloth ; alk. paper) | ISBN 9781469673929 (paperback ; alk. paper) | ISBN 9781469673936 (ebook)
Subjects: LCSH: Discrimination in medical care—Louisiana—New Orleans—History. | African Americans—Medical care—Louisiana—New Orleans. | African Americans—Segregation—Louisiana—New Orleans. | Slavery—Economic aspects—Louisiana—New Orleans. | New Orleans (La.) —Race relations.
Classification: LCC RA448.N3854 M37 2023 | DDC 362.1089/96076335—dc23/eng/20220912
LC record available at https://lccn.loc.gov/2022036485

Cover photo: Clinic patients at Flint-Goodridge Hospital, from Jay S. Stowell, *Methodist Adventures in Negro Education* (New York: The Methodist Book Concern, 1922). Courtesy of Schomburg Center for Research in Black Culture, New York Public Library.

To the memory of Michael Mizell-Nelson (1969–2014)

Contents

List of Illustrations ix

Acknowledgments xi

Introduction 1

CHAPTER ONE
Health and Health Care in the Era of Slavery, 1718–1843 17

CHAPTER TWO
The Growth of the Slave-Based Health Care Economy, 1800–1861 33

CHAPTER THREE
The Civil War, Reconstruction, and the Rise of Jim Crow Health Care, 1862–1900 51

CHAPTER FOUR
A White Medical District, 1900–1940 78

CHAPTER FIVE
Jim Crow Black Health Care, 1927–1950 99

CHAPTER SIX
Health Care in the Era of Civil Rights and Resistance, 1950–1968 123

CHAPTER SEVEN
Two-Tiered Health Care, 1965–1974 149

CHAPTER EIGHT
Black Health Care in the Age of Abandonment, 1975–2005 175

Conclusion: Black Health and Health Care after Katrina 193

Appendix 217

Notes 225

Bibliography 247

Index 261

Illustrations

FIGURES

4.1   The 1929 New Orleans Comprehensive Plan   87
5.1   Dedication of Flint Goodridge Hospital in October 1931   107
A.1   Charity Hospital prior to expansion in 1934   218
A.2   Aerial view of the recently completed Charity Hospital complex in 1940   219
A.3   Proposed HEAL plan for the New Orleans Medical District, 1969   220

MAPS

A.1   The Medical District in 1913   217
A.2   Select New Orleans medical institutions   221

TABLES

A.1   Population of New Orleans, 1769–2019   222
A.2   Number of Black and white medical doctors and ratio of doctors to population, 1791–1940   223
A.3   New Orleans mortality rates by race, 1810–2020   224

Acknowledgments

This work is only possible due to the aid of archivists. I wish to thank the staff at Amistad Research; the City Archives, New Orleans Public Library; the Ethel and Herman Midlo Center for New Orleans Studies, University of New Orleans; the Historic New Orleans Collection; the Howard University Archives; the Louisiana Collection, University of New Orleans; the Louisiana Research Center, Tulane University; the Louisiana State Archives; the Louisiana State Museum Historical Center; the Notarial Archives; the Rudolph Matas Library of the Health Sciences, Tulane University; and the Southeastern Architectural Archive, Tulane University. I am extremely grateful to Phillip Cunningham at the Amistad Research Center and John Kennedy at the Dillard University Archives. This project fittingly began and ended with visits to the archives at Dillard University, and John has been exceptionally kind and helpful.

My work as a historian started at the University of New Orleans. I could not have asked for a more supportive space to develop my academic skills and interests. I am forever grateful for the guidance of Connie Atkinson, Molly Mitchell, James Mokhiber, Andrea Mosterman, and Michael Mizell-Nelson. Molly Mitchell has continually been a mentor and supporter, and I am in her debt. Words cannot express how much Michael Mizell-Nelson has shaped my career and my life. Michael inspired my interest in public history and my desire to be a historian of New Orleans. He believed in me and my work and taught me that passion and kindness are the most important qualities in a teacher. He is deeply missed.

At UNO, I was fortunate to be in a cohort of wonderful people, primarily Graham Cooper, Jessica Dauterive, Lee Facincani, Emma Long, Brett Todd, and Pamela Walker. Lee, drinks at the German House are in order. Jessica, thank you for being such a great friend and colleague.

During my time as PhD student at Georgetown University, I learned from many incredible scholars. I wish to thank Katherine Benton-Cohen, Marcia Chatelain, David Collins, Michael Kazin, Joseph McCartin, Meredith McKittrick, Timothy Newfield, David Painter, Adam Rothman, and Jordan Sand. Timothy Newfield's Historical Epidemiology class made me want to be a historian of medicine and disease. No person is more responsible for this project than Marcia Chatelain. She is the rarest combination of brilliance and kindness, and the ultimate academic role model.

My cohort at Georgetown was filled with a group of talented individuals. I wish to thank Matthew Johnson, Matthew Lalime, Abhishek Nanavati, Trishula Patel, and Molly Thacker, and I look forward to reading their works and seeing where their paths take them. I especially want to thank Matthew Johnson for his encouragement and friendship.

Thank you to my colleagues at Nicholls State University. In particular, I am extremely grateful to Shae Smith Cox, who every day inspires me to be a better mentor, scholar, and teacher. I am also fortunate to work with fantastic students, principally those in the Clio History Club.

Thanks to all my friends, especially to those who have continued to ask about the progress of this work. To Anna Mahoney and Patrick Mahoney, my deepest gratitude for constant support and guidance. Saturday nights with Daria Dzurik and Graham Robinson are always a highlight, and Daria has been the biggest proponent of this book. Angela Grittman, Caleb Hicks, Kat Wampold, Morgan Wampold, Megan Webb, and Tyler White are a wonderful group, and I am fortunate to be in their company. Andreas Meyris, Jack Garratt, Sarah Roman Garratt, Kate Steir, Chelsea Tengels, Katherine Steir, Sarah Roman—it is always good to look upon you. To my Rutgers friends—George Alvarez, Mehmet Başoğlu, Brendan Finley, Brian Hartigan, John Ruff—thanks for many years of friendship. Shipra Pandya and Quinn Z. Edwards have helped sustain me with their much-needed phone calls. Special thanks to my family—my dad, my mom, my brother Mike, Jess (for the maps and for the continuous support), Duke, Dundee, Lottie, and Myrtle. Finally, I greatly appreciate Lucas Church and the team at UNC Press for their help in making this book a reality.

A City without Care

Introduction

In May 1974, M. A. Galathe knew something was seriously wrong with his fifteen-year-old daughter. For weeks, she had been repeatedly fainting. Galathe brought her to a private physician, but the doctor could not determine the cause of her problems. The doctor gave Galathe a referral to Ochsner Foundation Hospital, the leading center for medical research in the New Orleans area. Galathe, his daughter, and his wife took the referral to the hospital, and attendants asked them to sit in the waiting room. While waiting to be seen, the daughter again fainted. Galathe approached the desk staff and asked them to immediately have a doctor look at her; they refused. As the family even now more anxiously awaited their turn, Galathe's wife became severely ill, and started vomiting blood. This finally prompted a doctor to approach them, but instead of taking them for treatment, he informed them that they should go visit another hospital. Frustrated and angry, Galathe took his family to the car. However, as they reached the car, the daughter again passed out. Despite her illness, Mrs. Galathe ran inside and asked for help. In response, a doctor verbally accosted her and the nurses called security to escort her out of the building. The family went to East Jefferson Hospital, where a doctor prescribed treatment for a viral infection that had been causing the fainting spells. When Galathe called Ochsner Hospital for her medical records, the administrator told him they did not want "your type of people here."[1]

The experience of the Galathes, a Black family from New Orleans, was hardly an outlier in the period. From its origin as the Ochsner Clinic in 1942, the institution had a whites-only policy. Under the 1964 Civil Rights Act, discrimination at hospitals was forbidden. However, Black patients continued to experience racism at Ochsner and other hospitals in the New Orleans area. At the time of the Galathe's experience, the Department of Health, Education, and Welfare (HEW) was conducting a multiple-year investigation into Ochsner and other New Orleans–area hospitals for discrimination against Black patients and refusal to hire Black doctors.

The treatment of the Galathes exemplified a history of racial discrimination in health and health care that continues to this day, seen prominently in the ongoing COVID-19 pandemic. In summer 2020, ProPublica investigated the high rate of elderly people who died of COVID-19 at home, a rate of

17 percent in New Orleans compared to 4 percent nationwide. The reporters identified twenty-five cases of individuals who sought care at a New Orleans–area hospital and were subsequently involuntarily discharged and sent home on hospice to die. Families of patients alleged misdiagnoses, withholding of treatments that could have saved their lives, do-not-resuscitate orders signed without their consent, and pressure to remove their family member from the hospital. All twenty-five people were Black; Ochsner Hospital treated and then discharged most of these individuals.[2] Racial disparity in COVID-19 extended beyond these cases to significantly higher rates of Black COVID-19 mortality rates. As of June 2021, African Americans made up 59.74 percent of the city's population. However, Black residents comprised 72.38 percent of COVID deaths. Similarly, Black residents accounted for only 43 percent of vaccines initiated and completed.[3]

The disproportionate impact of COVID on African Americans in New Orleans mirrored trends seen in cities nationwide. In an April 2020 national briefing, Dr. Anthony Fauci, the head of the National Institutes of Health, told reporters that disasters like coronavirus could "shine a very bright light on some of the real weaknesses and foibles in our society." Fauci dismissed biological reasons for the higher Black death rate, and instead emphasized "underlying medical conditions—the diabetes, the hypertension, the obesity, the asthma"—as the primary cause of higher admittance rate to intensive care units and mortality rates. Ending his briefing, Fauci spoke of the need to address this problem: "when all this is over . . . there will still be health disparities which we really do need to address in the African American community."[4]

These comments on comorbidity matched the high prevalence of chronic health conditions afflicting Black residents in New Orleans: significantly higher rates of diabetes, heart disease, stroke, cancer, infant mortality, maternal mortality, asthma, lead poisoning, and HIV/AIDS than whites. Black New Orleanians in the 2000s and 2010s died at a rate twice that of whites and could expect significantly lower life expectancy. Individuals born in the late 1990s and early 2000s in the mostly Black and low-income Hoffman Triangle neighborhood had a life expectancy of only fifty-five years; individuals born five miles away in the mostly white and affluent Lakeview area had a life expectancy of nearly eighty years.[5]

Yet, focusing primarily on preexisting health conditions can be misleading, particularly without examining the historical, structural roots. Racial health disparities, seen in higher Black rates of disease and mortality, reflect social determinants of health, what the Centers for Disease Control and Prevention identifies as the "conditions in the places where people live, learn, work, and play" that "affect a wide range of health risks and outcomes." These conditions include income and economic security, access to healthy foods, neighborhood safety, conditions of the built environment, education, and access to health care.[6]

The last topic has received increasing attention in recent years, spurred by national conversations about the Affordable Care Act and Medicare for All. While just one of many components of social determinants of health, inadequate access to health care plays a large role in perpetuating racial health disparities. In the United States today, Black Americans have significantly lower access to health care than whites. The 19 percent rate of being uninsured for Black Americans is significantly higher than the 12 percent rate for whites. Over 23 percent of Black Americans have skipped seeing a doctor in the past year due to costs, compared to 15 percent of whites. Over 21 percent of Black Americans have no health care source other than the emergency room when sick, compared to 16 percent of whites. Finally, over 20 percent of Black Americans have made no health care visits at all in the past year, compared to 17 percent of whites. Nationally, this has helped account for racial health disparities, as seen in higher Black rates for many diseases than whites: children's asthma—14 percent vs. 6 percent; diabetes—11 percent vs. 7 percent; and HIV/AIDS—49.8 per 100,000 compared to 5.9 per 100,000. In turn, Black Americans suffer from higher disease mortality rates: infant mortality—11 per 1,000 vs. 4.7 per 1,000; diabetes mortality—38.7 per 100,000 vs. 18.8 per 100,000; heart disease mortality—204.2 per 100,000 vs. 167.3 per 100,000; and cancer mortality—178 per 100,000 vs. 157.9 per 100,000.[7]

These interrelated problems, lack of access to health care and racial health disparities, have deep historical roots. As in many cities, in New Orleans's racial inequality in health care started with the city's founding in 1718. In the colonial and antebellum periods, profit-driven treatment from enslavers and "slave hospitals" provided the limited medical care for enslaved African Americans, supplemented by care by lay and spiritual Black healers. Post-emancipation through the twentieth century, Black New Orleanians primarily relied on two hospitals: the Black-administered Flint Goodridge Hospital, opened in 1896 and closed in 1985, and Charity Hospital, the underfunded and overcrowded public hospital. After Flint Goodridge's closure, even though New Orleans had one of the nation's highest concentrations of physicians at a rate of more than 300 per 100,000 residents and contained twenty-five hospitals in the metropolitan area, Black residents predominantly used only Charity. That institution, in a dilapidated structure opened in the 1930s, provided medical care for 75 percent of Black New Orleanians. Fewer than

15 percent of the patients served by Charity earned over $20,000 annually; half of its in-patient services were designated for the uninsured. Charity provided most of the area's uncompensated and Medicaid and Medicare patient services. Despite the eight other acute-care hospitals in the city, Charity's emergency room, one of the busiest emergency rooms in the country and the only Level 1 trauma center in 300 miles, served most of the acute-care cases. Additionally, the hospital's clinics—the city desperately lacked clinics and primary care for low-income residents—served 350,000 patients annually.[8]

Despite this high usage, the state had been cutting support for the hospital for decades. Following the fiercely resisted battle over health care integration, Charity finally desegregated in the late 1960s after hundreds of years of segregation, discrimination, and mistreatment of African Americans, including nonconsensual medical experiments. After integration, the hospital became majority Black in its clientele as whites sought services at the city's private hospitals and surrounding suburban hospitals. Integration came to Charity, but money fled. The state continually cut the hospital's budget and reallocated federal funding meant to compensate the hospital for services for Medicaid and Medicare patients, resulting in repeated threats of closure and multiple episodes of accreditation loss. The funding cuts led to a decline in the quality of care, and years of backlogged repairs made the hospital unsafe. The institution treated patients with outdated technology and inadequate supplies. Physicians and interns initiated exoduses, and those who stayed dealt with overcrowding and the closing of beds and services. By 2004, the average wait time for emergency room services at Charity was up to twelve hours. The average waiting period for an appointment at a Charity clinic was six months. For many Black and low-income residents, the emergency room at Charity was their only source of health care.[9]

A remarkably different health care system with twenty-four mostly private hospitals served the white, middle, and upper class, those with insurance and options. These institutions, like Tulane University Hospital and Ochsner Hospital, were well funded, well equipped, and fully staffed. In lieu of the open wards in Charity, patients in these institutions had private rooms. Services for uninsured patients comprised an average of 4 percent of total services at these hospitals. Most patients at these hospitals—many of which had refused to admit Black patients until forced to do so by lawsuits and federal legislation in the 1960s—were white. Few patients used Medicaid or Medicare. In fact, many of these elite hospitals faced federal investigations by HEW and they spent years on class action lawsuits that lasted until the late 1980s because of discriminatory practices from illegally turning away

Medicare and Medicaid patients, treating Black patients poorly, and racist hiring and employment practices. In contrast to Charity, many of these hospitals thrived by the early 2000s. Ochsner, which had been established as a "white flight" hospital at midcentury, had become the region's largest hospital conglomerate and the area's largest single employer. Quality of care was generally high and wait times low. Perhaps more importantly, instead of relying on the emergency room at Charity as their main form of health care, these patients had access to primary care, clinics, and private practices, meaning many could avoid using the hospitals altogether.

The differences between Charity and the other hospitals in the area demonstrated the clear existence of a two-tiered health care system, one for the low-income and Black residents, and a second system for the non-indigent and whites. This system was not new.

As argued by historian Andy Horowitz in his award-winning work on Hurricane Katrina, there was not a "sudden turn towards capitalist practice, yoked to state power" in New Orleans after the hurricane; structural inequality and disaster capitalism "did not blow into the city with the storm."[10] Similarly, racial disparity in health care that has taken the form of the current two-tiered system—and the forces that produced it, including structural inequality and supportive state power—is a continuity, not a sudden manifestation in the post–World War II period when hospitals proliferated and the health care economy became a significant driver of the economy. Racialized health care had existed for hundreds of years in New Orleans. This work, the first to explore the historical development of one city's racialized health care system, traces that history.

This work defines a racialized health care system as one built on:

- Different levels of access to, and treatment for, whites versus nonwhites, based on the placement of individuals into racial categories, and often on ideas of scientific racism that define African Americans as biologically different from and inferior to whites.
- The embedding of racism into the structure of health care, seen most visibly in historically white health care institutions (hospitals, clinics, medical schools, etc.) that have carried out efforts of exclusion of African Americans as patients and practitioners and the exploitation of African Americans by white medical practitioners for profit and professional advancement.
- The perpetuation of racial health disparities.
- Support for the larger system of racist hierarchy, with whites at the top.

This framework draws heavily on the field of critical race theory, particularly the work of Eduardo Bonilla-Silva. Bonilla-Silva argued that racism is "embedded in the structure of a society," what many scholars call the concept of "structural racism." He labeled his perspective the "racialized social system" approach, which he defined as "societies in which economic, political, social, and ideological levels are partially structured by the placement of actors in racial categories or race," which are hierarchically ordered. He posited that the superordinate group—the racial category at top—develops views, practices, and social relations to preserve the hierarchy, and those at the bottom develop their own views and practices to challenge it. He also argues that racism changes over time, and has a "rationality," with actors supporting or challenging based on what benefits them. However, rather than focusing on the individual actors and their behaviors—"prejudice"—Bonilla-Silva argued that scholars of racism should employ a "materialist" focus on uncovering the "mechanisms and practices (behaviors, styles, cultural affectations, traditions, and organizational procedures) at the social, economic, ideological, and political levels responsible for the reproduction of racial domination." Bonilla-Silva argues that scholars need to further explore the racialization of space and organizations. His own scholarship examined the "racialization" of U.S. colleges and universities, and he labeled most institutions of higher education as "historically white colleges universities," arguing their history, demography, curriculum, climate, and symbols and traditions embody, signify, and reproduce whiteness and systemic racism.[11]

A City without Care heeds this call, and examines the racialization of health care, focusing on the racialized health care system in New Orleans from the city's founding in 1718 through the present and addresses several research questions. What factors led to the development and perpetuation of this system? What are the connections between racialized health care and a larger system of racist hierarchy? How has racialized health care impacted the health of Black residents? How have African Americans fought against this system and for improved health?

Racialized health care emerged as a key component of the slave-based economy in New Orleans, and then became institutionalized with the end of Reconstruction and the rise of Jim Crow. This system helped make segregation, and unfortunately a racialized health care system still exists today. The historically white medical system served white interests in ways that financially benefited members of the medical community, and it both accommodated and supported a racist economic system and hierarchy that survived from slavery, to Jim Crow, to the post–World War II liberal order of de jure segregation, and into the post-Katrina world of ascendant liberalism. Government policies at the local, state, and federal level helped the racialized health care system grow and sustain. Within these shifting institutional and power structures, Black New Orleanians fought for access to health care and improved health, including carving out their own health care institutions, but they always had to confront the limits imposed by the racist hierarchies.

The racialized health care system produced profit for its owners. In the period of enslavement, "slave hospitals" derived much of their income from enslavers paying for medical treatment for enslaved people. Doctors that conducted medical experiments on enslaved and free Blacks garnered accolades for innovating medical advances, amassed prestige, and attracted new clients when they applied their perfected techniques on white patients. For medical schools in which students practiced newly learned skills on the live bodies and cadavers of enslaved people, these practices helped boost their enrollments. After the overthrow of slavery, the removal of the profit motive—treatment paid for by enslavers—helped lead to the exclusion of African Americans, most indigent, from the health care system. Profit continued to impact the racialized health care system in the twentieth century as well. This is evident in the decision by private hospitals in the post-integration period to continue to deny Black Medicaid and Medicare patients, while admitting a small number of upper-income Black patients.

The racialized health care system also benefited the city's larger economic system. Doctors and hospitals played a key role in sustaining the slave-based economy; later, they would help fuel the emerging trade- and tourism-based economies; and finally, health care became its own economy with a proliferation of medical schools, hospitals, clinics, rehabilitation long-term care facilities, nursing homes, and biomedical companies that employed tens of thousands of residents and brought great wealth to the city in the later twentieth and early twenty-first centuries.

Yet, profit and economic impact alone cannot explain the persistence of racialized health care. The system endured in large part because of its symbiotic relationship with racial hierarchy. Even as whites in power caused racial health disparities by denying access and care, they used the rhetoric of scientific racism to justify their actions and pointed to higher Black rates of disease and mortality as an argument to maintain the very system that caused it. This created and sustained a self-perpetuating loop: the historically white health care system exploited or denied admission to African Americans, arguing they were inferior; whites then used the resulting higher disease and mortality rates as proof of their inferiority to justify the exclusion of African Americans not just in hospitals, but throughout the Jim Crow system.

Government policies and powers facilitated the growth of the racialized health care system. At the local level, the municipal government used its powers, particularly zoning, to promote historically white health care institutions and restrict Black ones. Beyond state-sanctioned slavery and Jim Crow laws, in the twentieth century federal programs like the Public Works Administration and the Hill-Burton Act helped segregated and whites-only health care institutions grow. Meanwhile, well-intentioned programs like Medicare and Medicaid financially damaged Black-owned and Black-serving health care institutions. The federal government also failed to enforce integration and protect equality in health care. At an even greater level, the decision in the United States to eschew state-controlled health care helped fuel the profit-driven and less regulated health care system in which discrimination perpetuated.

Despite these forces aligned in favor of racialized health care, Black New Orleanians have pushed for nearly 300 years for equal access to health care and health equality as part of the larger Black freedom struggle. These efforts have included self-help measures like establishing civic improvement leagues; the creation of a Black medical profession, with schools and hospital, and an alternate medical district; and efforts to gain access to and integrate the historically white health care system. While unsuccessful in dismantling the racialized health care system or eliminating racial health disparities, these efforts had a significant impact on quality of life.

The racialized health care system's survival was not inevitable. Although many factors facilitated its rise and perpetuation, there were moments when the racialized health care system could have ended. In his 1982 work *Making the Second Ghetto*, Arnold Hirsch identified several "crucial turning points," which he defined as "an opportunity for dismantling instead of expanding" residential segregation in Chicago in the postwar period.[12] Similarly, this work identifies several such crucial periods, particularly the period 1868–1877, the 1910s–1930s, and the late 1960s, when opportunities existed to dismantle, not expand, the racialized health care system in New Orleans. In 1868, Louisiana adopted a constitution that explicitly forbid whites-only institutions of higher education, including medical schools, and stipulated the protection of public rights, including the right to use hospitals. From 1868 until the return to power of the Southern Democrats in 1877, state and federal officials—who occupied New Orleans during Reconstruction—could have enforced these provisions, including the integration of hospitals and the medical schools, and could have broken the racialized health care system. In the 1910s and

1920s, New Orleans invested millions in municipal improvements including water, sewage, and drainage; carried out public health campaigns against diseases like tuberculosis; and experienced dramatic growth in medical institutions, with significant federal funding from sources like the Public Works Administration. The city did so to improve its image and bolster its growing tourism industry and trade with Latin America. These municipal, public health, and health care improvements could have significantly improved Black access to health care and Black health. In the 1960s, Civil Rights activists won key victories in integrating health care. With the passage of the Civil Rights Act of 1964, which included a provision that banned discrimination in hospitals, and Medicare and Medicaid in 1965; National Association for the Advancement of Colored People (NAACP)–initiated lawsuits that struck down the "separate but equal" part of the Hill-Burton Act in 1963; and subsequent successful lawsuits that mandated integration of hospitals and medical schools, government officials could have ended the racialized health care system.

All three turning points witnessed transformations in the city's health care system and increased roles of the federal government in health care. All three periods had increased health care access and declining death rates for whites. Yet, all three crucial turning points failed to end the racialized health care system. This happened partially because individual actors—doctors, hospital and medical school administrators, public health leaders, and local and state officials—used their powers to maintain the historically white health care system's ties to white supremacy. In these periods, doctors and others associated with historically white institutions explicitly endorsed their support for white supremacy, including leadership of organizations like the White League and the White Citizens Council. However, racialized health care continued as well due to the structural and institutional factors, practices (the placement of people into hierarchical racial categories; the teaching of scientific racism; the traditions, cultures, and symbols of white supremacy in medical schools and hospitals), and mechanisms, including state-sanctioned supported. In these periods, the federal government not only failed to enforce health care equality, but also perpetuated racialized health care by funding medical institutions that refused to serve Black patients or treated them in segregated spaces. The repeated failures in these turning points helped institutionalize racism in health care. Despite the fact that actors and institutions no longer explicitly endorse exclusion or segregation, racism is embedded in health care.

This work primarily makes contributions to historical scholarship on hospitals and health care, racial inequalities, and cities. It builds on the innovative work of historians Darlene Clark Hine, Vanessa Northington Gamble, David McBride, Todd Savitt, and Susan Smith, as well as more recent books by Gretchen Long and Thomas Ward Jr., who all explored the efforts in the late nineteenth and early twentieth century to create and expand Black hospitals and the Black medical profession.[13]

While this work explores these topics, it is purposely titled "Racialized Health Care in New Orleans" rather than "Black Health Care in New Orleans." Monographs and edited volumes about the history of American medicine, hospitals, and the medical profession often replicate the exclusions historically practiced by American health care. Because historically white health care institutions excluded Black patients and practitioners for much of their history, these works exclude African Americans in their pages. Another set of texts focuses on "Black health care history" and examines those excluded from the historically white health care system: the African Americans who created an alternate health care system. This work details the achievements and limitations of a Black medical school, hospital, medical district, and practitioners. However, I do not label this research as a piece solely on "Black health care history." Rather, I argue that two sets of texts must be in conversation, that the historically white health care system and the alternate Black health care system can be best understood in the context of the overall racialized health care system. As such, this work draws on groundbreaking techniques employed by historians like Keith Wailoo and Samuel Roberts Jr.[14] Only by detailing the exclusion, exploitation, and discrimination faced by African Americans in health care can we understand the limitations they faced as both patients and practitioners. Similarly, we must also understand how this same exclusion, exploitation, and discrimination of African Americans contributed to the development of the historically white health care system and medical profession and the upholding of white supremacy.[15]

While this book concentrates on health care and racial health inequalities, this is also a work of urban history. This book analyzes not only the factors that shaped the historically white health care system and the alternate Black health care system, but also how these institutions shaped the city, its economy, and its residents. Recent historical scholarship has explored the physical and economic impact of the expanding health care economy and its institutions in post-industrial cities.[16] However, the effect of health care on cities is not just a post-industrial story. As this work demonstrates, white leaders used health care and improving health—and preventing the spread of disease—as justification for displacement of African Americans from New Orleans's medical district in the 1930s, similar to the segregation of African Americans in Baltimore and the destruction of San Francisco's Chinatown in the early twentieth century.[17] As this book demonstrates, health issues and health care institutions have helped shape the development of cities since the colonial period.

I chose New Orleans as my case study for several reasons. I have lived in New Orleans for more than a decade. Familiarity with the city, and its archives, made the decision pragmatic, coupled with my desire to write about the city I am fortunate to call home. One of the dangers of focusing on New Orleans is the idea of the "exceptionalism" or "uniqueness" of the city. Proponents of this claim attribute this difference to the city's history—particularly the long control by the French, and later the Spanish—and creolized culture. Therefore, they argue, New Orleans is fundamentally different from other American cities. New Orleans is sometimes called the most Europeanized American city; others describe it as the Caribbean north. These ideas began propagating as the city increasingly turned toward promoting itself as a tourist destination in the early twentieth century. In the past two decades, scholars of New Orleans have challenged this notion of exceptionalism by detailing the similarities between the Big Easy and other American cities, or examining its connections and similarities to other global cities.[18]

While this work does not seek as its primary purpose to join the scholarly discourse on authenticity and exceptionalism, I do claim that a case study of health care in New Orleans offers insights into the history of many American cities. In other words, this work uses New Orleans not because of an exceptional history of health care, but because it shares similarities with other U.S. cities. Today in New Orleans the health care sector is the second largest employment sector, behind only the hospitality field, and hospitals and other health care buildings occupy large swaths of the physical landscape. New Orleans is increasingly becoming dependent on this kind of health care economy. This is perhaps most visible in the recently opened University Medical Center and the Veterans Affairs Hospital, both costing more than a billion dollars each, and part of the BioDistrict, an economic development area covering over 1,500 acres in the heart of downtown.

New Orleans is not unique in the focus on the health care economy. Many cities, particularly post-industrial ones, have increasingly turned to the health care sector to boost employment and public dollars, even as scholars warn of the dangers in relying on the health care field for economic growth and stability, and have detailed the role of the health care sector, particularly university hospitals, in gentrification.[19] But beyond this recent expansion, like New Orleans, cities throughout the United States witnessed significant growths in the health care economy, especially after the passage of the Hill-Burton Act in 1946. Even in earlier periods, hospitals played significant roles in many cities and their economic life. For example, "slave hospitals" existed in Charleston, Mobile, Augusta, and other southern hubs, not just the Crescent City. As in New Orleans, these institutions helped create powerful health care sectors that would drive city growth.

The health disparity that exists today in New Orleans, one which has persisted for hundreds of years, is not unique. The same social determinants of health and their negative impacts on Black health, permeate throughout the United States. As in New Orleans, African Americans in Atlanta, Chicago, Los Angeles, Milwaukee, Rochester, Trenton, and other cities face significantly higher disease and mortality rates due to inequality. Black residents in these cities have disproportionately relied on overcrowded and underfunded public hospitals, especially post-integration. The transformation of Charity Hospital from a space that primarily served low-income immigrants and enslaved people; to a Jim Crow, segregated hospital; to an overcrowded, understaffed, and underfunded public hospital utilized by most of the city's residents of color post-integration; to a university hospital that displaced hundreds of Black residents is echoed in the experiences of many American public hospitals. Similarly, many cities continue to have a separate, better-funded network of private, historically white hospitals that serve most white and upper-income residents. Racial health disparities and racialized health care systems exist in most American cities. While this work concentrates on New Orleans, the findings mirror the history and experience of many Black urbanites.

This book uses a variety of sources: government collections, including the documents of the city health and planning departments, the city council, mayoral administrations, and the state legislature; material from federal programs such as the Model Cities program; court records; health reports; material from many of the city's hospitals and medical schools; personal papers of prominent Black health care leaders; oral histories of local politicians, civic leaders, health care workers, and patients; newspaper articles; and demographic and neighborhood data, including census information and Sanborn maps.

This work explores the racialized health care system in the following nine chapters. Chapter 1 explores the origins of the racialized health care system in New Orleans. It details the creation and roles of early hospitals like the Royal Hospital and Charity Hospital, both of which enslaved people and provided invaluable medical care to many of the participants in the slave society. It examines the health requirements for enslaved individuals under the Code Noir and Black Codes, and the connection between the growing slave economy in New Orleans and the nascent medical field. The chapter details the role of physicians in promoting scientific racism used to justify the slave system. Finally, the chapter explores health problems of enslaved people and the limited health care provided by enslavers.

Chapter 2 details how the institution of slavery permitted the growth of the racialized health care system in the antebellum period, including private hospitals, Charity Hospital, two medical schools, and the practices of individual physicians. Private infirmaries called "slave hospitals" proliferated, buoyed by profits for providing care for enslaved individuals, paid by their enslavers. While not considered a "slave hospital," Charity Hospital strengthened its connections to slavery. The hospital continued to treat the increasing number of arriving enslaved people suffering from illness and bound for the slave market, used and sold enslaved laborers, and derived income from donations from large enslavers. This chapter also explores the growth of the medical schools and the emergence of New Orleans as the "medical metropolis of the South," a process deeply connected to slavery. Physicians derived prestige and wealth through exploitation and experimentation on enslaved people and passed down ideas of scientific racism to the next generation of doctors. Finally, this chapter examines the origins of an alternate Black health care field. Antebellum New Orleans was a Black health center, with Black doctors with medical degrees, others with informal training, and Black nurses, midwives, and folk and spiritual healers.

Chapter 3 examines one of the "crucial turning points" in the city's health care history. During federal occupation of New Orleans, an opportunity existed to end racialized health care. While Louisiana abolished slavery in 1864 and enfranchised Black voters, neither state nor federal officials enforced "public rights" by requiring integration of hospitals. Instead, the federal government created the short-lived and underfunded system of Freedmen's Hospitals for Black patients, which ended in 1869. From 1868 to 1877, Charity Hospital desegregated. However, with the end of Reconstruction and return to power of the Redeemers, medical leaders purposely chose to institutionalize racialized health care, with private hospitals and the University of Louisiana refusing to accept Black patients or students and Charity Hospital treating Black patients in separate wards. Excluded from health care and subject to many other aspects of discrimination, the racial health gap widened dramatically. This chapter also examines the early, unsuccessful attempts to create Black medical schools in New Orleans in the 1870s and 1880s, and the final successful creation of the Flint Medical College in 1889 and Flint Goodridge Hospital in 1896.

Chapter 4 explores the intersection of the segregation of health care and urban space in the early decades of the twentieth century. It examines how New Orleans's push for increasing trade with Latin America and tourism led to civic improvements, public health campaigns, and an expanding health care economy. As boosters promoted New Orleans as a healthy city, with a robust health care system, they also advocated for residential segregation and spatial concentration of Black residents in less-desirable areas, often using arguments of poor Black health as justification for removal. This chapter details the push by white leaders to evict Black medical institutions like the Providence Sanitarium, Flint Goodridge Hospital, and Flint Medical College from the medical district, and the role of municipal powers and federal funding—through programs like the Works Progress Administration (WPA)—in supporting the efforts to create a white medical district.

Chapter 5 explores the efforts of New Orleanians to create an alternate Black medical district in the Central City neighborhood. It details the attempts to create two hospitals, the unsuccessful Colored Hospital and a new Flint Goodridge Hospital, which became the anchor of the Black medical district. The chapter examines the initial challenges of the hospital—like fundraising and staffing—and the vision of Flint Goodridge as not just a hospital but a health center focused on three main goals: expanding hospital care for African Americans throughout the region, tackling the public health issues facing the Black community, and serving as a training center for Black medical professionals. Finally, the chapter explores two significant issues for the hospital: the deliberate effort of the municipal government to prevent the growth of the hospital with WPA-sponsored "slum clearance" and building of public housing units around the institution, and the post–World War II exodus of Black physicians from New Orleans.

Chapter 6 explores the decades-long struggle to desegregate health care in New Orleans, focusing on the period from the late 1940s through the late 1960s. It examines a seemingly paradoxical problem with Flint Goodridge Hospital: the desire to expand the Black institution—thwarted for years by the state's denial of federal Hill-Burton funding—occurring as Black leaders pushed for access to all hospitals. This chapter details the new strategies employed by civil rights leaders like A. P. Tureaud, who turned to litigation to desegregate medical schools, and the impact of federal court decisions and legislation like the Civil Rights Act of 1964, and Medicaid and Medicare, which mandated integration of health care institutions. This chapter also details the concentrated efforts of Charity Hospital and private hospitals to defy integration and the creation of "white flight" hospitals in the suburbs of New Orleans. As this chapter demonstrates, the late 1960s was another potential "crucial turning point" for the racialized health care system, and white municipal and health care leaders fought to preserve the racialized health care system.

Chapter 7 explores the post–Civil Rights period when the promise of an integrated health care system evaporated and the racialized health care system became re-entrenched, similar to what occurred in New Orleans a century earlier. This chapter starts with two juxtaposed stories: the simultaneous attempts to expand the white medical district, including the successful creation of Tulane University's new hospital, and the stymied work to expand Flint Goodridge Hospital, which entered into decline. It explores the creation of the state agency Health Education Authority of Louisiana (HEAL) and its "urban renewal" efforts to displace Black residents and businesses. This chapter also explores continued Black health activism, which took several forms. First, Black residents of Tulane Gravier organized against the expansion of the medical district and displacement. Second, Black residents and the NAACP initiated litigation against the formerly all-white hospitals that continued to discriminate, leading to investigations by the federal government, which were undermined by the failure of the federal government to enforce integration. Third, Black residents pushed for Health Department and federally funded Model Cities health clinics in public housing units and Black neighborhoods, and the Black Panther Party created their own People's Clinic in the Desire neighborhood; all the clinics proved short-lived. Finally, the chapter examines the transition of Charity Hospital to a "de facto" Black hospital and the accompanying decrease in state funding and quality of care.

Chapter 8 examines Black health care in New Orleans in the age of crisis, from the late 1970s until Hurricane Katrina. It explores the factors that led to the decline, sale, and closure of Flint Goodridge, primarily the hospital's declining finances due to low levels of reimbursement from Medicare and Medicaid, inability to attract donors or investors, and lack of government funding. This chapter also explores the growing corporatization of health care. While Flint Goodridge became a victim of this process, hospitals like Tulane and Ochsner that served a wealthier, whiter clientele thrived, buoyed by their support from hospital companies and continued aid from HEAL. Finally, this chapter details the further decline of Charity Hospital, principally caused by the state's continued reduction in funding. By the 2000s, Charity provided care for 75 percent of the city's Black hospital patients as both quality of care at the hospital and the racial health disparity worsened.

The concluding chapter explores the transformation of health care in post–Hurricane Katrina New Orleans, including Louisiana State University's controversial decision to keep Charity Hospital closed. Aided by political allies and federal funding, Louisiana State University succeeded in their long-desired plan to replace Charity Hospital with a modern university hospital. However, Black residents continued to suffer. The new university hospital did not open for ten years after the closure of Charity Hospital. Similarly, the predominantly Black New Orleans East neighborhood waited ten years for the reopening of a hospital in that area. Both of these waits disproportionately impacted Black residents, who made up the vast majority of patients at the two hospitals, and many African Americans had virtually no access to health care. Even when the university hospital opened in 2015, its abandonment of its mission to provide care for indigent residents in favor of becoming a "destination hospital" for individuals seeking cutting-edge medical practices resulted in the exclusion of many former patients. Additionally, the building of the university hospital as part of New Orleans's expansive BioDistrict, intended to foster the growth of the city's biomedical sector, led to further displacement of Black residents through eminent domain. Although the expansion of Medicaid funding and primary care clinics proved positive for low-income residents, racial health disparity and two-tiered health care remained, most visible in the disproportionate number of Black deaths during the city's COVID-19 epidemic.

This disparity in mortality from COVID-19 will hopefully serve as the impetus for an examination not just of racial health disparities, but also of the much larger and historically longer impact of structural racism. Racialized health care is just one part of the larger issue of negative social determinants of health that have plagued Black New Orleanians since the city's founding. But understanding its historical roots and evolution will help in understanding the continued problem of racial health disparity. I hope this work contributes to that understanding and the push for racial health equity.

CHAPTER ONE

Health and Health Care in the Era of Slavery, 1718–1843

In Washington, D.C. in 1841, enslavers kidnapped Solomon Northup, born in freedom in New York in 1807 or 1808, and shipped him to Richmond. There, Northup met Robert, another free Black man from Cincinnati. The slavers placed both men on board the brig *Orleans*, bound for New Orleans, the South's largest slave market. On board the ship, the slavers chained Northup, Robert, and others in the hold each night, even during three days of violent storms. All in the hold suffered from sea sickness, and the effluvia from the ill made the hold "loathsome and disgusting," Northup wrote in his autobiography *Twelve Years a Slave*. Sick and fearful of enslavement, Northup wished at that moment for the release of death. "It would have been a happy thing for most of us," Northup wrote, "had the compassionate sea snatched us that day from the clutches of remorseless men."[1]

Northup survived, but his torment only intensified. Several days later, Northup, Robert, and a third man planned to seize control of the ship. However, Robert became ill. The sailors announced Robert had smallpox, a highly contagious and deadly affliction. Robert died, and Northup and the others on board "were all panic-stricken." When the ship arrived in New Orleans, many of those on board too became ill. A physician came to inspect them, and Northup related the death of Robert and his belief that all on the ship now suffered from smallpox. The physician sent the afflicted to Charity Hospital, designated by municipal law as the hospital for those suffering from contagious disease. Northup recalled that he was "entirely blind" for three days. Northup also described his feeling about the potential of dying in the hospital: "I thought I could have been resigned to yield up my life in the bosom of my family, but to expire in the midst of strangers, under such circumstances, was a bitter reflection." After sixteen days recuperating, enslavers sent Northup and the other survivors to the slave market. Subject to a physical examination to determine his health, and his corresponding worth, Northup noted he was "bearing upon my face the effects of the malady"—meaning he had scars or pockmarks on his face, telltale signs of smallpox. Northup speculated that his bout of smallpox may have lowered his price from an original $1,500 to a final of $1,000 dollars.[2]

Northup labored on a series of plantations in Louisiana, forced to construct buildings, clear land, and pick cotton. Northup's health deteriorated due to overwork, beatings, malnutrition, and poor housing conditions. In 1843, Northup became severely ill, suffering from chills, high fever, weakness, and dizziness. Nevertheless, as he noted, the overseer "compelled" him to "keep my row." As he became sicker, and less productive, the overseer continually whipped him. After months of illness, Northup could not leave his cabin, but enslaver Edwin Epps provided no care until he believed Northup close to death. As noted by Northup, Epps's motivation was potential profit loss; Epps, "unwilling to bear the loss, which the death of an animal worth a thousand dollars would bring to him," finally "concluded to incur the expenses" of sending for a doctor. Dr. Hines diagnosed the cause of his maladies as the "effect of the climate." Hines ordered Northup to eat no meat, and to "partake of no more food than was absolutely necessary to sustain life." Despite this dubious treatment, Northup slowly recovered over several weeks, owing more to rest than to Hines's prescribed treatment. Epps soon ordered Northup back into the fields, although Northup felt it was "long before I was in proper condition to labor." Northup, unlike many in his position, survived.[3]

Northup's experiences have become famous in recent years, especially after the Oscar-winning film *Twelve Years a Slave* came out in 2013. His memoir provides firsthand accounts of the precarious condition of African Americans in the antebellum United States, even those born into freedom, and the brutality of the slave system.

Northup's experiences also illustrate the health problems experienced by enslaved individuals and their interaction with doctors. Like many, Northup became severely ill during his forced journey. Upon arrival, officials quarantined Northup and others suffering from smallpox to prevent an outbreak, a constant concern in the period. Paid by enslavers, physicians treated Northup to prepare him for sale at the slave market. The examination of Northup and others, often done by physicians, showed the further role of medical professionals in converting the physical body of the enslaved individual into a commodity. His subsequent illness on the plantation demonstrated the toll of slavery on the health of enslaved people, planters' reluctance to call for costly physicians, the financial motivations of medical care, and the limited knowledge of doctors.

Northup was witness to the early stage of the racialized health care system in New Orleans, explored in this chapter. It details the creation and roles of the Royal Hospital and Charity Hospital, both of which enslaved people and provided invaluable medical care to many of the participants in the slave society. It examines the health requirements for enslaved individuals under the Code Noir and Black Codes, and the connection between the growing slave economy in New Orleans and the nascent medical field. The chapter details the role of physicians in promoting scientific racism used to justify the slave system. Finally, the chapter explores health problems of enslaved people and the limited health care provided by enslavers.

Origins of Racialized Health Care

In the eighteenth and early nineteenth centuries, members of a family primarily cared for the sick. Only about 4,000 physicians practiced nationwide by the American Revolution, with a mere 200 possessing medical degrees. The first medical school, what would become the University of Pennsylvania, started in 1765, and the first medical school in the South began in 1807. Most physicians received training as apprentices rather than formal education, and few states had medical societies or licensing boards. The number of large hospitals nationwide was relatively few. Most Americans distrusted hospitals, perhaps rightfully so with their high mortality rates due to limited medical knowledge. As a result, many felt that care at home was safer. The state's involvement in health care was limited. Some cities had charity hospitals, and most had state-funded facilities for those afflicted by mental disorders. Most Americans viewed hospitals as places for the destitute, those without a family to take care of them, and attached a stigma to those who used hospitals.[4]

Early New Orleans reflected these health care trends. No sustainable medical society existed, and the city's first medical school did not open until 1834. The small number of physicians received training in Europe or through apprenticeships. The French Company of the Indies created the Royal Hospital in 1720, administered by Ursuline nuns until 1770. Initially only soldiers and employees of the Company of the Indies could use the space; however, in 1724, the local council voted to allow the hospital to treat paying civilians and provide free care for indigent residents.[5] In 1731, with the collapse of the Company of the Indies, the French crown assumed control of Louisiana. The Crown cut back on funding for the hospital and pressured the institution to primarily provide for royal administrators and soldiers, not civilians. The few private physicians offered care for wealthier colonists, but most people primarily relied on family and friends. The indigent and sailors far from home had no such support system.[6]

This changed with the opening of Charity Hospital. In January 1736, French shipbuilder Jean Louis died and bequeathed the money made from the sale of his property "to serve in perpetuity to the founding of a hospital for the sick of the City of New Orleans." The sale netted 10,000 livres used to create the twelve-bed Hospital of St. John, also known as L'Hospital des Pauvres de la Charite, opened on May 10, 1736, six weeks after Bellevue Hospital in New York City, the nation's longest continually operating hospital. Like the Royal Hospital, the Ursuline nuns administered Charity Hospital.[7]

Due to fears of spreading contagion, the hospital was situated in several locations on the periphery of the expanding city. Originally in a former residence on Chartres Street, it moved in 1743 to Rampart Street. The hospital suffered from overcrowding and underfunding, with no support from the French and little from the colony, instead relying on donations from wealthy patrons. By 1763, the hospital board of administrators comprised business leaders as well as clergy and government officials.[8] That year, the Spanish gained control of Louisiana and pledged to continue to provide support for Charity Hospital.[9] In 1779, a hurricane destroyed the building. Don Andres de Almonaster y Roxas, a wealthy landowner and city councilman, donated 114,000 pesos for the construction of a new brick hospital, completed in 1786, on the previous site. Almonaster also bequeathed an annual gift of $1,500 to maintain the institution, now known as the New Charity Hospital of St. Charles. The hospital contained twenty-four beds for a population of 9,756 and, while primarily focused on care for the indigent, allowed paying patients as well.[10]

The Royal and Charity hospitals contributed to racialized health care and the growth of the burgeoning slave system from their inceptions. During the early colonial period, the number of enslaved people in Louisiana remained relatively low. Colonial officials enslaved few Indigenous people due to their need of maintaining relationships with local tribes for trade and military support, as well as white views that enslaved Indigenous people were not productive and could easily escape. As a result, Louisiana turned to the transatlantic slave trade. From 1719 to 1743, the French transported 5,761 enslaved Africans to Louisiana. Most of the enslaved people arrived in the 1720s. While the Louisiana colonists wanted larger numbers of enslaved laborers, competition with other European powers, priority placed on the plantation colonies in the Caribbean, and initial scarcity of enslaved Africans kept their numbers in Louisiana low. Colonists forced many of the enslaved Africans to work on indigo and tobacco farms and plantations. Others labored in New Orleans as enslaved domestics, in skilled trade positions, or on the city's roads, canals, and levees, helping not just to generate wealth for whites but also the infrastructure that would sustain the city's growth.[11]

The hospitals in New Orleans played a crucial role in this early slave system. No existing records from the hospitals document the treatment of enslaved Indigenous people, but based on the relationship between the hospitals and enslaved Africans, it is likely the institutions treated some Indigenous people enslaved by colonial officials. Enslaved Africans often arrived in New Orleans suffering from severe health problems, if they survived at all. Historians estimate that as many as half of the Africans ensnared in Atlantic slaving died before leaving the continent, during capture or the forced march to slave holding areas, or waiting in pens and fortresses.[12] From 1719 to 1723, the mortality rate of enslaved Africans on ships for Louisiana was relatively low at 3.6 percent. As the captivity period in Africa prior to embarkation lengthened and the number of enslaved people on each ship increased, so too did deaths. The mortality rate of enslaved Africans during the Middle Passage to Louisiana from 1726 to 1731, the peak years of the slave trade in French Louisiana, was 15.7 percent, similar to the estimated average mortality rate of 15–20 percent on Middle Passage voyages during the transatlantic slave-trading period.[13] Those that survived arrived exhausted, underfed, and ill, often suffering from severe problems like dysentery, scurvy, and yaws. Many died—on average, about 4.3 percent of all enslaved Africans newly arrived in the Americas—after they first arrived and before they were sold.[14]

Colonial officials had several concerns over the health issues of newly arrived enslaved Africans. First, administrators feared the importation of disease and the spreading to whites. In 1724, the French government ordered health inspections for all enslaved people before they were allowed to disembark from ships, and sent many of those to the colony's "smallpox hospital," an isolation space.[15] In 1728, the company built a hospital on its 4,000-acre plantation located on the west bank across the Mississippi River from the French Quarter; this space also served as an isolation space for enslaved Africans suffering from disease.[16]

Second, officials feared lost profits. France granted the Company of the Indies a monopoly on the slave trade from several ports in Africa, primarily Senegal, and most of their ships in the late 1720s sailed to Louisiana. The high sickness and mortality rate cut into profit from sales of enslaved people and production on their plantation. Ships that arrived in the late 1720s often had large numbers of severely ill enslaved Africans. For example, the *Duc de Noaille* arrived in 1727. Of the 362 Africans forced to embark to Louisiana, only 242 disembarked in New Orleans, for a mortality rate of 33.1 percent. One hundred and ten of the 242 required hospitalization at the Royal and smallpox hospitals. At the company-sponsored auctions, colonists often refused to purchase sick enslaved Africans. Some colonists purchased enslaved Africans and then returned them to the company within days due to illness. This led Governor Étienne Perier to offer colonists a one-month guarantee. Enslavers could bring enslaved Africans they purchased for treatment at the hospital and if necessary return the enslaved individuals—branded to avoid substitution—to the company for a full refund within the first month. This policy became the basis of Louisiana's redhibition policy, discussed in the following section.[17]

After purchase, medical treatment of enslaved people remained a significant issue. Historian Gwendolyn Midlo Hall estimated that nearly 20 percent of enslaved Africans forced to Louisiana from 1719 to 1723 had died by 1726, and the mortality rate increased in the late 1720s and 1730s. For example, *La Venus* departed Gorée in April 1729 with 450 captives on board. Only 320 survived to reach New Orleans, and an estimated two-thirds had died by August.[18] While perhaps an extreme example, the high death rate demonstrated the poor health conditions during captivity and adaptation to a new environ, and the harsh working and living conditions on plantations. Early slave codes mandated access to medical care for enslaved people. In 1724, France instituted the Code Noir in Louisiana, which required enslaved people "be properly fed, clothed, and provided for by their masters" (XX); and "slaves who are disabled from working, either by old age, disease, or otherwise, be the disease incurable or not, shall be fed and provided for by their masters; and in case they should have been abandoned by said masters, said slaves shall be adjudged to the nearest hospital" (XXI).[19] Although historians have challenged earlier arguments that the Code Noir led to better treatment of enslaved people in Louisiana than in other colonies and the provisions of the statute seem to have been rarely enforced, enslavers did provide some medical care for enslaved people, including hiring doctors and building hospital buildings on plantations such as the space constructed by the Company of the Indies on its plantation in 1728. Some enslavers may have brought enslaved people to the Royal Hospital—during at least the Spanish period, Charity appears to have explicitly forbidden the treatment of enslaved people. A dearth of documents from the hospitals and physicians in the colonial period limits this discussion, but records from the later American period document the treatment of enslaved people by physicians and "slave hospitals"; this is addressed in the following section.

The slave system in New Orleans was still in its early stages in this period and would not transition from a "society with slaves" to a "slave society" until the late eighteenth century. However, the health care institutions from their origins were tied to slavery and played an integral part in helping the slave system start and develop. Beyond treating newly arrived enslaved Africans, the Royal Hospital provided care for company and colonial officials and Charity treated sailors involved in the transport of enslaved Africans and agricultural products grown, harvested, and refined by enslaved laborers. These services proved vital to the slave-based system for a city nearly abandoned in the 1720s due to the high death rate.

In turn, the growing slavery system directly financially supported the hospitals. The 1724 Code Noir stipulated that enslavers pay eight cents a day for elderly and infirmed enslaved individuals unable to work and sent to the Royal Hospital; if they did not pay, the hospital would place a lien on their plantation (Section XXI). Section XXXIV forbid anyone from helping enslaved people escape to freedom and required free people of color to pay to enslavers thirty livres for each day they hid an enslaved person who self-emancipated, and, if unable to pay, the colony would enslave and sell the free person of color, with any excess amount of the sale (minus the thirty livres a day owed to the enslaver) going to the Royal Hospital. Section LLII forbid whites from gifting or bequeathing money to manumitted people and free people of color; the colony would seize any such donation and give it to the Royal Hospital. These policies accomplished two simultaneous goals of establishing rules for the burgeoning slave system in Louisiana and supporting the fledgling hospital.

The hospital also established ties to slavery through the utilization of enslaved Africans as laborers. As part of the contract with the Ursuline nuns to run the Military Hospital, the Company of the Indies gave the religious order eight enslaved people. At the hospital, which the sisters operated with the aid of a physician and three physician's assistants, the nuns used four of these enslaved individuals as laborers. This may have been the first instance of a hospital in what would become the United States using enslaved laborers.[20] Section VI of the Code Noir forbid marriage between whites and African Americans and interracial children, and stated if an enslaver had a child with a women he enslaved, the enslaved woman and their children would be sent to labor at the Royal Hospital and "shall be forever incapable of being set free."

Charity Hospital also used enslaved individuals throughout its history, starting with the Ursuline nuns in the 1730s. In 1737, François Tiocou, a free Black man who had previously earned his emancipation in exchange for his defense of the Louisiana colony during the 1729 Natchez revolt, signed a contract with the hospital. Tiocou agreed to work for the hospital for a period of seven years for no pay, and at the end of the term the administrators granted freedom to his wife Marie Aram, an enslaved woman, who would also work for the hospital for the period. The administrators freed Aram in March of 1744 "in reward for the good services she has given to said hospital"; Aram and Tiocou stayed on at the hospital as paid laborers.[21] The hospital continued to buy, sell, and use enslaved people under Spanish rule of Louisiana, from 1763 to 1802, a period when the number of enslaved people in New Orleans tripled—and in all of Louisiana increased tenfold—with the proliferation of plantations and the legalized importation of enslaved people from British-controlled Jamaica. For example, Charity's administrator purchased Rosette, aged 28, from Thimoleon de Chataubaudaux in 1770 for 1,000 livres.[22] Benefactor Almonaster personally gave five enslaved people for use at the hospital in 1786, including Domingo, described in the hospital's 1793 constitution—written by Almonaster—as a "phlebotomist"—an individual trained to collect blood—"instructed in surgery," and stated Domingo would "exercise the function of the head of the surgery ward." The document did not detail where Domingo received training, and no surviving records indicate if Domingo ever acted as a surgeon or directed the surgery ward—which would have been remarkable for the period and made Domingo perhaps the first Black surgeon in an American hospital. In addition to Domingo, Almonaster forced Paugi, Magdalena, and Juana to work in service roles at the hospitals, and Gayllard was charged with running the kitchen and the garden.[23] The 1791 city census documented the hospital enslaving eight unnamed individuals, including three children.[24] A 1794 inventory listed three enslaved men who labored as carpenters—Pedro, aged fifty-five; Joseph, aged thirty-five: and Phillip, aged sixty—as well as four children—Andres, fourteen; Maria, eleven; Luis, three; and Francisco, two.[25]

Records on the medical care of Indigenous people and free people of color in New Orleans are lacking, limiting analysis. Under more lenient policies, including the practice of coartación, which allowed enslaved people to work on their free time and purchase their freedom, the number of free people of color increased from 99 in 1769 to 1,566 in 1805 (see table A.1). No records yet identified by the author detail the treatment of free people of color at the Royal or Charity Hospitals. Some free people of color may have paid for medical services from local physicians, including James Durham, who with the opening of a practice in New Orleans in 1783 became the nation's first Black doctor (detailed in chapter 2).

Americanization, Scientific Racism, and Expansion of Racialized Health Care

In 1803, Napoleon sold Louisiana to the United States to help pay for his continued military aims, including his hope to put down the insurrection of enslaved people in Haiti. By that time, a racialized health care system had already been established in New Orleans and was tied to slavery. Under the American period, racialized health care expanded and became more entrenched, more profitable, and more closely linked to the growing slave-based economy. Demand for enslaved people in Louisiana intensified with the transition to large-scale sugarcane production in the early 1800s. The end of the international slave trade in 1808 witnessed a more significant role for New Orleans as a slave market, as slavers resold enslaved individuals brought from the Upper South for sale to planters in the Mississippi Valley region. At its peak, New Orleans contained fifty-two slave markets and an estimated 135,000 enslaved people came through the port.[26]

Simultaneously, and intricately connected to New Orleans's increasing role as a slave market, the city's historically white medical field expanded. The emerging health care needs of the city were evident in the creation of two medical schools, the growth of Charity, and the flourishing of private physicians and hospitals. The growth of the medical establishment proved fundamental to the city's rise in population and significance as a slave port. New Orleans had one of highest mortality rates of any American city in the first half of the nineteenth century. The mortality rate ranged from a low of 36 deaths per 1,000 at the end of 1820s to a peak of 1 in 15 in 1853. Endemic malaria and outbreaks of smallpox and yellow fever accounted for the high death rate. Yellow fever was actually a direct by-product of the slave-based system. Slave ships introduced the virus and the main vector, *Aedes aegypti* mosquitoes, from Africa to Louisiana. The transformation of the landscape with wide-scale sugarcane cultivation aided its spread, with new canals, cisterns, and other open bodies of water serving as breeding grounds for mosquitoes, which fed on sucrose from the sugarcane for nutrition. Starting in 1796, and occurring nearly biannually after 1817, New Orleans suffered epidemics of yellow fever that killed more than 100,000 people throughout the nineteenth century. While physicians lacked the knowledge to eliminate these scourges until the late nineteenth and early twentieth centuries, the medical establishment provided a necessary service by providing treatment to the afflicted, which helped sustain the city's growth.[27]

Medical doctors also helped provide justification for the institution of slavery. In the second half of the eighteenth century, British physicians in the Caribbean plantation colonies began disseminating the idea that people of African descent had an innate immunity to tropical diseases like yellow fever and malaria, an idea picked up by American doctors in the early nineteenth century.[28] By the mid-nineteenth century, many physicians in New Orleans pushed this view, repeatedly writing about the issue in medical journals like the *New Orleans Medical News and Hospital Gazette*.[29] Physicians also argued that Africans had a naturally stronger countenance to field labor. Writing in the *Medical News and Gazette* in July 1859, Dr. Anthony Peniston, professor at the New Orleans School of Medicine, stated there was "no doubt" that Africans were of a "different species of the *genus homo*," an "intermediate between the Caucasian race and the anthropoid apes." He noted their bones were harder and denser and their "resisting power" was much greater, which was offset by smaller brains. He continued that their development of "animal and physical properties" occurred "at the expense of the intellectual." According to Peniston, these properties made them ideal as enslaved plantation laborers.[30] By the late eighteenth and early nineteenth centuries, this belief in Black resistance to disease, need for less sleep, and predisposition for physical labor had become a widely accepted and institutionalized aspect of the dogma of racialized difference in the white Atlantic World.[31]

One of the most significant advocates of these beliefs about races was New Orleans's Samuel D. Cartwright. A popular physician invited to give addresses to various medical groups and schools throughout the region, Southerners used his 1851 report "How to Save the Republic" as scientific proof of the physiological inferiority of African Americans and the need for slavery. Cartwright argued that planters must take care of infantile enslaved people, who suffered from drapetomania, a mental illness that caused them to flee if an enslaver was either too cruel or attempted to "oppose the Deity's will, by trying to make the negro anything else than 'the submissive knee-bender,' (which the Almighty declared he should be), by trying to raise him to a level with himself, or by putting himself on an equality with the negro." Cartwright infused this argument with the supposed biblical role of enslaved individuals, the "position of submission," and the "curse of Ham," God's punishment upon Canaan in the book of Genesis. Christian proponents of slavery argued that Africans were the descendants of Canaan, and differentiated by their black skin, which marked them for slavery. Many proponents of slavery used Christian beliefs to support the institution of slavery, and the Christian church was a large-scale enslaver in many parts of the United States.[32]

Cartwright also claimed that African Americans suffered from dysaesthesia aethiopica, an affliction brought about by their inherent "rascality" or laziness, particularly in free Blacks—he labeled it the "natural offspring of negro liberty." Cartwright argued that African Americans were naturally lazy and possessed "so great a hebetude of the intellectual facilities, as to be like a person half asleep." Based on his studies, Cartwright found evidence that African Americans afflicted by dysaesthesia aethiopica unintentionally committed acts of "mischief" like the destruction of "everything they handle" due to their "stupidness of mind and insensibility of the nerves induced by the disease." He also stipulated that African Americans naturally suffered from health problems like skin lesions that they would not take care of when free due to their inherent laziness. Again, Cartwright's solution was enslavement based on the need for "some white person to direct and to take care of them."[33]

The claims of Cartwright and others helped legitimize the notion of benevolent slavery. Due to their biological differences, including disposition to the diseases he studied and their low intelligence, African Americans needed the care of enslavers. Many argued that enslaved African Americans were better treated than poor white laborers in the North, and that they enjoyed their forced labor. Charity Hospital's Dr. Warren Brickell wrote in 1856 in the *New Orleans Medical News and Hospital Gazette* that Africans were not only more physically inclined to work in the fields, but they also did so "not from compulsion, from choice" even when they suffered from illness, which helped account for their high mortality rate, as they deceived slave owners about health problems—because they wanted to continue field work—until too late.[34]

While arguments like these by physicians justified the slave trade, doctors and historically white medical institutions continued to play a key direct role in fostering the slave system's growth. As happened under French and Spanish rule, ordinances in the American period required traders of enslaved people to report diseases of newly arrived enslaved people to the city council and send the ill to Charity Hospital.[35] Slave traders like J. A. Beard, the largest in the city, brought sick enslaved people to Charity and later to Touro Infirmary (founded in 1852). Bernard Kendig, another significant slave trader, purposely bought sick enslaved individuals for low prices, and then brought them to Touro in hopes that physicians could return them to full health. Then he could sell them for full value. As a result of his schemes, buyers repeatedly sued Kendig for selling them enslaved individuals that were ill or had some kind of hidden medical affliction.[36]

In slave markets, traders employed physicians as part of their effort to boost their profits, with values determined by the concept of "soundness." As argued by historians Sharla Fett and Herbert Covey, enslavers looked for "soundness," the health of the enslaved individual as related to their ability to do work, to measure their worth.[37] Enslaved individuals that appeared the "soundest" fetched the highest prices. To boost value, and thus their profits, slavers attempted to improve the superficial appearance of enslaved individuals for sale—allowing them to wash, dying hair, trimming beards, giving them more food, and applying oil to make their skin shine. However, the unhygienic conditions of the slave pens further worsened the situation of the already weakened and sick enslaved people. The March 1854 edition of the *News and Hospital Gazette* noted that many enslaved people kept in pens were suffering from pneumonia, bronchitis, catarrh, diarrhea, dysentery, measles, cholera, and whooping cough.[38] Some traders paid physicians to treat enslaved people to boost their profits. Historian Walter Johnson described the care taken before sale as "speculations" on the traders' part, "tactical commitments to slaves' bodies that were underwritten by the hope of their sale." Potential profit motivated care; those deemed less valuable, traders sold quickly rather than provide care as the investment of paying for a physician was not worth the potential return.[39]

While sellers attempted to present enslaved people to maximize their profit, buyers subjected enslaved individuals to intense physical examination before purchase to minimize their risk. Buyers often required enslaved individuals to strip to inspect their bodies for signs of maladies and asked them questions about their health histories and current physical conditions. Medical conditions or previous illnesses discovered by buyers or disclosed by the enslaved individual themselves could lower the price or prevent the sale altogether. Physicians wrote pamphlets for buyers on what they should look for on their bodies. Some buyers purchased enslaved individuals "on trial," for periods ranging from a few hours to several months, during which the owner could view their ability to work and take them to a physician for an examination. However, this also presented an opportunity for enslaved individuals to fake some affliction to prevent their sale to an undesirable owner.[40]

The redhibition laws, part of the Louisiana Civil Code, helped protect buyers from buying enslaved individuals with health problems. Traders were required to disclose physical ailments and illnesses, if known, prior to the sale. An 1855 advertisement for the auction organized by the firm of J. A. Beard & Company of 178 enslaved people from the Waverly and Meredith Plantations identified Sarah Moore as having "tonsils occasionally inflamed"; Jack Turner, "slightly affected with gleet"; Henry Cozey, "subject to piles"; Cely, Jacob Turner, Jinks, Kitty, Militia, and Lizzy as "sickly"; Barbara Ann, "crooked knee"; Modesty, "injured slightly in the head"; John, "asthmatic,"; Harry, "afflicted with palpitation of the heart"; Ezekiel, "slightly rheumatic"; and John Moore, "back injured." The assortment of injuries detailed the physical toll of labor on cotton and sugar plantations, seen in injuries like the damaged back and crooked knee, as well as afflictions like rickets and respiratory problems—detailed more in the following section—caused by factors like malnutrition and poor housing conditions.[41]

Enslavers and traders risked lowered sale prices for disclosing problems as described above, but also could face potential lawsuits for failure to detail the information. If a trader brought an enslaved individual to Touro Infirmary, the hospital could issue a certificate of health that guaranteed the individual's medical soundness. Buyers could return an enslaved individual to a trader within a year if they discovered the enslaved individual had an unknown severe "vice" like epilepsy or leprosy. However, the code also placed limitations on the returns and "warranty suits" against traders and taking a trader to court was often a long and costly process, emboldening traders to sell unhealthy enslaved individuals. Physicians often testified in these suits, with the doctors employed by the traders serving as key witnesses for the defense and physicians also testifying for the plaintiff to discuss a "vice" discovered after sale.[42] In addition to physical health problems, buyers looked for "vice of character" as well. Medical journals detailed the biological predisposition of Africans toward "vice of character," like Cartwright's alleged "drapetomania," the psychological compulsion to seek freedom. Buyers looked to avoid enslaved individuals with these "vices of character," looking for physical signs, such as whipping marks that indicated punishment for problems like running away.[43]

Physicians themselves purchased enslaved individuals. The 1791 city census documented that all eight doctors were enslavers.[44] The 1830 federal census listed eighteen New Orleans physicians as enslavers, with a total of 144 enslaved individuals.[45] Some doctors enslaved people suffering from an illness for relatively cheap in the hope of curing them and then selling them again for a large profit.[46] Other physicians purchased enslaved individuals to conduct medical experiments. In Louisiana in the 1850s, a doctor bought a man named John Brown to conduct sunstroke experiments on him, and later developed a pill that he sold for large profits based on this work.[47] As detailed in a subsequent section, medical experimentation on enslaved people became a common practice, with many such incidents occurring in the hospitals of New Orleans.

The roles of hospitals and physicians in this stage of the slave trade—from arrival through sale—demonstrated the deep ties and mutually beneficial relationship between the medical and slavery systems. Charity Hospital protected white residents from the spread of contagious disease from newly arrived enslaved people. Touro Infirmary and private physicians treated enslaved people to boost the sale price for traders, and it supported the redhibition policies that helped sustain sales. Through these actions, the medical establishment contributed not only to the slave economy, but also directly to the commodification of enslaved people as the medical treatments helped turn their bodies into sale prices and wealth. In turn, the medical establishment benefited financially from this commodification, receiving payment for these services.

This relationship continued after the sale of enslaved people, as hospital and physicians provided medical care for enslaved laborers on plantations. Enslaved individuals on plantations suffered from severe health problems and a high mortality rate. As many as 25 percent perished during the "acclimation period," the first eighteen months as their bodies adjusted to new locations, climates, and diseases.[48] The Black infant and childhood mortality rate was double the rate for whites. More than half of all Black children were born severely underweight, due to the poor treatment of and lack of nutrition for pregnant enslaved women; many miscarried or gave birth to stillborn babies. On average, Black mothers could only nurse their babies for three to four months, compared to eight months for white babies. The early weaning, and the same horrid living conditions and lack of proper nutrition that affected pregnant women, resulted in more than half of Black infants dying before the age of one.[49] For enslavers, this represented an economic problem, particularly after the ban on the importation of enslaved Africans in 1808, as they desired to increase their wealth through enslaved women giving birth to children enslavers could use as laborers or sell. As a result, enslavers often hired physicians to increase the birthing of enslaved children.[50]

The mortality rate remained higher for African Americans than whites beyond childhood. Mortality rates varied by location and by the type of plantation; enslaved people died at higher rates on sugar plantations, common in southern Louisiana, than on cotton plantations in northern Louisiana and elsewhere.[51] A host of health problems afflicted survivors. A low-quality supply of food resulted in "protein hunger" and deficiencies in thiamine, niacin, calcium, vitamin D, and magnesium.[52] The cramped and poorly constructed cabins, contaminated water sources, physical punishments including whipping, harsh working conditions, and constant stress and trauma exacerbated malnutrition, which led to higher susceptibility to disease and developmental problems.[53] Many enslaved people suffered from rickets, bowed legs, dysentery, respiratory ailments, cholera, typhoid, worms, skin problems, dementia, blindness, seizures, and swollen abdomens.[54] The lack of record-keeping at many plantations makes it difficult to know exact numbers, but scholars estimate that due to the high infant and childhood mortality rate, the average life expectancy for an enslaved individual came to between eighteen to thirty-eight years old compared to white rates of forty to forty-two during the antebellum period.[55]

After Louisiana became a U.S. territory, the legislature passed its own Black Code in 1806, modeled after the earlier French regulations and existing customs, with a mixing in of new American-inspired provisions. Like the previous documents, the 1806 Black Code contained the following provisions on medical care: "SEC. 4. Slaves disabled by old age, sickness or any other cause, whether their disease be incurable or not, shall be fed and maintained by their masters, in the manner prescribed by the second and third sections of this act, under the penalty of a fine of twenty-five dollars for each offence against this provision. SEC. 5. It shall be the duty of the master to procure for his sick slaves all kinds of temporal and spiritual assistance which their situation may demand." The government rarely enforced these health care requirements. Instead, officials focused primarily on stipulations that increasingly restricted enslaved and free people of color, who made up over one-third of the population. Under American rule, Louisiana attempted to change from the tri-caste system, with a large population of free people of color, to a binary of free and enslaved based on race. Shaken by the Haitian Revolution, the 1811 German Coast uprising, and fears of the abolition movement, white leaders created new policies that restricted the rights of free people of color. The 1806 Black Codes ended the right of coartación—self-purchase; denied all people of color the right to vote and serve in office or on juries; and made it illegal for an African American to insult or show disrespect to a white person. An 1816 theater segregation ordinance followed. In 1830, an order claimed that all free people of color who had come to the city after 1825 had to leave. As white leaders attempted to solidify race-based slavery in Louisiana, conditions for free and enslaved African Americans worsened.[56]

However, enslavers had economic incentives to provide some medical treatment for enslaved people due to the high costs of purchase. On plantations, when an enslaved individual became sick or injured, enslavers had several options, all done at their discretion and with no consent from the enslaved person. The enslaver or the overseer could apply whatever basic treatment they knew to assist the person and they often relied on pamphlets like *Ewell's Planter's and Mariner's Medical Companion*. Companies in New Orleans sold powdered drugs like ipecac, herbs, teas, and concoctions with names like "Speed's Tonic" and "Minor's Magic Fever Cure" for enslavers to administer.[57]

Enslavers could call upon an enslaved individual who had some knowledge of medicine from their plantation or a neighboring one. Black men and women used practices they had learned in Africa before slavery—including Cesarean birthing and inoculation for smallpox—or from other enslaved members, passed down orally. Black women predominantly served in this role and functioned as midwives for other enslaved women and even whites. However, many enslavers worried about allowing enslaved individuals to occupy positions of knowledge and power like healers and refused to utilize their skills.[58]

Many plantations had a space that was used as a "hospital" for the sick or injured. Most were poorly constructed and unhygienic.[59] William Howard Russell described one such "hospital" he visited on a sugar plantation owned by Governor Andre Roman outside of New Orleans in 1861. An elderly, enslaved woman ran the space, which held several beds in "naked rooms." Five patients occupied the hospital when he observed it. He described the patients, who "sat listlessly on the beds, looking out into space; no books to amuse them, no conversation—nothing but their own dull thoughts, if they had any. They were suffering from pneumonia and swelling of the glands of the neck: one man had fever."[60]

Enslavers could request a physician come to the plantation; some enslavers had yearly contracts with a specific doctor. However, few physicians possessed formal education in medicine, and often relied on traditional practices like bloodletting that only worsened afflictions. The lack of success, and costs, prevented many enslavers from employing physicians. Finally, in the early nineteenth century, enslavers could send enslaved individuals to a growing number of "slave hospitals" that proliferated in New Orleans. The growth of these institutions—explored in the following chapter—helped strengthen the ties of the nascent medical field to slavery, further creating a racialized health care system.

CHAPTER TWO

The Growth of the Slave-Based Health Care Economy, 1800–1861

In April 1860, Dr. Erasmus Darwin Fenner wrote a brief notice in the *New Orleans Medical News and Hospital Gazette*. Fenner discussed the Museum of the New Orleans School of Medicine, which he cofounded in 1856. Fenner detailed the "valuable specimens" sent to the museum by physicians in the region. He highlighted "the foot of a negro, a perfect specimen of elephantiasis" contributed by a Dr. D. R. Cole, who also submitted a "uterus in state of fibrous degeneration." Fenner also noted intestines, a mole, and a placenta contributed by three other physicians, and "a large number of diseased organs collected by Professor Flint and others from that inexhaustible storehouse—Charity Hospital."[1] Most of the "specimens" Fenner described came from the bodies of enslaved men and women, taken by physicians after their deaths and submitted to the medical school for display and anatomy lessons for students. This practice, and many other cases of exploitation of and profit from Black bodies, helped fuel the success not only of the New Orleans School of Medicine, but also of the larger medical system in what would become known as the "medical metropolis of the South."

While chapter 1 examined the ways the nascent medical profession supported the institution of slavery, this chapter details how the institution of slavery permitted the growth of the historically white health care institutions in the antebellum period, including private hospitals, the state-administered Charity Hospital, two medical schools, and the practices of individual physicians. Private infirmaries called "slave hospitals" proliferated, buoyed by profits for providing care for enslaved individuals, paid by their enslavers. While not considered a "slave hospital," Charity Hospital strengthened its connections to slavery. The hospital continued to treat the increasing number of arriving enslaved people suffering from illness and bound for the slave market, used and sold enslaved laborers, and derived income from donations from large enslavers. This chapter also explores the growth of the medical schools and the emergence of New Orleans as the "medical metropolis of the South," a process deeply connected to slavery. Physicians derived prestige and wealth through exploitation and experimentation on enslaved people, and passed down ideas of scientific racism to the next generation of doctors. Finally, this chapter examines the advent of New Orleans as a Black health center, with a sizable number of Black doctors, nurses, midwives, and folk and spiritual healers.

Private Hospitals and Slavery

When enslaved individuals suffered from medical problems, enslavers could bring them to a hospital or clinic in New Orleans; other major Southern cities like Charleston, Mobile, and Savannah had "slave hospitals" too.[2] In the first half of the nineteenth century, private hospitals began to flourish in New Orleans, part of an expanding political economy of slave health care. Part of the impetus for the growth in private hospitals came from white patrons who wished to avoid using Charity Hospital. Charity suffered from a poor reputation due its overcrowding and high mortality rates, which regularly exceeded 20 percent annually in the period.[3] Beginning in the early nineteenth century, physicians began operating clinics that skirted the city's earliest area, on the border of the French Quarter and in the Tremé and Central Business District neighborhoods. Beyond the patronage of wealthy white patients for their own health care, these physicians and clinics depended heavily upon enslavers and slave traders for financial support. In slave-trading ports like New Orleans, the institution of slavery created economic opportunities for physicians. Some doctors advertised directly in newspapers and offered their services to enslavers, and they viewed the work as a steady source of income.

As the slave-based economy and the ensuing wealth of Louisiana grew in the antebellum period, "slave hospitals" proliferated. At many of these institutions, enslaved people made up a large percentage or even a majority of patients, and were kept in separate spaces from whites.[4] In 1835, Dr. C. A. Luzenberg opened the Franklin Infirmary across from the Pontchartrain Railroad station, with the first floor containing private rooms for whites for five dollars per day; the second floor, a ward for whites for two dollars a day; and the third floor, a ward for the care of enslaved people, with their care paid for by enslavers at a charge of one dollar per day.[5] In 1839, Dr. Warren Stone started an infirmary based out of his home on the corner of Canal and Claiborne Streets. The hospital had the same division of space and rates for whites and enslaved patients as the Franklin Infirmary. By 1860, enslaved individuals made up nearly 62 percent of Stone's patients.[6] In 1852, the Sisters of Charity began to administer the hospital, renamed the Maison de Santé.[7] In 1858, the sisters moved to a location on Tulane Avenue, several blocks from Charity, and opened their own separate hospital named the Hotel Dieu, with the same setup—white rooms, a white ward, and an enslaved ward on ascending floors—as the Franklin and Stone infirmaries.[8] During the hospital's first five years in its new location, more than a third of the patients seen there were enslaved people.[9] Slave traders too were significant clients, bringing in 22.6 percent of the enslaved patients.[10] In 1841, Dr. G. W. Campbell, Dr. J. Monroe Mackie, Dr. Stanford Chaille, and Dr. Alfred Mercier opened the Circus Street Infirmary in the Central Business District, with a ward and private rooms for enslaved patients.[11]

These hospitals shared several things in common. Physicians that were founders and teachers at the city's first two medical schools—discussed in the next section—started the clinics, a reflection of the burgeoning community of medical professionals in New Orleans. Almost all had worked at Charity Hospital, which gave the doctors opportunities to develop their reputations and a network of clients during two-year residencies but offered little or no financial compensation for their services, except for the position of house surgeon. Instead, they made their money by starting private practices and hospitals for paying clients including enslavers, a steady source of income that allowed the hospitals to survive and the physicians to become wealthy. Through this wealth and status, physicians purchased large homes and attained positions of political power including sheriffs, states representatives, and senators.

Touro Infirmary was the largest of the "slave hospitals," and perhaps most demonstrated the connections between medical institutions and the slave economy. Philanthropist Judah Touro founded the space in 1852, after purchasing a mansion in the Warehouse District and converting it into a twenty-eight-bed infirmary. When Touro died, his will bequeathed funding to sustain the hospital as a charitable institution. Although primarily designed for indigent patients, Touro also admitted paying patients, including enslaved individuals with care paid for by enslavers. From January 1855 to April 1861, nearly 52 percent of Touro's patients were enslaved people, treated in a segregated space.[12] Enslaved people suffered a mortality rate of 6.3 percent compared to a white mortality rate of 23.4 percent at Touro during the period, at first a seemingly remarkable gap, considering their general poorer health. However, this difference illustrated the financial calculus that enslavers applied to medical care for enslaved individuals. As detailed by economists Jonathan Pritchett and Myeong-Su Yun, the mortality rate reflected two main factors. First, many of the white patients were newly arrived immigrants suffering from yellow fever. In contrast, most enslaved individuals suffered from diarrhea and dysentery, respiratory afflictions, and accidents. Pritchett and Yun argued that enslavers usually only sent to hospitals enslaved individuals that they expected to recover, not those they expected may die, in comparison to many whites fatally suffering from yellow fever. With a median stay of nine days at a cost of one dollar per day plus other expenses, enslavers were loath to pay for care. Additionally, the justified fear of an individual becoming ill or dying from a stay in the hospital—Touro's overall mortality rate exceeded 15 percent in the period—made the financial expenditure even riskier. However, enslavers also weighed the potential financial losses, including labor and the initial investment or cost of replacement. The cost for an enslaved, prime-aged male in New Orleans in 1860 was $1,800, the equivalent of over $50,000 today.[13] Like at Hotel Dieu, a dozen major slave traders were significant clients of Touro. Thomas Foster had sixty-one enslaved individuals treated at the hospital in 1857 and 1858; A. O. Sibley, thirty-six in 1857; and Bernard Kendig twenty-five from 1855 to 1857.[14]

Dr. Joseph Bensadon, the hospital's chief surgeon, brokered the hospital's relationships with slave traders and exemplified the economic opportunities for physicians with the institution of slavery. Prior to his role with the hospital, the firm of Walter Campbell, a large slave trader in the city, paid Bensadon to treat enslaved individuals they sold and testify on their behalf in court cases when sued for violation of redhibition policies. When Bensadon became chief surgeon at Touro, the doctor brought his connection with the firm to the hospital, as Campbell brought enslaved people to Touro for treatment prior to auction. Bensadon provided certificates for slave traders like Campbell that attested to the health of enslaved individuals as part of the redhibition guarantees. Bensadon also worked part time as a medical examiner for the U.S. Life Insurance, Annuity and Trust Company; in this capacity, he conducted exams on enslaved individuals for slave owners' insurance policies. Through his treatment of enslaved individuals on the behalf of slave traders and owners, Bensadon advanced professionally and became wealthy, and helped the hospital remain financially solvent. Even after Judah Touro's endowment ran out and the hospital provided many indigent patients with free care, Touro Infirmary prospered due to the payments from slave owners and traders; like other private hospitals, Touro likely would not have survived if not for the income from the slave system.[15]

Charity Hospital and Slavery

Although private hospitals flourished, Charity Hospital remained the largest hospital in the city. In 1811, the Almonaster family turned control of Charity to the Louisiana legislature, which ordered construction of a new hospital after a fire destroyed the previous building in 1809. From 1810 to 1815, the legislature rented a plantation to house patients. The new hospital first existed on Canal Street, and then in 1831 moved to its lasting location in the Tulane Gravier neighborhood (see map A.1 in the Appendix). Overcrowding problems persisted, requiring continual expansion. When the building opened, administrators estimated the space could hold 400 patients; by 1849, that number had been increased to 1,000 patients. In 1833, the Board of Administrators asked the religious order Sisters of Charity to manage the hospital and serve as nurses.[16]

Like the other hospitals, Charity's connections to the slave system grew in the first half of the nineteenth century, although its ties were often more indirect than institutions like Touro and Hotel Dieu. Charity treated some enslaved patients, although the number of Black patients rarely exceeded 1 percent of the total number of users. Most of the enslaved individuals received care at Charity due to city ordinances which mandated that all enslaved people would be inspected for contagious disease on arrival and treated at Charity.

Charity also maintained ties to the slave system through medical care for white laborers and sailors. From the 1830s through the Civil War, many of Charity's patients were recently arrived immigrants, many of whom found work in expanding the levees, canals, and other infrastructure projects, or in the warehouses and docks in the city that had become what historian Rashauna Johnson calls "Slavery's Metropolis."[17] Throughout this period, Charity also continued to provide care for thousands of sailors involved in the slave trade or the exportation of agricultural goods produced by enslaved people, not just from New Orleans, but from throughout the country and the lager slave-trading Atlantic World.

More directly, Charity continued to buy, sell, and use enslaved laborers. The hospital purchased at least eleven named enslaved individuals from 1817 to 1844.[18] Hospital records also document Charity purchasing four unnamed enslaved individuals for $2,600 in 1832, when the hospital moved into its larger home; and enslaving a man named Andrew, valued at $1,200, from 1857 to 1862.[19] Administrators bought enslaved people from some of the city's largest enslavers and businessmen involved in the slave trade and slave-based economy. The hospital sold enslaved people as well. The 1849 annual report included the sale of three people for a total of $1,925 from July to August.[20]

Additionally, the hospital derived income from donations by enslaver benefactors. Jean Etienne de Boré, the city's first American mayor, a large-scale enslaver, and a plantation owner who ignited the production of sugarcane in Louisiana in 1795, bequeathed $1,000 to the hospital. The 1824 will of Julien de Lallande Poydras, a chief political figure in the American purchase and early government of Louisiana, owner of multiple plantations, and enslaver of many people, donated real estate that the hospital sold for $35,000. John Burnside, a wealthy Irishman who owned the largest home in the city, multiple sugar plantations, and enslaved more than 750 people, gave $10,000.[21] In 1850, Stephen Henderson donated the Union Cotton Press to the hospital, which allowed the hospital to lease out the property for a steady source of annual income.[22]

One of the most complex ways that Charity financially benefited from slavery is illustrated by an event in 1818. In February, Renato Beluche, a New Orleans–born Venezuelan privateer, captured the Spanish slave ship *Josefa Segunda*, which was sailing from Africa to Havana with more than 200 enslaved people onboard. Beluche sold some of the enslaved people in Cuba, then the ship sailed for the Island of Margarita (off the coast of Venezuela), but was forced to stop in La Balize, Louisiana, for supplies. An inspector of revenue from La Balize boarded and seized the vessel in April 1818 for violating the 1808 ban on importation of enslaved people. With the aid of a Navy ship, customhouse officials brought the vessel and 175 enslaved people onboard to New Orleans. Federal law allowed states to enact their own bills that stipulated how the state dealt with captured, enslaved people. In 1810, Louisiana enacted a law that ordered the enslaved people sold at auction in New Orleans, with the money going to the state treasury. The legislature updated the law in March 1818, splitting the proceeds between whoever captured the ship and Charity Hospital. Officials sent 152 enslaved individuals from the *Josefa Segunda*—twenty-three had presumably died after the initial seizure—to Dr. William Flood, a Louisiana planter and physician. Flood held the group for eighty-one days and put them to work in his fields. He later successfully requested $4,000 for housing and feeding costs associated with the seizure, and another $1,570 for providing medical care.

The Cuban owners of the vessel, the firm of Caricabura, Arrieta, and Company, came to New Orleans and filed suit for return of the vessel and the enslaved people, claiming its capture to be illegal and in violation of international law. Additionally, multiple individuals—Beluche, the naval officer involved in bringing the vessel to New Orleans, the customs collector in New Orleans, and the surveyor of the port of New Orleans—all filed claims to receive money from the upcoming sale. All the claimants pushed for immediate sale of the enslaved people even before settling legal ownership as the value decreased due to illness and death during the "seasoning period" on Flood's plantation. Charity too supported the immediate sale as it would earn half of the profit. The auction on July 30th earned $95,000, less $14,000 in costs like the physician's charges. The Louisiana courts and later the Supreme Court ruled that the seizure was legal and the naval officer, the customs collector, and the port surveyor could split half of the net of $81,000, with the other half—more than $40,000, about $850,000 in today's money—going to Charity Hospital.[23]

Slavery proved vital in sustaining Charity Hospital in the decades preceding the Civil War. Money from the sale of the enslaved individuals in the *Josefa Segunda* case; financial support from enslavers; income from the cotton press; the use of enslaved people as laborers; and other ties to slavery sustained its operations. Without this revenue, the institution likely would have closed as it regularly struggled to remain financially solvent. In 1843, for example, administrators reported the hospital owed a cumulative debt of $79,898 to creditors and vendors. Administrators that year and nearly every year asked for more funding from the state legislature. The legislature never established a set amount to annually award the institution, and some years provided less than $1,000.[24] Costs at the hospital soared in the late 1840s and 1850s with large-scale immigration from Europe. Patient numbers, which had averaged 2,000–3000 annually in the early 1830s jumped dramatically, reaching a peak of 18,031 in 1852 due to immigration and the continuous epidemics of smallpox, cholera, and yellow fever, which killed tens of thousands in the period. To meet this increasing usage, the hospital relied on fluctuating sources like fees for dancing and gaming licenses, money bequeathed in wills by dying patients, charges for patients that exceeded the maximum income threshold, and a tax imposed on disembarking passengers. However, the financial support from the slave system proved to be the steadiest source of income.

Medical Schools and the "Medical Metropolis of the South"

Like the doctors and hospitals of New Orleans, medical schools established early connections to the slave system. In 1834, seven young physicians—John Harrison, Thomas Hunt, Charles Luzenberg, J. Monroe Mackie, T. R. Ingalls, August Cenas, and E. Bathurst Smith—founded the Medical College of Louisiana (later Tulane University School of Medicine), the first medical school in the state, and one of fourteen opened nationwide in the 1830s, although many proved short-lived. Many young doctors started medical schools to financially support themselves.[25] The founders stated in the annual circular that they started the Medical College of Louisiana "with the express view of educating Southern physicians, and under the conviction that a more eligible site for a great medical school could nowhere be found." They argued that city's qualities—low cost of living, "most healthful and agreeable climate from November to July," and status as the "great Commercial Emporium of one half of the Union"—made it the ideal location for a medical school.[26]

The state legislature granted a charter to the school in 1835. The school used several temporary locations, including Charity. In 1843, the legislature granted a lot near Charity to construct their own building and included the Medical College as the medical school for the newly created and state-funded University of Louisiana. In exchange, the medical school agreed that faculty and students would serve as attending physicians and surgeons at Charity for free for a period of ten years; the school also pledged to take one indigent student from each parish per year. Beyond direct funding each year, the state legislature also appropriated $40,000 for construction costs in 1847 and $25,000 in 1850 for a museum. In 1847, the institution formally became the University of Louisiana, the state's first public university.[27]

Dr. Erasmus Fenner, a founding member of the American Medical Association and the editor for the *New Orleans Medical News and Hospital Gazette*, along with several other local physicians—notably Samuel Choppin, Cornelius Beard, Anthony Peniston, and D. Warren Brickell—started a second school, the New Orleans School of Medicine, admitting students starting in 1856. To support the school, the state legislature appropriated $20,000. Like the University of Louisiana, all students—seventy-six the first year—trained at Charity, with professors having privileges at the hospital. Fenner foresaw great things for the school and the city. He posited that New Orleans would soon become the South's leading "medical center."[28]

Fenner's prediction appeared to be coming true in the following years. By 1859, the University of Louisiana's medical program had 333 students and the New Orleans School of Medicine had 164 students, making them the fifth and ninth largest U.S. medical schools; New Orleans joined New York City and Philadelphia as cities having two or more of the ten largest medical schools.[29] By 1860, the New Orleans School of Medicine was the seventh largest medical school with 216 students hailing not just from Louisiana, but eleven other states and South America.[30] The makeup of the student body at the University of Louisiana was similar.[31] By 1861, the New Orleans School of Medicine educated 247 students, with another 400 enrolled at the University of Louisiana, the third largest medical school in North America at the time.

More than 4,000 had matriculated at the latter since its opening in 1835. In the words of Dr. D. Warren Brickell, in the span of a few years New Orleans had gone from a "fifth-rate point for medical students"—behind Louisville, Charleston, Augusta, and Nashville—to the "medical metropolis of the South."[32] The transformation was deeply tied to New Orleans's simultaneous emergence as "slavery's metropolis." Both schools relied heavily upon state appropriations derived from the slave-based economy. Sons of enslavers made up large percentages of the medical students, providing the other source of income, tuition.

Funded by the slave system, these schools supported that same system in multiple ways. Both schools maintained the color line by refusing to admit Black students. At both institutions, instructors like Brickell, Fenner, Beard, and Peniston—all of whom published accounts of experiments on African Americans—taught lessons based on notions of scientific racism, used to propagate both the slave system and the racialized medical system. As part of their training, instructors distilled ideas similar to Samuel Cartwright, on biological differences among the races, including lower levels of Black intelligence, higher levels of pain tolerance, and immunity to diseases like yellow fever. Students learned anatomical lessons and practiced procedures on cadavers from Charity, mostly Black, and taken without seeking the consent of families.[33]

Taking a step further in the macabre, at the New Orleans School of Medicine, Dean Fenner created the afore-described "museum" to display cadavers. Initially, Fenner purchased them from Europe, but starting in 1857 white physicians in the region began to send him cadavers and body parts of enslaved people, many of whom had displayed unusual medical conditions. For example, in August 1857 a Mississippi physician named Dr. John Butts shipped the arm of an enslaved Black woman that was suffering from elephantiasis. In his correspondence with Fenner, Butts stated the disease would slowly kill the woman, but noted his excitement on discovering the case and wrote that he would be "pleased" to have Fenner's opinion on the noteworthiness of the case. Other white physicians followed suit, which allowed Fenner to amass a large collection.[34]

To give students an even greater advantage in their training, both schools offered the opportunity to practice on live patients at Charity, making them among the first institutions nationwide to provide hands-on experience in a hospital. Administrators at both schools highlighted access to Charity as one of the key draws for students. In his opening lecture to the incoming class of 1857, Brickell stated that Charity's greatest "resource" was its "superabundance of anatomical material," including enslaved patients and free people of color.[35] The taught lessons of racial inferiority and the view of African Americans as "anatomical material" resulted in generations of physicians that imbibed and propagated these ideas. One example could be seen in dissection of Black bodies. White physicians in the period knew that many African Americans did not want the bodies of themselves, friends, or family dissected. Brickell noted in the *New Orleans Medical News and Hospital Gazette* in 1856 the "utter abhorrence which negroes have for cutting up a dead body."[36] Yet, the hospital continued to dissect Black bodies over their objections.

Many New Orleans physicians also experimented on enslaved people, and a large number of the city's doctors—and physicians from throughout the region—published these experiments in the *New Orleans Medical News and Hospital Gazette*, edited by Brickell and Fenner. In 1854, Charity's head surgeon, Samuel Choppin, attempted the nation's first blood transfusion on an enslaved person suffering from cholera. European physicians started carrying out blood transfusions in the 1850s, and Choppin witnessed one performed in Paris in early 1854. Despite only witnessing the procedure once and never assisting in the complicated operation, Choppin tried a blood transfusion upon his return to New Orleans. During this trial, Choppin made four unsuccessful attempts of transfusing the blood, and the enslaved patient died. Nevertheless, Choppin published about the event in the *New Orleans Medical News and Hospital Gazette* to claim the first attempt of blood transfusion in the United States.[37]

In the same issue of the journal, Dr. A. P. Jones described his experiments on enslaved people suffering from smallpox on a plantation outside of the city. Jones detailed how he put ointment on half of one man's face and one hand to see if would prevent pitting—it did not work. With others, he tried different procedures, including excluding light, applying nitrates of silver, and prescribing masks of oiled silk. Dr. Cornelius Beard, who ran the Beard Eye Infirmary, noted in July 1859 that he developed his procedure for the removal of cataracts by experimenting on enslaved people.[38] In the July 1856 edition, H. J. Richard described the removal of a polyp from the uterus of an enslaved woman in Atchafalaya. Richard noted that the polyp itself had "nothing singular in its size or structure"; only the method of removal—using a silken cord—which deviated "from that recommended and normally practiced" made the case notable.[39]

Like Richard's procedure, many of the experiments occurred on enslaved women. As argued by historian Deirdre Owens Cooper, white physicians in the pre–Civil War period pushed for advancements in the fields of obstetrics and gynecology for white women by experimenting on enslaved women first.[40] New Orleans's D. Warren Brickell was one significant example and reaped great professional benefits. Brickell began his career as a visiting physician at Charity. He regularly carried out experiments on enslaved people, both men and women. In the February 1856 edition of the *Gazette*, Brickell wrote of how he attempted to find a cure for typhoid pneumonia, which he noted "could only be attained by experiment." To this end, Brickell detailed the following procedures he tried on enslaved Charity patients: bleeding, enemas, opium, brandy, carbonate of ammonia, and quinine—which he argued worked best.[41] However, it was his experiments in the fields of obstetrics and gynecology that led to his greatest acclaim and career advancement. In 1858, Brickell detailed in the journal how he tested various treatments on several enslaved women for vesicovaginal fistula, a hole that develops between the vagina and bladder and leads to leaking of urine into the vaginal canal. He did so, he noted, because of his "surprise" when a fellow doctor informed him that a case of vesicovaginal fistula had never been cured in the city. Brickell considered the fact to be a "stigma on the profession of so large a city." Although he noted that he had "no experience in the matter of operating" and had never even observed the procedures, Brickell nevertheless sought to remove the "stigma on the profession." He read about the works of other physicians, ordered medical instruments, and then he had to "get a case on which to operate." His first patient was an enslaved woman "considered incurable" an enslaver allowed him to operate on in one of the city's private hospitals. Brickell noted that it was an "ugly case for a beginner," but he was "determined to try it." Brickell tried two methods made famous by other surgeons, notably a procedure promoted by J. Marion Sims. Sims, who owned and operated the largest hospital for enslaved people in the state of Alabama, experimented with the method on twelve enslaved women—all received no anesthesia and several died—at his private hospital from 1845 to 1849. Upon finally reaching success, Sims published the procedure in 1852 and became revered as a medical pioneer as the "father of gynecology."[42]

Like Sims, Brickell did not administer anesthesia, and like Sims's early work, he "failed signally." Brickell then tried a method advocated by Nathan Bozeman, a rival of Sims who pushed for another way to repair fistulas that he had developed through experimentation on enslaved women in Montgomery. This too failed and Brickell "abandoned" the woman, thinking her "incurable" and likely to die. The woman's enslaver brought her to Bozeman, who successfully operated; Bozeman later moved to New Orleans in 1859, working as a visiting surgeon at Charity and operating the Bozeman Hospital for the Disease of Women, where he continued to experiment on enslaved women. Brickell, after two other failed attempts, finally succeeded on his fourth patient.[43] After three more successful efforts on enslaved women and feeling confident after he had practiced on enslaved Black women, Brickell operated for the first time "on a very respectable white woman" in 1859.[44] Brickell continued to experiment on Black women, for example, trying a new method for draining an ovarian tumor on a free woman of color in March 1858. She died, which he blamed on the woman waiting too long for medical treatment. He then attempted the procedure again in April 1858, with success, on an enslaved woman. Brickell parlayed his experiments into a highly successful career, including his role as coeditor of the *Gazette*, cofounder of the New Orleans School of Medicine, and professor of obstetrics. In many ways, Brickell was one of the leading pioneers in the field of gynecology and obstetrics. The New Orleans School of Medicine's first annual report in 1856 proudly highlighted that the school was one of the first in the country to offer coursework in obstetrics and the "diseases of women," taught by Brickell and largely based on the procedures he attempted and perfected on Black bodies. He and Fenner, who carried out his own experiments on enslaved women, also provided paid medical advice to enslavers on methods of "breeding" enslaved people, which again shaped his teaching of obstetrics.[45]

Doctors like Choppin, Brickell, and others saw no problem with experimenting on enslaved people, often without administering anesthesia and frequently resulting in death. Scientific racism, including the idea that African Americans did not experience pain like whites, guided these practices. Doctors were leading proponents of ideas of Black racial inferiority, and even status as subhumans. Many saw the high rates of disease and mortality—caused by the very system of slavery they supported—as proof of Black inferiority and justification for slavery. And despite their experiments killing many Black patients, they castigated others for their own attempts at treatment, including enslavers, midwives, and folk healers. In the same article in which he described his myriad of attempts to cure typhoid pneumonia—including bleeding, which only weakened sufferers and may have facilitated death, and opium—Brickell lambasted enslavers for trying to cure the medical problems of enslaved people themselves. Brickell said of these enslavers and overseers: "their knowledge is complete, or, at any rate, sufficient in their own estimation, to warrant such efforts for the restoration of the sick man as they would not, on any account, have exerted on the simple and comparatively worthless cart wheel."[46] Ideas about physicians' superiority and self-importance littered the writings that appeared in the *New Orleans Medical News and Hospital*

Gazette. Writing in an editorial in 1855, Brickell and Fenner wrote of how enslaved people viewed white physicians with respect and practically as deities. The two wrote: "As he (a physician) plies his toilsome way, there is not a negro he meets but has a ready bow and grin for him whom he looks upon as akin to the Gods, as his doctor and special friend." Furthermore, they argued that physicians like themselves worked harder than the enslaved people they provided care to: "The veriest slave toiling in the galleys or in the mines has not a more laborious task than he."[47] These statements fed into a notion of physician paternalism akin to that espoused by the enslavers themselves, with doctors as benevolent and almost heroic figures, and enslaved people as fortunate recipients. As teachers at the medical colleges and supervisors at the hospitals, these men instilled lessons of scientific racism to subsequent generations of doctors, ensuring this self-reinforcing cycle of medical racism and the larger system of white supremacy continued after the end of slavery.

These medical practices—of white students viewing and practicing on Black bodies as "anatomical material," and white physicians experimenting, killing, and dissecting Black patients—had several significant results. First, they greatly benefited the physicians as individuals and as a profession. These practices helped turn what had often been seen as a largely unorganized, nonlucrative, and part-time pursuit—many doctors in the colonial period were either wealthy or had other careers to support their medical endeavors—into a profession that provided wealth and social status by the mid-nineteenth century.

Second, doctors played an integral role in sustaining slavery and white supremacy. The hundreds of physicians that graduated from the University Louisiana and the New Orleans School of Medicine in the decades before the Civil War worked at Charity, Hotel Dieu, Touro, and the private "slave hospitals," providing medical care for enslaved people and the sailors and working-class members of the slave-based port economy. As physicians hired by enslavers, they treated enslaved people and offered advice on how to promote reproduction of enslaved people. As medical consultants, they helped slave traders achieve the highest sale price in the city's slave markets. As medical examiners for insurance companies, they backed life insurance policies taken by enslavers on enslaved individuals. As private physicians, they cared for whites who gained great wealth from the slave economy. These roles became even more important in the first half of the nineteenth century as the value of enslaved people increased with the expanding slave-based economy and the end of the international slave trade to the United States. The medical establishment in New Orleans played an integral role in supporting the system of slavery, and in turn the slave system played an integral role in supporting the medical establishment. Both benefited from each other, and both grew in the period at least partially due to the other.

Black Health Care

While both the medical establishment and the supporters of the slave system benefited from this reciprocal relationship, African Americans, both free and enslaved, suffered. As previously detailed, enslaved individuals suffered from numerous health problems due to the conditions of slavery. For enslaved people, the financial interests of the enslaver primarily dictated the medical care they received. Due to neglect and fear of white physicians and enslavers, enslaved individuals provided care for themselves. On plantations, enslaved Black men and women used folk medicine they had learned in Africa before slavery—including plant-based and herbal remedies, Cesarean birthing, and inoculation for smallpox—or from other enslaved members, passed down orally. Black women predominantly served in this role and functioned as midwives for fellow enslaved people and even white women. Medical care also often involved spiritual elements like prayers, charms, songs, and conjuring.[48]

African Americans also provided care for themselves in New Orleans. Most physicians and hospitals refused to treat free people of color, who made up 34.6 percent of the city's population in the 1810 census. Some free people of color worked as physicians, providing care for other members of their community. James Durham is believed to be the nation's first Black physician. Durham was born in Philadelphia in 1762. His enslaver, Dr. John Kearsley Jr., a throat specialist, trained Durham as a child and used him as an assistant in treating patients. When Kearsley died in 1777, a British surgeon, Dr. George West, became Durham's enslaver and used him as a physician's assistant. West sold Durham to Dr. Robert Dove of New Orleans. Durham continued his medical training under Dove and bought his freedom in 1783 for 500 pesos. Durham established his own medical practice in the Spanish-controlled city, treating both white and Black patients, earning an estimated $3,000 a year, placing him among the city's wealthiest residents. Durham briefly returned to Philadelphia in 1788, where he befriended Dr. Benjamin Rush, a leading physician, Founding Father, and opponent of slavery. In speeches and letters in support of abolition, Rush held up Durham as an example of the intelligence and capability of African Americans, stating of Durham: "I expected to have suggested medicines to him; but he suggested many more to me." Durham moved back to New Orleans in 1789, where he continued to practice medicine until at least 1802. Although Durham cared for many patients during yellow fever outbreaks in 1794 and 1800, new Spanish rules permitted him to only treat throat ailments in 1801 due to his lack of a formal medical degree. After 1802, Durham either moved—some speculated he returned to Philadelphia—or died, as his record trail ends in that year.[49]

Several other Black doctors followed Durham, although they were few in number. The first free person of color from New Orleans to earn a medical degree was Dr. Joseph Chaumette. Chaumette studied medicine and interned in Paris in the 1840s and returned to New Orleans in 1845. White physicians required that Chaumette pass an examination they administered prior to being allowed to practice in Louisiana, a stipulation not mandated by law nor applied to white doctors. Oscar Guimbilotte too earned a medical degree in Paris and opened a practice in New Orleans in 1858.[50]

Charles Louis Roudanez was another Black physician. His mother, Aimee Potens, was a free woman of color, born to an enslaved woman in Saint Domingue. Potens fled the Haitian Revolution and gave birth to Charles in Louisiana in 1823. After her husband's death, Potens moved with her children to New Orleans. Potens worked as a midwife and healer. Roudanez received his early education in New Orleans and earned a considerable amount of money through investments in municipal bonds. He then traveled to Paris, where he earned a medical degree at the Faculty of Medicine of Paris in 1853. Returning to the United States, he earned a second medical degree at Dartmouth College in 1857 and opened a prosperous medical practice in New Orleans, reportedly with both Black and white patients. Roudanez also cofounded and personally financed *L'Union* (1862–1864), the first Black newspaper in the South, and in 1864 started the *New Orleans Tribune* (1864–1870), the South's first Black daily newspaper. Roudanez used the newspapers to advocate for ending slavery, and Joseph Chaumette wrote pro-abolition essays and poems for the *Tribune*. Roudanez and Chaumette joined James McCune Smith and David Peck as Black doctors who used their positions of prominence to promote abolition.[51]

Chaumette, Roudanez, and Guimbilotte were Creoles of color, a community of free people in New Orleans that was predominantly Catholic, Francophone, and educated. Due to the legacy of less restrictions on manumission and Black property ownership under the French and Spanish, free people of color—who made up 23 percent of the city's population in 1840—had 23 percent of the city's wealth.[52] Their positions of relative prosperity allowed the Creoles Chaumette, Roudanez, and Guimbilotte to attend medical school, a rarity for most African Americans in the antebellum period. Few opportunities to train in the United States existed for African Americans—David Peck became the first Black graduate of an American medical school, Chicago's Rush Medical School, in 1847. Most aspiring Black physicians sought training in Europe—following James McCune Smith, who became the first Black medical school graduate in 1837 with a degree from the University of Glasgow. Chaumette, Roudanez, Guimbilotte, and possibly a fourth man named Joseph Joly chose this path, all studying in Paris before returning to practice in New Orleans.[53] In addition to these men with medical degrees, at least three other individuals had informal training as doctors. The 1860 census identified two "mulatto" men, Nicola Joly—Joseph Joly's father—and Charles Page, as "Indian doctors," a term for folk healers and herbalists.[54] Similarly, the 1860 and 1870 census listed John Montane as a physician, followed by the 1880 census, which identified him as an "Indian Doctor."[55]

The number of Black doctors in New Orleans was relatively small. As documented in Table A.2 in the Appendix, there were four Black physicians in 1850, and six in 1860, for a ratio of 1 doctor to every 7,007 Black residents in 1850 and 1 per 4,254 in 1860. In comparison, 224 white doctors practiced in New Orleans in 1850, and 301 in 1860, for ratios of 1 per 408 and 1 per 495 white residents in each respective year. Still, with less than two dozen Black doctors nationwide with medical degrees by the Civil War, New Orleans, with likely four individuals with medical degrees and others involved in health care, was home to a sizable Black medical community that also included numerous Black women. The city directory from 1851 listed ten Black women with their occupation as nurse, and three women as midwives.[56] Other free women of color operated as folk and spiritual healers, like Aimee Potens, Roudanez's mother. Perhaps the most famous healer was Marie Laveau, the so-called Voodoo Queen of New Orleans. Born as a free person of color, Laveau rose to prominence as hairdresser for the wealthy and also for providing nursing care. Laveau became a practitioner of voodoo, a syncretism of Catholicism and West African folk beliefs, part of the Afro-Creole culture that developed in Louisiana.[57] She sold powders created from herbs and roots to cure afflictions and reportedly had thousands of followers and clientele, both Black and white, who used her medical services, including business leaders, planters, and politicians.[58]

Most white physicians viewed Black physicians, healers, and midwives with scorn. The labeling of the aforementioned John Montane provides some insight. Montane was born in Africa with various listed birth years of 1801, 1808, and 1813. By 1860, Montane was a wealthy doctor, with real estate valued at $12,000. Despite this success, the 1860 census taker wrote their own word of judgment in parenthesis next to physician in the occupation column: "quack." This term revealed not just derision by whites, but also how white doctors viewed Black healers as potential competition for their services. In an 1860 article in the *New Orleans Medical News and Hospital Gazette* entitled "Quackery Rampant," Dr. Cornelius Beard noted that "the sick of high and low degree flock for relief" to folk healers. He warned that the city was "infested with these miserable imposters" and that prescriptions made by Black healers would either provide no cure or potentially make the ailment worse.[59] Similarly, D. Warren Brickell complained in an 1857 article in the same journal of Black midwives, whom he considered to be the "curses of communities in which they are found."[60]

The role of Black physicians, healers, and midwives was not just a problem for white physicians fearful of competition. Black positions of knowledge, power, and wealth threatened the racialized system that rested on notions of Black inferiority and white supremacy. Thus, whites required Black but not white physicians to pass examinations to practice medicine as part of an effort to curtail their professional success; some Southern states banned Black doctors altogether. This mirrored other restrictions increasingly placed on African Americans as sectionalism spread. In 1840, the city banned whites and enslaved people from attending balls for free people of color and prohibited interracial baseball games. In the following two decades, the city banned interracial gambling, ended emancipation of any kind, banned free people of color from owning businesses that sold alcohol, required segregation of brothels, and increasingly pushed for residential segregation.[61] As a result, many free people of color also left New Orleans, fleeing the increasing restrictions. From a peak 23,348 in 1840, by 1860 only 10,939 free people of color resided in New Orleans (see table A.1 in the Appendix).

Nevertheless, free people of color in New Orleans, particularly Creoles of color, faced significantly better conditions than other Black Americans, including in terms of health care and overall health. New Orleans's antebellum status as a Black health center, with the significant number of health care practitioners, led to relatively lower mortality rates. As documented in table A.3 in the Appendix, until 1856, Black New Orleanians had a lower mortality rate than whites.[62] As noted by historian Kathryn Meyer McAllister Olivarius, yellow fever may have played a significant role.[63] "Unseasoned" immigrants, having no previous exposure to the disease, died at the highest rates. Thus, the large influx of immigrants in the 1830s and 1840s to New Orleans, a population that died from yellow fever at high rates, may have significantly lowered the overall white life expectancy—immigrants made up 55.7 percent of the city's white population in 1850. Still, the longer life expectancy for free people of color is remarkable, particularly as non-Creoles of color, American Blacks, had less education, wealth, and access to health care as many could not afford to utilize Black doctors or other healers. This group suffered from some of the same health problems that afflicted enslaved people on plantations, including malnutrition and tuberculosis due to poor living conditions; most lived in low-quality housing in the "back part of the town," closer to the swamps and more flood-prone, or near the wharves. They also worked on jobs that exposed them to greater risks of injury.[64]

The health conditions for all African Americans in New Orleans declined dramatically with the Civil War. However, the years after the Civil War offered the promise of significant change. With a new constitution adopted in 1868, all African Americans gained access to health care for the first time. This proved to be a short-lived period, lasting until only 1877 and the return to power of proponents of white supremacy. Chapter 3 explores this crucial turning point for racialized health care.

CHAPTER THREE

The Civil War, Reconstruction, and the Rise of Jim Crow Health Care, 1862–1900

On July 3, 1864, an enslaved man named Valsin entered the Hotel Dieu Hospital. Valsin's enslaver was Christopher Toledano, a wealthy cotton broker and president of the Merchants Insurance Company. Suffering from an unknown ailment, Valsin stayed at the hospital for twenty-three days, with Toledano paying for his treatment at a cost of twenty-three dollars. On July 25th, the hospital released Valsin to return to his enslaved labor.[1]

Valsin's case is notable due to his status as the last documented enslaved person treated at a New Orleans hospital. When Valsin entered the hospital on July 3rd, delegates were meeting to discuss a new state constitution. That constitution, adopted on July 22nd, formally abolished slavery in the thirteen Union-held parishes of Louisiana, although it did not go into effect until approved by voters in September. The end of Valsin's treatment marked the end of the practice of "slave hospitals" in New Orleans. Valsin was also one of the last Black patients treated in a private hospital until integration a century later.

This chapter examines one of the crucial turning points in the city's health care history. During federal occupation of New Orleans, an opportunity existed to end racialized health care. After Louisiana abolished slavery in 1864, the state's new constitution in 1868 guaranteed protection of "public rights," including the right to use hospitals. However, state and federal officials refused to enforce this right or mandate integration at hospitals or in the medical colleges. Instead, the federal government created the short-lived and underfunded system of freedmen's hospitals for Black patients, which ended in 1869. Additionally, from 1868 to 1877, Charity Hospital desegregated. While falling short of integration, this change marked the first time that many Black New Orleanians could use a hospital. However, with the end of Reconstruction and return to power of Southern Democrats, white leaders purposely chose to institutionalize racialized health care. Hospitals adopted the policy of only hiring members of the Orleans Parish Medical Society, founded in 1877 with a whites-only membership clause. The University of Louisiana, which became Tulane University in 1884, formally adopted a whites-only clause as well, backed by Louisiana law in 1884. White physicians also played leading roles in paramilitary, white supremacist organizations like the White League. Subject to terror from this and other groups, the discrimination that became institutionalized with the advent of Jim Crow laws, and exclusion from the historically white health care system, the racial health gap widened dramatically. This chapter also examines the unsuccessful attempts to create Black medical schools in New Orleans in the 1870s and 1880s—undermined by the legislature's illegal refusal to fund the programs—and the successful creation of Flint Medical College in 1889 and Flint Goodridge Hospital in 1896.

Health Care in Crisis and the Freedmen's Hospital

Changes in the New Orleans medical field occurred as soon as the Civil War started. Nearly every physician and medical student joined the Confederate Army, leading to the closure of both medical schools and all hospitals except Charity and Hotel Dieu. When the Union Army captured New Orleans in May 1862, the forces occupied the closed medical schools and several hospitals. A year into the Civil War, the historically white health care system was mostly shuttered.

The medical field's ties to slavery lingered, though. Hotel Dieu continued to serve enslavers by treating enslaved people brought in and paid for by enslavers through July 1864. Federal policy allowed this connection between health care and slavery to continue. Lincoln's Emancipation Proclamation exempted federal-occupied territories including southern Louisiana. Slavery remained legal until the state ratified its new constitution in September 1864. Even after this change, Hotel Dieu did not admit its first non-enslaved African American until December 1865. Thus, federal occupation did not upend racialized health care.[2]

Some African Americans gained access to health care through military service, fighting against the Confederacy and their former enslavers. In September 1862, the Union Army created the Louisiana Native Guard, which eventually comprised three regiments and nearly 4,000 free people of color and individuals who self-emancipated. These regiments, which became part of the Corps d'Afrique in 1863, received care at the Corps d'Afrique Hospital in New Orleans. Although the army provided little funding to this hospital in comparison to hospitals for white troops, the space treated hundreds of Black soldiers during the war.[3]

The hospital also opened its doors to non-soldiers in response to the health crisis caused by the influx of thousands of other African Americans who self-emancipated. By the summer of 1862, more than 10,000 formerly enslaved individuals lived in and around New Orleans; two years later, the number exceeded 30,000 people, and many had no housing. As they did elsewhere as federal forces gained territory and advanced, the military created refugee camps, known as "contraband camps," at Camp Parapet, St. Phillip, and Fort Jackson, all near New Orleans. Over 6,000 people lived in these camps.[4] Life in the camps was difficult. Residents were considered "contrabands of war," no longer enslaved but required to work for wages as manual laborers, teamsters, and laundresses for the army. Confederate guerillas regularly raided the camps in Louisiana, capturing for enslavement or killing residents.

Living conditions were poor, including lack of adequate food and housing. The army constructed temporary housing—mostly tents or huts—but, as officer F. S. Nickerson detailed, "very few of any suitable materials has been provided of which to construct." Nickerson described the conditions of the existing structures as "brutish": "Nearly all of the huts are open and leaky—incapable of protecting either from rain or cold. Many of them are much more suitable for hog-pens than for human beings to inhabit."[5] Conditions gradually improved, as the army constructed better shelters and commandeered buildings within the city to house people. Still, many suffered, and hundreds in the camps around New Orleans died of disease, including epidemics of cholera and smallpox, but also dysentery and diarrhea.[6]

Those who lived outside of the camp in the city—New Orleans's Black population more than doubled in the 1860s to 50,456 by 1870—also faced hunger, malnutrition, disease, and physical violence. Many arrived destitute, with no money, food, or shelter, and the federal government compounded this misery with discrimination in aid. Although African Americans made up 25 percent of the population, the government distributed over 90 percent of relief—food and direct monetary payments—to white families. Thousands settled in tenement buildings in the Central Business District; flood-prone areas in the swampy back-of-the-town regions; or along the industrializing riverfront, mostly all in poor-quality housing. Most African Americans struggled to find work, exacerbated by the postwar economic downturn. Many white employers refused to hire African Americans, and some unions refused to admit Black members. This discrimination forced African Americans to take positions as unskilled laborers and servants; in 1870, for example, while African American men made up only 23 percent of the city's labor force, they made up 52 percent of unskilled laborer and 57 percent of servant positions. The collapse of the Freedman's Saving and Trust Company in 1874 wiped out the savings of many who were able to find jobs and save money.[7]

Most of the refugees suffered from a lack of formal education. During occupation, the Freedmen's Bureau and the American Missionary Association established Black schools. In 1868, the state's new constitution forbid segregation in the Orleans Parish schools, although some schools resisted for several years; an estimated 500 to 1,000 Black students attended school with white children annually from 1870 to 1874.[8]

Black New Orleanians also faced everyday acts of violence from whites. In March 1867, General Samuel Thomas, in charge of the Freedmen's Bureau in Louisiana, reported that from July 5, 1865, to February 20, 1867, whites shot, stabbed, or physically assaulted 210 formerly enslaved individuals and murdered at least seventy others statewide. Thomas stated that parish officials also underreported many acts of violence and estimated that the number of murders of African Americans by whites was probably at least double the official statistic. Thomas noted that no white man was punished for any of the attacks or murders, with the coroners or juries acquitting most whites charged.[9]

The combination of these factors—poverty, violence, poor nutrition, inadequate housing, lack of education, and unemployment—resulted in high rates of disease and mortality. Until the 1850s, free people of color had a lower mortality rate than whites. In 1861, the first year of the Civil War, the Black mortality rate of 37.16 per 1,000 slightly exceeded the rate of 31.58 per 1,000 for whites. By 1864, the growing health disparities resulted in a Black mortality rate of 81.75 per 1,000 compared to 42.14 per 1,000 for whites (see table A.3).[10]

Facing this mounting health crisis, the federal government made a fateful decision that limited the push for equality in the medical system. Rather than force the existing hospitals—Charity and Hotel Dieu—to admit Black patients, the federal government created separate and federally administered Black hospitals. They were all intended to be temporary, and the government underfunding, lack of supplies, and other problems plagued these hospitals. The first such space in New Orleans was the aforementioned Corps d'Afrique Hospital, a 1,700-bed institution funded by the military that primarily treated Black soldiers, but also treated Black civilians. A register from the hospital from September 30, 1863 to January 28, 1864 listed 108 patients labeled as "contrabands." Of these patients, thirty-nine suffered from intermittent fever, thirty-two from diarrhea, seven from scurvy, and four from smallpox, all common afflictions due to the poor living conditions in the refugee camps and in the city. Thirteen of these patients died in the hospital.[11]

Services expanded when the newly created Freedmen's Bureau took over the hospital in December 1865. Established by Congress as the Bureau of Refugees, Freedmen and Abandoned Lands in March 1865, the agency focused on several components in aiding recently emancipated individuals: education in the form of schools; distribution of clothing, food, and other supplies; securing labor contracts; settling formerly enslaved people on confiscated and abandoned land; helping Black soldiers secure pay and benefits including pensions; protecting African Americans from violence; and providing legal representation. In June 1865, the head of the Freedmen's Bureau, Oliver O. Howard, created the agency's Medical Division, which established freedmen's hospitals throughout the South.

When the Freedmen's Bureau assumed control of the Corps d'Afrique Hospital in New Orleans in December 1865, the agency transferred all patients to the vacant Marine Hospital, which then became the city's Freedmen's Hospital. The hospital, which had cost half a million dollars during its construction from 1856 to 1858, had never been fully occupied prior to the Civil War due to continual problems, including the sinking of the building caused by its cast-iron framework. During the war, Confederate forces used it as a hospital and an arsenal. Union forces too used it as a hospital for white troops, until the Freedmen's Bureau assumed control of the space. The building also contained the Dependents Home Branch—for African Americans too ill or disabled to live on their own—and an orphan asylum for Black refugee children.[12]

The 600-bed Freedmen's Hospital in New Orleans was one of three hospitals established by the Freedmen's Bureau in Louisiana in 1865 and 1866, with the other two in St. Charles Parish and Shreveport, as well as smaller dispensaries in Gretna, Algiers, Carrollton, St. John the Baptist, Gretna, Assumption, and two in New Orleans. The Freedmen's Hospital in New Orleans treated thousands of Black patients during its four-year existence. Freedmen's Hospital in New Orleans had the highest death rate, but this also reflected the fact that the bureau usually sent those most ill to that hospital. From January to November 1866, the hospital provided care for 2,030 individuals, with 547 deaths, a 27 percent mortality rate. An outbreak of cholera that year drove up the death rate—the hospital treated 239 cases of cholera, with 141 fatalities.[13] However, other ailments remained the most significant killers. For example, during the summer of 1867, physicians listed dysentery and diarrhea as the most common cause of death, followed by tuberculosis, pneumonia, smallpox, and cholera.[14] In 1866, the bureau's hospitals and health stations statewide treated 5,106 African Americans, with 762 deaths statewide, for a 15 percent in-hospital mortality rate.[15]

Health care for African Americans from the Freedmen's Bureau suffered in many ways. First, the bureau did not distribute enough rations to the hospital.

Second, army supply officers refused to turn over promised articles of clothing and supplies. Third, the bureau provided little care in the rural districts of Louisiana, refusing to treat Black laborers on former plantations—considering it "impolite" to place physicians on these fiefdoms, noted a bureau official. The plantation owners promised to provide medical care for laborers, although few did.[16]

Fourth, many of the bureau's administrators, agents, and doctors adhered to the same racist ideas as the proponents of slavery. In his 1866 annual report, Freedmen's Hospital head surgeon E. H. Harris noted that the number of treated cholera cases that year was "remarkable" in "view of the of the filthy conditions of the city & the general habits of the freedpeople as a class." Harris also wrote that African Americans were "naturally indifferent to the suffering of others." Thus, Harris, and many of the officials that worked for the bureau, continued to hold beliefs similar to those purported by Cartwright and others, that African Americans were by nature unhygienic and unable to properly care for themselves.[17]

Fifth, and perhaps most significantly, bureau and other federal officials did little to push local and state officials to aid formerly enslaved people, including admittance to hospitals. Harris wrote in his 1866 report:

> The civil authorities in this state do not seem inclinded to take any care of sick & destitute refugees and freedmen, not do I believe they intend to do so . . . In this city the civil authorities made no provision whatever to relieve sick and destitute freedmen. They are not admitted to the Charity Hospital unless it be some exceptional cases of more than usual interest to the medical profession. The same feeling is exhibited throughout the state generally. Cases are sent to the Freedmen's Hospital in this city from all parts of the state, on the grounds they are burdens to the Parish & authorities refuse to care for them and turn them over to the Bureau agents.[18]

Although they asked for local officials to admit formerly enslaved people to public hospitals, they did nothing when institutions like Charity refused to comply and allowed parishes statewide to send African Americans to the Freedmen's Hospital in New Orleans rather than treat them in their local hospitals. This occurred even as the bureau began to close down its operations in the South; thus, bureau officials knew that African Americans would soon be largely shut out of health care in Louisiana.

This also occurred as African Americans continued to face violence, which exploded in the form of the Mechanics' Institute Massacre of 1866. That July, white supremacists attacked and murdered supporters of the constitutional convention marching in favor of African American suffrage. The perpetrators, many of them former Confederate soldiers and members of the New Orleans police force—as well as the city's mayor—killed as many as 200 African Americans. Only blocks away from the attack, Charity Hospital treated white victims, but refused to admit Black patients; the Freedmen's Hospital, still located across the river in Algiers, treated the 119 African American patients.[19]

Despite this event and other similar acts of violence and the continued refusal of hospitals to admit Black patients, the Louisiana Medical Division of the Freedmen's Bureau began shuttering operations in 1867, two years after opening. Many hospitals lasted for only months. The department established temporary dispensaries in 1867 in Assumption, Monroe, New Iberia, New Orleans, and Vidalia, primarily in response to outbreaks of epidemics of cholera, smallpox, and yellow fever, and shut them down after the outbreaks subsided. As the bureau closed these dispensaries and the other hospitals—shuttering their hospital in St. Charles Parish in January 1867 after less than a year of operation—the patient load at Freedmen's Hospital increased. In 1867, the institution treated 5,918 patients, with 468 deaths, an 8 percent mortality rate. Epidemics of cholera, smallpox, and yellow fever accounted for 12 percent of cases and 27 percent of deaths, but most patients continued to be admitted for problems like diarrhea, dysentery, tuberculosis, and pneumonia. The hospital also treated 110 white refugees of war; it is not indicated in the records if white and Black patients were treated in separate wards.[20]

Although the hospital witnessed increased admissions, the bureau attempted to reduce personnel and funding, which had already been low and had led to rationing and medicine shortages in 1866. The hospital's chief surgeon Charles Warren noted in his 1867 report that the hospital "is conducted with a view to promote economy compatible with efficiency." One way the administrators attempted "economy" was reducing the number of nurses and having convalescents carry out their duties. The chief surgeon also had disabled patients engage in manufacturing baskets, which the institution sold. The surgeon further believed that this work "would be of benefit to the dependents." This again reflected stereotyped views of African Americans that Freedmen's Bureau employees accepted. In this case, hospital administrators warned of freedmen as "lazy" and "malingerers," and the danger of them becoming dependents. In his May 1868 report, he stated that "hospitals have a tendency to degenerate into almshouses," which he tried to prevent.[21] In August 1868, he noted that he had orated "stringent and repeated instructions" to doctors to reduce the number of sick by only admitting the "deserving"—the "indigent sick"; treating most as outpatients; and discharging patients as quickly as possible.[22] Warren viewed it as his role to teach African Americans how to take care of themselves, which enslavement had left them unable to do. He wrote in his December 1868 report: "Freemen are beginning to see the merit of relying upon their own efforts for support in sickness as well as in health to learn that industry and thrift are the best preventatives for want and suffering and only sure preservatives of manhood and independence." Warren believed that labor on plantations would best serve formerly enslaved individuals. He argued that planters were mostly fulfilling their contracts by paying wages and providing medical care—negating the need for bureau doctors. He further posited that the work was instilling self-sufficiency.[23]

Warren's attitudes revealed one of the fundamental problems with the Medical Division, and the Freedmen's Bureau in general. At a period when formerly enslaved people most needed assistance, the agency provided inadequate and increasingly dwindling resources, and instead emphasized the need for African Americans to provide for themselves, even though few opportunities existed in the white supremacist South. Bureau officials and the Andrew Johnson administration argued that securing employment would help prevent health problems, and thus freedmen's hospitals would not be needed as long-term solutions. As formerly enslaved people struggled to find employment and housing and suffered from severe health problems, Congress increasingly cut funding to the bureau. This resulted in further shuttering of medical institutions in Louisiana and increased pressure on the Freedmen's Hospital in New Orleans. The bureau closed the Shreveport hospital in May 1868, and by September 1868 only a medical dispensary and the hospital in New Orleans remained open for the whole state. The bureau shuttered the smallpox and cholera wards at Freedmen's Hospital and cut the physician staff to seven—down from a peak of fifteen—despite the number of patients climbing 45 percent from the previous year to 8,759.[24]

Even more consequentially, the Freedmen's Bureau did not mandate that public and private hospitals accept Black patients. Warren and other bureau officials repeatedly asked local officials to pledge to provide medical care for Black patients with little success. The bureau closed its dispensaries and hospitals with some municipal promises to offer treatment in their absence, but these appeared to have been empty words. For example, when the bureau closed the Shreveport hospital in May 1868, local officials pledged to care for Black patients. However, Warren wrote on September 30 of that year that "nothing had been done by authorities to care for the indigent sick." The following month he complained that he had repeatedly written to the mayor of

New Orleans to pledge to treat patients "regardless of race or color," with no reply.[25] Despite these failed assurances that Black patients would receive medical care in hospitals, the bureau slowly closed the remaining hospital in New Orleans. Originally, the department intended to shutter the space by January 1869, the official end date for the Freedmen's Bureau. However, the hospital remained open until June 1869—with one physician treating over 130 patients on expenditures of less than forty-five cents per patient per day— because the local hospitals in New Orleans refused to accept Black patients.[26]

Ultimately, the Corps d'Afrique Hospital and its successor, the Freedmen's Hospital, were both successes and failures. While hampered by poor supplies, rations, underfunding, lack of personnel, overcrowding, and racist attitudes of some officials, these spaces presented the first access to hospitals for most Black New Orleanians. Their service from 1863 to 1869, as well as the desegregation of Charity Hospital from 1868 to 1877—discussed in the following section—represented an opportunity to end racialized health care.

Charity Hospital under Occupation

For a period lasting from 1868 to 1877, Charity Hospital was fully integrated, despite its refusal to do so during the early years of federal occupation. During the war, Charity declined sharply, as a naval blockade reduced the number of immigrants to the city. This population loss meant a decline in revenue because of the corresponding tax on passengers that helped fund the institution, as well as a loss in access to medicine, rations, and supplies. Charity also provided care for Confederate soldiers, with no compensation from the Confederate government, which further drained the hospital's scarce resources.[27] With the city's capture, hospital leaders initially refused to treat federal soldiers. However, upon discovering that the hospital provided care to Confederate soldiers, federal troops assumed control of the hospital and triggered a forced removal of the board of administrators and the voluntary resignation of most of the hospital staff. The hospital lost the revenue from renting out the Union Cotton Press, as the army used the building for housing of occupying troops. The number of patients served declined to a low of 4,857 in 1864. The federal government provided rations, medicine, and other supplies, but the hospital was severely underfunded. Administrators asked for at least $100,000 in appropriations from the state legislature in 1864 for needed repairs to the building, which they described as "falling into decay."[28]

Patient numbers began to increase after the war ended as the port slowly regained some of its prewar trade and immigration. With the closure of the

Marine Hospital in 1869, the federal government temporarily awarded the contract for care of merchant seamen to Charity, providing over half of the hospital's budget in the 1870s. Still, the hospital continually struggled financially, as state aid proved inadequate and debts mounted. Administrators repeatedly cut expenditures, lowering the quality of care, and even had patients help with upkeep. Annually, the hospital board asked the state for more aid and to establish a state almshouse as they argued Charity had become the de facto facility for the poor, not just for New Orleans and Louisiana, but for states throughout the region.

However, Charity's most significant change during occupation was integration in 1868. Despite federal occupation, many former Confederates regained political power in 1865 and the state legislature passed restrictive Black Codes, including legislation that barred African Americans from voting. These laws combined with white violence helped maintain white supremacy in Louisiana. State leaders permitted Charity to continue to deny access to Black patients. However, Republicans in the state began gaining political power in the fall of 1866, aided by federal actions including the ratification of the Fourteenth Amendment and the Reconstruction Acts, which divided the South into military districts and placed greater federal control and military presence in the former Confederate states to protect Black male suffrage. With these measures, Republicans elected H. C. Warmoth as governor in 1868 and gained control of the state legislature. In 1868, the Republican-majority legislature ratified a new constitution that removed the Black Codes and enfranchised all men over the age of twenty-one residing in the state for a year. The constitution also guaranteed "public rights," which it detailed in Article 13: "All persons shall enjoy equal rights and privileges upon any conveyance of a public character; and all places of business, or of public resort, or for which a license is required by either State, parish or municipal authority, shall be deemed places of a public character, and shall be open to the accommodation and patronages of all persons, without distinction or discrimination on account of race or color." Hospitals were considered "places of public character" under this provision.[29]

With this radical change in the state constitution that included the concept of political rights and public rights, in 1868 the legislature ordered Charity Hospital to implement a nondiscrimination policy, over the objection of Democratic representatives. That September, the hospital board adopted a resolution "that in admitting sick persons to the benefits of this hospital no distinction be founded on race, color, or previous condition."[30] With the closing of Freedmen's Hospital in June 1869, the institution's remaining 400 Black patients were transferred to Charity. The number of Black patients from 1868 to 1876 at Charity Hospital is unknown, as the annual reports did not count patients by race. In 1877, when Charity again began segregating patients, the hospital had total admission of 1,039 Black patients, out of 6,695 total. While admission numbers rose in the early to mid-1870s, administrators noted that the hospital had not witnessed an increase in Black patients; thus, it is likely that the 1877 figure of 1,039 closely matches the number of Black patients in the preceding years.[31]

In addition to admitting Black patients, in 1871 Charity Hospital also permitted the first Black doctor. Born in New Orleans in 1846, James T. Newman received his medical education in Canada before establishing a practice in Chicago. Newman returned to the Crescent City to run the American Missionary Association's Hathaway Home for the Poor and Friendless, which provided free care for indigent patients, white and Black, from 1870 to 1871. As a member of the visiting staff at Charity, Newman performed surgeries on Black patients—administrators refused to allow him to treat white patients—and trained Black students of Straight University's short-lived medical program—detailed in a following section—in lessons in the surgical wards. Although only allowed to practice on Black patients, Newman and his medical students' presence in the hospital represented a significant break from the medical system of the past.[32]

The Postwar Health Care System

This Reconstruction-era opening of health care for African Americans proved short-lived and only occurred at Charity Hospital. Despite federal occupation and the "public rights" provision of the 1868 state constitution, which required hospitals to treat all patients, private hospitals continued to refuse to admit African Americans. After the abolition of slavery in 1864, Hotel Dieu, which had treated hundreds of enslaved people brought by slave owners, treated only thirteen individuals that hospital records identified as Black. The first patient, Josephine, was treated for burns from December 14 to 15, 1865; the last, Ben Osetors, received care for seizures from May 30 to June 8, 1869. After that date, every patient in the hospital's records is identified as white.[33] Touro Infirmary admitted no Black patients after reopening in 1869. The city's other smaller private hospitals followed suit and denied admission to African Americans. Administrators chose to do so, even though many badly needed patient revenue. New Orleans's economic system in the postwar years nearly collapsed due to the end of slavery and trade in slave-produced goods. Unlike other cities, New Orleans had not invested in railroads, and instead continued to believe that steamboat trade would remain dominant. With changing trade patterns, New Orleans's role as a commercial center declined. Similarly, manufacturing was underdeveloped. Finally, the state was hurt by the depression of 1873. Due to these factors, New Orleans's economy suffered a depression until the late 1870s.[34]

Recognizing the symbiotic relationship between the city's economy and the health care field, physicians tried to boost the economy, much as they had earlier for the slavery-based antebellum economy. In 1875, a committee of doctors met with a trade delegation from England. They presented a report on the sanitation and health of the city to convince them to increase investments and trade partnerships. The report attempted to defend the health reputation of New Orleans, still known as the "City of the Dead" for the continued outbreaks of yellow fever. The physicians argued that the large number of sufferers of tuberculosis who came to the city each winter and outsiders afflicted by other ailments that used Charity Hospital drove up the mortality rate. They stated that deaths from malaria and yellow fever had decreased in recent years due to improvements in drainage. They also posited that "great allowances should be made for disparity in mortality between the white and colored races." They argued the higher Black death rate, particularly the infant mortality rate, unfairly ruined New Orleans's reputation in comparison to other cities: "if the negro mortality rate was eliminated from the death rate of New Orleans the comparison would be more favorable."[35] New Orleans's leaders would use many of these same arguments, particularly the necessity of excluding the high Black death rate, to promote the city's burgeoning trade with Latin America and the tourism industry in the early twentieth century, discussed in chapter 4.

As the economy foundered through this period of uncertainty, so too did the historically white health care field. The abolition of slavery ended a significant source of income for many hospitals. The fact that most private hospitals did not reopen after the war, and the struggle of those that did, demonstrated the reliance on the slave-based economy. Because enslaved people comprised more than half of the patient base, many hospitals simply could not survive the ending of slavery. Even the larger hospitals that treated high numbers of enslaved people—Hotel Dieu and Touro—struggled to overcome this funding loss. Like at Charity Hospital, newly arrived immigrants made up the vast majority of patients in the postwar decades at Touro and Hotel Dieu, although different social strata used different hospitals. The indigent, working poor, and sailors made up a large percentage of patients at

Charity, whereas middle-class workers used Touro Infirmary and Hotel Dieu.[36] With the economic depression, many private practices and hospitals never reopened, and others took years to return. In 1866, only three private hospitals had returned to operation: Stone's Infirmary, the Circus Street Infirmary, and the Luzenberg Hospital, which functioned primarily as the smallpox and isolation hospital.[37]

As the overall economic situation slowly started to improve with increasing river and port trade due to physical improvements to channels and the Mississippi River, several other hospitals opened or reopened: DePaul Hospital (operated by the Sisters of Charity of St. Vincent de Paul, who cared for patients suffering from mental illnesses at Charity Hospital starting in 1841) in 1863 in Uptown; the French Hospital (operated by the French Benevolent and Mutual Aid Society) in Tremé in 1867; Nathan Bozeman's Surgical and Women's Hospital, started in 1860 as a "slave hospital" and reopened in 1869; and the Orleans Infirmary, founded in 1869 by D. Warren Brickell, Samuel Choppin, Cornelius Beard, and J. Dickson Bruns and located in the Central Business District. All four hospitals chose not to admit Black patients. Most white physicians also refused to accept African Americans as patients at their private practices.

Even at Charity, the only hospital open to African Americans, Black patients faced discrimination and exploitation. Men who previously promoted slavery and scientific racism, and fought for the Confederacy, returned to their positions at Charity after the war. While the Republican-controlled legislature pushed for equality for African Americans and ordered nondiscrimination at the hospital, the physicians and surgeons who worked at Charity actively fought against these same ideals. These individuals still viewed Black bodies as subjects for experimentation and dissection, and "anatomical material" for white medical students.

The hospital's head surgeon, Andrew Smyth, set the tone through his exploitation of Black patients. In 1864, chief surgeon Smyth operated on William Banks to remove a tumor on his neck. A decade later, Banks returned with another tumor on his neck. Smyth did not operate this time, as he felt Banks's condition was terminal. When Banks died, Smyth wanted to dissect Banks's corpse, and keep the upper part of the body in his anatomical collection as the operation in 1864 on the pulsating tumor was the first such surgery of its kind on record. However, Banks belonged to a Black fraternal organization that demanded the hospital turn over his body for burial in accordance with Banks's wishes. Smyth ordered his assistant Edmond Souchon to dissect the body and sneak out the desired section while Smyth argued with the fraternal organization in the waiting room as a distraction. Years later, Souchon recalled with pride the incident, describing it as a "living legend throughout the medical world" and spoke amusingly of the appalled looks on Banks's friends' faces upon finally seeing his body: "But judge of their shock and horror when they saw all that was left of their saint, two legs with the viscera and a left arm without being able to find where the balance had gone." Souchon gleefully told friends that Banks's compatriots never found out what happened to the rest of his body.[38]

These same men also taught at the medical schools, which, like the private hospitals, slowly recovered in the postwar period. Union troops occupied the campuses of both the University of Louisiana and the New Orleans School of Medicine until the end of the war. After forced exile due to his unwillingness to sign a loyalty oath to the Union, E. D. Fenner returned to New Orleans and worked for months to secure the school's return and reopened it in November 1865. However, Fenner died in May 1866 and the college found it difficult to attract students who could afford medical school; the college closed in 1870.[39] The University of Louisiana struggled as well to attract students when it reopened in 1866, with only thirty-two graduates that year; in comparison, 134 had graduated in 1861. The numbers slowly increased but were still at slightly more than half of the prewar peak by 1871, with seventy-two graduates that year.

Despite financial difficulties due to low enrollment, both colleges refused to admit Black students in explicit violation of Article 135 of the 1868 state constitution, which forbade the establishment of colleges "exclusively for any race." Like the private hospitals, these institutions faced no punishment from state or federal officials. This inaction was a further failure in a potential turning point for the racialized health care system. Under the 1868 constitution, hospitals and medical schools should have integrated. When they failed to do so, state or federal officials should have enforced this mandated integration.

Instead, proponents of white supremacy directed the hospitals and the medical schools that produced the next generation of physicians. Brickell led the New Orleans School of Medicine after Fenner's death. After the school closed in 1870, Brickell founded and headed the short-lived Charity Hospital Medical College from 1874 until it too closed in 1877. The former head surgeon of the Confederate Army, Tobias Richardson, served as dean of the medical program at the University of Louisiana, and former Confederate officers filled nearly all teaching positions at both medical schools. Both schools continued to receive Black cadavers for dissection and anatomy lessons from Charity; in 1869, the year that Charity began admitting free people of color, the New Orleans School of Medicine's annual report noted that the "anatomical material is always abundant." Students also continued to utilize Fenner's anatomical museum, comprised primarily of body parts of enslaved people donated by white physicians. In the late nineteenth century, Edmond Souchon started his own such museum at the University of Louisiana, one that reached national renown.[40]

While smaller in size than in the prewar period, the University of Louisiana dominated the medical profession in New Orleans. By 1872, graduates of the school comprised two-thirds of all physicians in the city. Graduates also worked as physicians in other parts of Louisiana and in other Southern states and served as sheriffs and state representatives and senators, demonstrating the school's prominence. A high percentage of these doctors—over 60 percent in the decade after the Civil War—had fought for the Confederacy. In medical school, their teachers instilled lessons of scientific racism. As physicians, these men applied these lessons at hospitals and in private practices, while simultaneously many participated in the White League—discussed in detail in a following section—and other white paramilitary organizations of terror; both activities ensured the continuance of white supremacy and racialized health care.[41]

Black Medical Schools and Physicians

Illegally excluded from medical schools in New Orleans and most medical schools nationwide, African Americans found some opportunities for higher education with a series of Black colleges. Several of these colleges included medical programs. In New Orleans, two schools attempted to initiate medical programs, following the lead of Howard University, which created the first Black medical school in 1868. Black and white civic and religious leaders founded three Black institutions of higher education, creating Straight University in 1868, Leland University in 1870, and New Orleans University in 1873. Albeit briefly, both Straight and New Orleans University established medical programs, the third and seventh Black medical colleges in the country.[42]

Funded by the American Missionary Association and the Freedmen's Bureau, Straight University included medicine as one of eight initial programs. In January 1870, the legislature appropriated $35,000 to start and house the medical department.

White legislators may have been motivated by a desire to circumvent Article 135 of the 1868 state constitution. Fearing a push for the integration of Louisiana State College and the University of Louisiana, politicians supported state funding for Straight University to address Black higher education without integrating white institutions. However, Governor Henry Clay Warmouth vetoed the bill. While the school awaited the outcome of a lawsuit to receive the funding, Straight established a medical program under James Newman. As Straight waited to see what would happen with state funding, Newman began preparing the medical program and officials hoped to buy a lot for the medical building near Charity Hospital. The Louisiana Supreme Court ruled against Straight and upheld the governor's veto, stating that as a private institution it was ineligible to receive state funding. Nevertheless, when the state colleges continued to refuse integration in violation of Article 135, the legislature awarded limited funding for Straight, which was open to both Black and white applicants, although not enough to fully support the medical program.[43]

Undeterred, Newman pressed for the opening of the medical program, which finally occurred in 1873 with ten white and Black students. Newman served as the only instructor and trained students in the medical and surgical wards at Charity Hospital, where he had attending privileges. The opening of the program, the Deep South's first medical program for Black students, was a notable achievement, and again could have led to significant changes in the medical system. However, foreshadowing many of the limitations imposed by the racist hierarchy and the city's power structure, the medical program faced insurmountable obstacles. The state's meager allocation of funding for Straight only provided $1,000 to establish the medical program, far too little. As a result, Newman was unable to hire any other instructors and Newman paid for all the students' educational material out of his own salary.

Additionally, Newman faced institutional opposition within the school and the American Missionary Association (AMA). Anticipating twentieth-century debates about the creation of separate Black medical institutions versus the push to integrate, Straight University president Samuel S. Ashley and other board members openly opposed the creation of the Black medical program. They favored a push to integrate the University of Louisiana's medical programs instead. Facing an economic recession in 1873 and mounting costs for educational programs throughout the school, the board refused to grant Newman additional funding to purchase a separate medical building—the medical program operated out of the school's main building on North Esplanade and North Derbigny Streets—but approved his plan to raise money to purchase a lot on Common and Villere Streets. Told not to solicit religious groups, Newman instead approached sympathetic physicians for financial support. However, a group of white doctors led by D. Warren Brickell bought Newman's desired lot and there started the Charity Hospital Medical School. Newman then proposed purchasing a hospital building on the corners of Claiborne and Canal, one block from Charity Hospital. Again, the AMA allocated no funding but approved Newman's plan to fundraise $5,000. However, Newman failed to secure the money, as few Black doctors practiced in the city and white doctors refused to contribute. In 1874, Straight University discontinued its medical classes.[44] A second medical college started as part of the founding of New Orleans University in 1873, an institution funded by the Methodist Episcopal Church (MEC). School leaders envisioned a large medical college that would attract Black students from throughout the region. However, similar to Straight University, the program sputtered at first. Classes did not begin until 1878, with eight students and five faculty, including James Newman, who served as dean of the faculty. Akin to Straight, the college discontinued medical classes after the first year due to financial difficulties.[45]

The limitations, particularly financial, imposed by the existing power structure that derailed both attempts at establishing a Black medical school and permitted the illegal exclusion of Black students at the University of Louisiana severely limited the Black medical system in New Orleans. Some private Black physicians practiced in New Orleans in the postwar years and played significant roles in the Black community. Louis Charles Roudanez remained the most prominent example. In addition to his practice, which he maintained until his death in 1890, Roudanez continued to advocate for equality with his newspaper the *New Orleans Tribune*. Although criticized by some African Americans as elitist and representing the views of the wealthier Afro-Creoles, the publication identified itself as the "organ of the oppressed." White supremacists also attacked the newspaper, perhaps the most radical in the country, as it championed Black enfranchisement, wages for formerly enslaved African Americans, integrated schools, and the civil rights codified in the state's 1868 constitution. Two of Roudanez's sons became physicians, and a third became a dentist.[46]

Other Creoles of color also became doctors, including Eugene Dubuclet. Eugene's father, Antoine, was the wealthiest and largest enslaver among free people of color in the state by the Civil War, and afterward he served as Louisiana's Secretary of Treasury from 1868 to 1878. Antoine sent all twelve of his children to France for education, including Eugene, who studied medicine in Paris before operating a practice out of his residence in the Marigny neighborhood of New Orleans.[47]

Dubuclet and Roudanez—and his two sons who both became doctors—were part of a small group of physicians that came from the ranks of Creoles of color and primarily served this clientele. In the mid- and late nineteenth century, while whites attempted to solidify a white–Black binary, Creoles of color attempted to distinguish themselves from formerly enslaved people, including where they resided. While many formerly enslaved people settled in Central City and the back of town, Creoles of color still lived predominantly in Tremé and the Marigny. Many of this group maintained jobs in skilled labor, such as plasterers, masons, carpenters, and longshoremen. Some owned businesses like tailor and clothier shops, groceries, and cigar factories. Others continued in professional positions. With higher incomes, they could afford to send their children to one of seven private schools established in the 1860s and 1870s. With their wealth, they also used the services of the handful of Black medically trained physicians who had practices in Tremé and the Marigny.

Other Creoles of color relied on health care provided by fraternal organizations. In the late nineteenth century, a number of proto life and health insurance companies formed. For example, the Les Societé des Jeunes Amis, founded in 1867, paid death benefits of $100, gave access to a physician to visit, and provided pharmaceutical drugs for sick members and weekly cash relief of three dollars if they missed employment due to illness. The society employed three physicians and a pharmacist to treat members. To join the exclusive organization, a current member had to vouch for an applicant, and all the members had to vote on admission. Members paid one dollar a month in fees and had to obtain a health certificate from a society physician before admission. A society physician had to also confer a certificate of illness for a member to receive medical care and sick benefits.[48] La Concorde provided the same benefits for its members, including care by a society physician. Similarly, the Young Female Benevolent Association provided members—that paid fifty cents per month—sick benefits of two to four dollars per week and one dollar for doctor's visits, in addition to fifty dollars in death benefits.[49]

Even for Creoles of color, though, health care was limited. Only fourteen Black physicians practiced in the city in 1870, and sixteen in 1880, for a ratio of 1 doctor per 3,604 Black residents in 1870 and 1 per 3,601 in 1880; this compared to 1 doctor per 590 and 1 per 619 white residents in each year, respectively (see Table A.2). Of these, few had formal medical education. Men like Roudanez and Dubuclet were outliers. Although it is impossible to determine the training of all the doctors, of the twenty-eight individuals listed in the 1870 and 1880 census (two were listed in both), the census identified six as "Indian Doctor," likely signaling no medical degree. Additionally, at least eight of the twenty-eight were labeled as illiterate.

These individuals and other folk healers served 57,617 Black residents by 1880. Most African Americans could not afford the services of a private physician like Roudanez or to receive care from benevolent organizations like Les Jeunes Amis. With the closing of the Freedmen's Hospital in 1869, their only option was Charity Hospital. However, Charity struggled in the 1870s to remain open due to lack of funding and was staffed by physicians that openly advocated for white supremacy. By the end of Reconstruction in 1877, African Americans made up 15.5 percent of the hospital's patients. African Americans were underrepresented at the hospital, as they made up 26.7 percent of the population; white foreign-born immigrants were overrepresented, as they made up 18.2 percent of the city's population but 51.8 percent of patients. At the hospital, African Americans had a mortality rate of 22.8 percent, more than double the white rate of 11.3 percent. One factor was the disproportionately high numbers of respiratory problems like tuberculosis and pneumonia, which were all symptomatic of poor housing conditions and nutrition. Strikingly, even at Charity, the hospital used by whites with the most negative social determinants of health—predominantly impoverished immigrants forced to live in low-quality housing, among other factors—African Americans still fared significantly worse, revealing the sharp racial disparity in health care.[50]

Rise of the Redeemers and the Institutionalization of Jim Crow Health Care

In the 1870s, the power of the Republicans waned and an already precarious situation for Black residents declined even further. Although a Republican, Governor Henry Warmoth backed away from his initial support for Black equality to secure more white electoral support. This move included his vetoing of legislation that would have enforced the protection of "public rights" by fining owners of public accommodation—which would have included hospitals—for discrimination or denial of admittance to African Americans. In 1872, Democrats disputed the election results that awarded the governorship to Republican William Pitt Kellogg. Whites formed paramilitary organizations to challenge the results of the election and Reconstruction in general and to carry out a campaign of terror and violence against African Americans. In Opelousas in April 1874, the white supremacist "White League" formed, and a New Orleans chapter started in June with Fred Ogden as the head and Drs. J. Dickson Bruns, Samuel Choppin, and Cornelius Beard as leaders and members of Ogden's inner circle. On September 13, 1874, Bruns published a circular titled "Citizens of New Orleans" in the city's newspapers.

Bruns called for whites to assemble the following day at 11 A.M. at the statue of Henry Clay on Canal Street to protest the "outrage after outrage heaped upon you by an usurping government" and to "Declare That You Are of Right, Ought to Be, and Mean to Be, Free."[51] On September 14th, approximately 6,000 whites, many armed, gathered to hear the leaders of the White League and voted en masse to adopt a resolution that called the 1872 election a "fraud," argued the "usurper" Kellogg's refusal to resign presented an "imminent danger of republican institutions throughout the entire country," and called for his immediate abdication and the installation of John McEnery, the Democratic candidate who lost the gubernatorial race. The leaders designated five men, including Dr. Samuel Choppin, to present the resolution to Kellogg, demand his immediate response, and present that response to the crowd. The committee reported back at one o'clock that Kellogg refused to receive the resolution and called for the dissolution of the crowd, which Kellogg described—accurately—as armed and a "menace." Upon hearing the report, Dr. Cornelius Beard called on whites to return to their homes, gather their weapons, make the city an "armed camp," and drive out Kellogg and his supporters. The head orator Robert Marr directed the crowd to meet at Canal Street at 2:30 P.M. In what become known as the Battle of Liberty Place, over 5,000 supporters of the White League—including the three aforementioned physicians, as well as Drs. D. Warren Brickell, Howard Smith, Charles Tebault, and Samuel Logan—attacked the Metropolitan Police. Sixteen members of the White League, thirteen policemen, and six bystanders died, and dozens were injured; Choppin led a medical corps that provided aid to the injured White Leaguers. The White League successfully deposed Kellogg and installed McEnery as governor for three days until federal troops arrived on September 18. While the coup proved short-lived, the event—which shocked many Northerners and convinced them that Reconstruction would never succeed—helped end Reconstruction.[52]

While largely absent from historical scholarship, white doctors played key roles in facilitating the failure of Reconstruction in Louisiana. Many of the doctors who participated in the Battle of Liberty Place were part of the first generation of graduates of the University of Louisiana. Their instructors instilled lessons of scientific racism, with practice on Black bodies and cadavers from Charity Hospital. They worked at Charity and the "slave hospitals," where they applied the learned lessons of scientific racism on Black patients. They accumulated wealth through this work that allowed them to become enslavers themselves; for example, the 1860 census listed Cornelius Beard as living in a mansion with five enslaved domestic laborers, and Samuel Choppin and Warren Stone enslaving six people each in their homes. They volunteered to support the Confederate Army as doctors. After the war, they ran hospitals and clinics that denied admittance to Black patients. They served as professors at the University of Louisiana and the New Orleans School of Medicine and instilled the same lessons of scientific racism in the succeeding generation of doctors.

Their support of white supremacy extended far beyond the field of health care. While not elected officials, they used their standing to support white supremacy and anti-Black violence and to question and undermine the legitimacy of the democratically elected officials and the constitution lawmakers created to protect Black rights. Several served as leaders of the Democratic clubs that helped elect politicians who enacted the Black Codes and other policies that curtailed Black freedom. They led the White League, Confederate veteran groups like the United Confederate Veterans, and paramilitary organizations like the Crescent City Regiment, all of which carried out campaigns of terror and violence against African Americans. They also led groups like the Southern Historical Society—Bruns and Dr. Joseph Jones (chair of the chemistry department at the University of Louisiana and physician at Charity) were cofounders—that promoted the Lost Cause ideology. As men of significant social standing—educated, wealthy, revered as Confederate officers, and active in prominent social organizations like the Boston Club—these men gave the veneer of intellectual credibility and respectability to claims of white supremacy, Black biological inferiority, and the righteousness and patriotism of white supremacist violence. A celebrated orator, Bruns perhaps best captured these ideas in a keynote address he gave to a crowd of 4,000, including the mayor and other city and state leaders, commemorating the first anniversary of the Battle of Liberty Place. Bruns lamented the North's "lust of conquest" that produced the Civil War and posited the federal government "created the domestic violence to quell" during Reconstruction. He blasted the "fraud" that produced the Thirteenth, Fourteenth, and Fifteenth Amendments and the 1872 election results. He described the election of Black officials as "crime against nature itself which subjected the high and ancient civilization of free born Anglo Saxon commonwealths to the rule of debased and ignorant Africans." He denounced the despotism of the federal government and the "carpetbaggers," including the confiscation of Confederate weapons, which left whites vulnerable to the "oath-bound league of the blacks." Whites were subjected to Black crimes including "murder, arson, and rapes which began to run riot in the parishes"; these acts "warned us that a war of races, which of all horrors we were most anxious to avoid and the Radicals to precipitate was imminent, and we had either to avert it or perish by it." The White League formed to protect whites against this threat and to "maintain and defend the Constitution of the United States of the State." He described the Battle of Liberty Place as the defense of the "spirit of liberty," the three-day rule of the White League as a "saturnalia of freedom," and the White Leaguers who died as the "patriot sires of Lexington and Concord."[53] Doctors like Bruns, Choppin, and Beard never achieved the prominence of figures like McEnery and Ogden, but nevertheless played significant roles in hastening the end of Reconstruction.

Boosted by these individuals and the message of white supremacy they explicitly endorsed, Southern Democrats, known as "the Redeemers," returned to power in the election of 1876. Under Democratic rule, local and state leaders began institutionalizing racialized health care. Governor Francis Nicholls—a former Confederate general—appointed Samuel Choppin as president of the Board of Health. The new state legislature approved funding for the Nicholls Home for Soldiers, which provided medical care for Confederate veterans. Also in 1877, physicians formed the Louisiana and Orleans Parish Medical Societies (OPMS), headed by Choppin, Brickell, Bruns, and Beard. OPMS proudly embraced its members' roles in the Battle of Liberty Place and other efforts to end Reconstruction, with founders writing that "white patriots" created OPMS as part of the "offspring of the hard-won liberty gained" against "scalawags and free negro slaves."[54] OPMS instituted a whites-only membership clause. OPMS also mandated that all hospitals in New Orleans only hire OPMS members, ensuring that no hospitals would integrate their staff until OPMS did so—which did not occur until 1965. Additionally, all private hospitals pledged to continue to deny admission to Black patients. Only Charity and the Marine Hospital admitted Black patients. However, the Marine Hospital only admitted dues-paying merchant seamen, a small portion of the city's Black population.[55]

Outside of the merchant seamen, Black New Orleanians could only use Charity Hospital. However, Charity also embraced Jim Crow in the period. In violation of the 1868 constitution, Charity began segregating patients by race in 1877 and started treating African Americans in a separate ward in 1881; the new 1879 state constitution endorsed the practice. In 1877, the hospital fired James Newman, the hospital's only Black doctor, who had served as a visiting surgeon since 1871. Charity's brief period of integration lasted only nine years; it would be another ninety years before the hospital integrated again.[56]

Rather than being a harbinger of increasing equality in health care, Charity's integration instead was as an outlier, a sampling of the promise of Reconstruction snuffed out by white supremacy. The historically white health care system reasserted itself, with judicial backing. The U.S. Supreme Court endorsed segregation, first with the Civil Rights cases (1883), which allowed states to permit discrimination in private establishments like New Orleans's private hospitals, which continued to deny admittance to African Americans, and then with *Plessy v. Ferguson* (1896), which legalized the segregation Charity had been carrying out for nearly two decades. With the University of Louisiana's legal transition to Tulane University in 1884, the school officially adopted a whites-only clause, encoding its discrimination that dated back to the school's opening in 1834. As it did before the Civil War, the school continued to receive "anatomical material" from Charity, primarily the cadavers of African Americans. Like E. D. Fenner at the New Orleans School of Medicine, Edmond Souchon, who served as a professor of anatomy for decades at the University of Louisiana, created a museum of anatomy, filled primarily with specimens from Black bodies, for medical students. Souchon developed a national reputation for his museum, with other medical schools throughout the country asking for his consultation in establishing their own anatomical museums. In 1909, the *New York Medical Journal* described Souchon's collection as "the finest room of its kind in this country or abroad." Medical groups across the country borrowed Souchon's collection for display at their medical school or conference for medical professionals; the Louisiana Board of Health utilized it in the 1910s as part of a traveling "Health Exhibit Train" that toured the state.[57]

Beyond access to health care, Black residents continued to suffer from health disparity due to several factors, including educational inequality in the underfunded and decaying buildings that served as Black schools.[58] African Americans continued to live in low-quality, overcrowded, and flood-prone housing that perpetuated high rates of tuberculosis, mosquito-borne afflictions like yellow fever and malaria, and other health problems. Everyday discrimination, intimidation, threats, and violence continued, and in some ways intensified. From 1882 to 1936, whites lynched at least 333 African Americans in Louisiana, including at least fourteen in the New Orleans area.[59] In July 1900, Robert Charles shot a police officer who harassed and assaulted him. In retaliation, mobs of thousands of white New Orleanians burned Black schools and businesses. They pulled African American riders off the streetcars and shot them and beat Black residents in the streets and in their homes. Whites murdered at least twenty Black residents; the city later arrested nine whites, but never tried or convicted anyone.[60]

New city and state laws intensified the restrictions, including the segregation of baseball games in 1890 and of boxing matches in 1892 in New Orleans;

the 1892 state segregation of railroads; disenfranchisement through the state's 1898 constitution, which included a literacy test, poll tax, and grandfather clause; the 1902 segregation of New Orleans streetcars; and the 1908 state ban on cohabitation. While strict enforcement of the segregation of public venues like bars, restaurants, and music venues did not occur until the period during and after World War I, the late nineteenth century nonetheless witnessed the further decline of Black rights in New Orleans.

Racial health disparities accompanied the growing push for a culture of segregation. In 1880, African Americans citywide suffered from a mortality rate of 34.3 per 1,000, compared to a rate of 22.96 per 1,000 for whites (see table A.3). Tuberculosis remained the largest health problem. From 1877 to 1880, an average of 362 Black residents died from the disease, accounting for 16.4 percent of Black deaths. While more whites died from the disease, an average of 502 per year in that same period, tuberculosis disproportionately killed African Americans, who made up 28 percent of the population but 42 percent of tuberculosis deaths. Additionally, tuberculosis only accounted for 7.2 percent of white deaths, with yellow fever still the largest single cause of death for whites. African Americans had an infant mortality rate of 450 per 1,000 in 1880, and those who survived the first year could expect to live to an average of thirty-six years compared to forty-six for whites. The fact that many of the city's Black residents were formerly enslaved, with the lasting medical problems from years of abuse and medical neglect, partially accounted for these figures, compounded by the problems and medical neglect they encountered in New Orleans after the end of slavery. While medical advances lowered the white mortality rate in the following decades, accompanied by a decline in the immigrant population more susceptible to yellow fever, the Black mortality rate increased as Jim Crow intensified, reaching a rate of double that of whites by the end of the century.[61]

The decisions over health care made in the 1860s and 1870s directly resulted in this racial health disparity. The federal government's choice to operate a separate freedmen's hospital for Black New Orleanians rather than enforcing integration at the city's hospitals; and the decisions of individual white doctors, hospitals, and medical schools to not admit Black patients, students, and doctors—with no enforcement of antidiscrimination laws by state and federal officials—paved the way for the institutionalization of racialized health care after the end of Reconstruction. In the Jim Crow period, racial health disparity continued as the historically white health care system expanded. However, two affiliated institutions, Flint Medical College and Flint

Goodridge Hospital, would make remarkable strides in addressing Black health problems and the lack of Black physicians.

Flint Medical College and Flint Goodridge Hospital

While the state's illegal denial of funding doomed the first two efforts at a Black medical program, a third attempt finally succeeded. In 1889, under the auspices of the MEC, New Orleans University reopened its medical program as the New Orleans Medical College, again under the leadership of James Newman. School leaders imagined New Orleans not just as the site for a new medical college—the only one for hundreds of miles—but as a leading Black medical hub. Administrators hoped to raise $200,000 for a new building; $75,000 in endowments; $10,000 for endowed professorships; and $25,000 for an endowed deanship. Although never able to meet these lofty goals, Bishop Willard Francis Mallalieu successfully lobbied MEC parishioner and cotton manufacturer John Flint to fund the purchase of a lot and three-story building on Canal and South Robertson Streets, plus an endowment of $10,000. The college used the first floor for lectures, the second for clinic rooms and operating rooms, and the third for laboratories. The school graduated its first class in 1892.[62]

The students of the school—renamed Flint Medical College in 1901—initially could gain no experience working in a hospital as all hospitals in the city barred Black physicians. In 1894, a New Orleans chapter of the Phyllis Wheatley Club formed with the intention to create a Black hospital for those patients who exceed the maximum income restrictions at Charity. Black women's clubs originated in the late nineteenth century as benevolent organizations. During the Progressive Era, Black women's clubs like Phyllis Wheatley clubs focused on social reform issues including improving Black public health. These clubs—composed primarily of upper-income members—carried out neighborhood cleanups and health education campaigns and started Black hospitals and nursing schools, including New Orleans's Phyllis Wheatley Sanitarium and Training Hospital for Nurses.[63]

The New Orleans Medical College initially allowed the club to use one room with beds for seven patients, starting in 1896. The club also started a training program for nurses and provided an opportunity for medical students to gain practice on patients in a hospital setting. Due to financial problems, the club was unable to maintain the hospital and nursing program after the first year. New Orleans Medical College took over the sanitarium and the nursing program. The two-year nursing program offered full-time students free tuition and board in exchange for serving as nurses at the hospital; non-resident part-time students took three hours of class weekly and paid three dollars a month, which could also be reduced in exchange for nursing work at the hospital. Students from throughout the country and abroad attended, the only such program for African Americans in Louisiana or the three adjoining states.[64]

As he did with John Flint, Bishop Mallalieu successfully lobbied MEC member Mrs. Caroline Mudge of Boston to pledge several thousand dollars to buy land to establish a separate hospital in a two-story building purchased in 1901. Mudge also gave a $25,000 endowment in the form of cotton mill stocks. The school named the new sixteen-bed hospital Sarah Goodridge Hospital in honor of Mudge's mother.[65]

The opening of Sarah Goodridge—later renamed Flint Goodridge—following the establishment of the medical school marked a significant achievement for Black health care in New Orleans. Black students from throughout the region could now become nurses and doctors. Black patients—both paying and indigent, as the hospital offered free care for low-income residents—could now access a hospital, the only hospital in the Deep South to have Black doctors. The medical school and the hospital were also the region's only truly integrated institutions. The medical school admitted both Black and white students, and the hospital treated Black and white patients—not just from New Orleans, but from throughout the country and as far away as Switzerland, with many traveling to the hospital to use its services. The hospital employed no full-time physicians and instead all Black and white doctors with private practices could treat patients as visiting staff. While dwarfed in size by the larger Charity and nearly every private hospital, Flint Goodridge treated hundreds of Black patients annually.

Flint Medical College produced leading Black physicians not just for New Orleans, but also for Black communities throughout the United States. Forty-two individuals from six states—Arkansas, Louisiana, Mississippi, Oklahoma, Oregon, and Texas—and one from Honduras graduated Flint Medical College by 1900. Emma Wakefield-Paillet (class of 1897) became the first Black woman in Louisiana to earn a medical degree and established a practice in the Marigny.[66] Following the tradition of Black Creole physician-activists like Roudanez and Joseph Chaumette, Louis Martinet graduated from the inaugural class of 1892. Born in 1849 in St. Martinville, Louisiana, Martinet served in the state legislature from 1872 to 1875; was a teacher and board member for Straight University; published *The Crusader*, a leading newspaper advocating

African American rights; and cofounded the Comités des Citoyens, which challenged segregation ordinances, resulting in the *Plessy v. Ferguson* case.[67]

By the turn of the century, New Orleans had become one of the country's leading Black medical centers. Eighteen Black physicians practiced in New Orleans in 1890—representing 6 percent of the city's physicians at a time when African Americans accounted for less than 1 percent of doctors nationwide—and twenty-one in 1900; ten of the twenty-one were Flint graduates.[68] As earlier, the 382 white doctors, and ratio of 1 doctor per 548 white residents, far exceeded the twenty-one Black doctors and ratio of 1 doctor per 3,701 Black residents. Regardless, New Orleans had the fourth most Black physicians of any American city behind Washington, D.C., Baltimore, and Nashville, the only three cities that exceeded New Orleans in total Black population. Additionally, New Orleans was one of only five cities in the country with a Black hospital, a Black medical college, and a Black nurse training program—Washington, D.C., Nashville, Raleigh, and Louisville were the others. While five other cities in the Deep South—Atlanta, Charleston, Montgomery, Savannah, and Tuskegee—had Black hospitals, Flint Medical College and nurse training program set New Orleans as the region's most significant city for the Black medical profession.[69] However, in the early twentieth century white leaders pushed for the removal of Flint Medical College and Flint Goodridge Hospital to make the medical district a white space, an effort examined in chapter 4.

CHAPTER FOUR

A White Medical District, 1900–1940

In 1925, Dr. James Newman was seventy-six years old and writing his memoirs, deemed by the *Louisiana Weekly* as a "very valuable addition to medical information." Seemingly, few men could have been better qualified to write such a work. The *Weekly* called Newman "the Dean of Negro Physicians." The *Times Picayune* labeled him as one of "the best known among the negro race in the country." For fifty years, Newman had been involved in nearly every important venture in Black health care in New Orleans. He had been a renowned surgeon, the dean of the city's first Black medical school, a professor for over twenty-five years, the director of the state's first program for Black nurses, a mentor for multiple generations of Black physicians, the first Black doctor at Charity, the first Black member of the city Board of Health, the head of surgery at the city's first Black hospital, and the chief of his own hospital. He was also a much-requested orator and civic leader, heading fundraising drives for Black institutions like the city's first Black YMCA.[1]

Yet, despite his feats, no figure better represented the limitations faced by the Black medical profession than Newman. The whites-only University of Louisiana had refused admission to Newman, a native of the Crescent City, forcing him to study medicine in Canada and initially start a practice in Chicago. Brought back to New Orleans to run a medical dispensary, Newman had led both Straight University and New Orleans University's initial efforts, doomed by the legislature's illegal refusal to provide funding. He had been the only Black physician at Charity from 1871 to 1877 and was dismissed when the hospital segregated. In 1878, the city removed him from the Board of Health. He had served as a professor of surgery at Flint Medical College before the Flexner Report shut it down in 1913—detailed in this chapter.

With the closing of the medical school, Newman concentrated on running his own hospital, the Provident Sanitarium and Nurse Training School. Newman started the institution with support from the First District Baptist Association. Opened several blocks from Flint Goodridge in the heart of the Medical District, the hospital offered several wards for patients—both Black and white. Newman served as the chief surgeon and head of the nurse training program, with two graduates of Flint Medical College as assistant surgeons and instructors for the program. Although the hospital received support from the Baptist Association and Black donors, like Flint Goodridge, it struggled financially. Through the lobbying of Newman and the Board of Directors, the hospital secured an annual allocation from the city council. However, the council only gave $200; in comparison, they awarded $2,000 and $2,500, respectively, to the similar-sized New Orleans Dispensary and the Ear, Eye, Nose, and Throat Hospital, and over $10,000 to the Touro Infirmary.[2]

In 1916, the hospital attempted to move to a new, significantly larger location on Third Street in Central City. Under a city ordinance, the hospital had to secure permission from the city council, which granted the request that October. However, in January 1917, a group of white leaders and residents, described by the *Times Picayune* as "bitterly opposed," came to the city council meeting to protest their decision. Benjamin School principal Ellen Murphy spoke on "behalf of the school children." The president of the Playgrounds Commission, Olive Stallings, spoke on "behalf of the children of Taylors Playground." The newspaper noted the women "based their objections upon the white children having to pass the sanitarium, and upon the possibility of the sanitarium leading to trouble between the races." Both women suggested placing the hospital in "more of a negro neighborhood," with Murphy arguing for a location in the area bounded by Freret, South Rampart, Toledano, and Washington Streets, and Stallings pushing for a site opposite the Thomy Lafon playground, both further into Central City. State Senator Stafford and Assessor James Mallow spoke on "behalf of their constituents of the Eleventh Ward," who believed the "institution would depress property values." Others spoke to oppose the building "because it was a negro institution and others solely because it was a hospital."[3]

Attorney Richard B. Montgomery and U.S. customs inspector Walter L. Cohen represented Newman and the hospital at the meeting. They presented a map to the council that showed that most of the homes on the 2800 block of Third Street were Black-occupied. Speaking on behalf of the council, member Philip Newman stated that although "the majority of residents in the neighborhood are negro and sanitariums must be placed somewhere," he was "impressed" that a location in a "more thoroughly defined negro neighborhood might be found" and also that the proposed location—and its current location in the white Medical District—"might lead to conflict between the races." Swayed by the arguments of the protestors, the council rescinded the hospital's permit.[4]

In February, Newman appeared before the council again, asking for permission to build the hospital on Delachaise Street, in the area Ellen Murphy argued was "more of a negro neighborhood."[5] The council granted the permit in March 1917, and Newman set to fundraising.[6] That summer, the Moose Lodge purchased the building that housed the Provident Sanitarium. In the seven years since the hospital had opened, the surrounding blocks had increasingly become more valuable as the nearby Central District grew and the white presence in the surrounding area expanded. Upon acquiring the building, white neighbors immediately petitioned the Moss Lodge to evict the Provident Sanitarium; as described by Black physician L. B. Landry, Newman was "driven from pillar to pest by dissatisfied neighbors."[7] The Moose Lodge—which had a whites-only membership clause—complied, evicting the hospital. Newman turned his sole focus to the fundraising for the proposed hospital in Central City.

Newman and Landry launched a fundraising campaign that raised several thousand dollars in four months, with support from Walter Cohen and Dr. George Lucas, president of the local NAACP chapter.[8] The group, which named itself the Colored Hospital Association, also approached white leaders, including Mayor O'Keefe, who publicly endorsed the project, and the editor of the *Times Picayune*, Daniel Moore. Moore urged white readers to give, and personally pledged $100,000 if, he told the Colored Hospital Association, "their people and medical men proved worthy." With an initial $14,000, the Colored Hospital Association built a small structure on the Delachaise property, but no white business leaders gave any money and fundraising stalled. Moore withdrew his pledge and the hospital efforts collapsed in 1921. An empty building stood on the Delachaise Street lot for several years as a vestige of the effort. In 1925, Newman died, his memoirs uncompleted and the building on the Delachaise Street lot unoccupied.[9]

Newman's struggles and the demise of the Providence Sanitarium are not just tragic stories of a forgotten vanguard physician and Black hospital. The removal of the hospital from the Medical District demonstrated a new phase of racialized health care in the first decades of the twentieth century. This chapter examines how New Orleans's push for increasing trade with Latin America and tourism led to civic improvements, public health campaigns, and an expanding health care economy. As boosters promoted New Orleans as a healthy city, with a robust health care system, they also advocated for residential segregation and spatial concentration of Black residents in less-desirable areas, often using arguments of poor Black health as justification for removal. This chapter explores a second crucial turning point for racialized health care, the 1910s and 1920s, a period when Flint Medical College was a leading producer of Black physicians, and Flint Goodridge Hospital, Provident Hospital, and other Black health care providers had carved out space in the Medical District to serve the health needs of Black residents. However, as detailed, proponents of white supremacy used their powers—including federal funding—to evict these institutions and create a white Medical District.

A Growing Health Care Economy and Public Health

The growing medical profession—Black and white—in New Orleans was part of the city's expanding health care economy and mirrored a national trend. Throughout the United States, the perception of hospitals had changed. Previously viewed as charitable spaces for the care of the indigent, by the turn of the twentieth century hospitals were increasingly seen as a necessary component of health care. Important changes included increasing professionalization of practitioners, including standardized education, testing and clinical instruction, professional administration, advances in medical knowledge and treatment, and improvements in medical equipment and sterilization resulting in declining hospital mortality rates. Middle- and upper-class Americans were more willing to use hospitals. In particular, surgeries for acute conditions, which were more profitable than long-term care, increased. As a result, private hospitals proliferated, relying not on charity or philanthropic support, but on patient fees. By the 1900s, hospitals had become business enterprises.[10] Although much of the South lagged behind this trend, New Orleans's health care economy grew in the late nineteenth and early twentieth century. As was the case in the antebellum period, small, private hospitals and infirmaries still existed for private physicians to treat their wealthier clients unwilling to use larger hospitals. Several new, small hospitals opened in the period.[11] However, the number of these infirmaries would gradually decline because they were unable to compete with larger hospitals like Charity, Hotel Dieu, and Touro. Three new, large hospitals joined these ranks, all started by religious organizations: the Presbyterian Hospital in 1910, Mercy Hospital in 1924, and Southern Baptist Hospital in 1926.

With the city's geographic and population growth in the same period, hospitals opened in new neighborhoods along the city's expanding urban periphery. Wary of the spread of disease, most residents still did not want hospitals in their neighborhood. When the Southern Baptist Convention announced plans to build their hospital in 1924, white residents unsuccessfully petitioned to halt the placing of the hospital on Napoleon Avenue, but they did successfully petition the city council to only permit the structure to extend into the Black-majority blocks of the Freret neighborhood, rather than the white-majority blocks of the Broadmoor neighborhood. This fight over space—with the designation of Black areas, but not white ones, as acceptable for "hazards"—would characterize the period as the city sought to foster racial segregation, including areas around medical institutions, particularly the Medical District. Additionally, as discussed in greater detail in following sections, the expansion of hospitals would be linked with disruption of Black neighborhoods and displacement of Black residents.[12]

The area around Charity Hospital (the Tulane Gravier/Central Business District neighborhoods) was still considered the medical district in the early twentieth century. When Charity Hospital relocated there in 1831, the area was largely undeveloped. In the mid- and late nineteenth century, commercial and later industrial enterprises concentrated there, earning the lasting moniker of the Central Business District. In addition to these businesses, medical institutions proliferated there as well, drawn primarily by Charity Hospital—where many of these institution's leaders were staff members. The Medical College of Louisiana opened close to Charity in 1834, followed by several smaller, private hospitals including Warren Stone's infirmary in 1837, the Circus Street Infirmary in 1841, and Hotel Dieu in 1858. In the late nineteenth century and early twentieth century, other institutions joined the Medical District: the Ear, Eye, Nose, and Throat Hospital in 1889, Flint Medical College in 1889, Flint Goodridge Hospital in 1896, the city's Isolation Hospital in 1905 (for quarantining patients with contagious diseases), the aforementioned Presbyterian Hospital in 1910; the City Hospital for Mental Diseases in 1911, the Illinois Central Railroad Hospital (open to employees of the Illinois Central Railroad) in 1913, and the Lying-in Hospital (a municipal maternity hospital) in 1917. In addition to following national trends, the expansion of the health care economy reflected city leaders' recognition of the contributions of the health care sector—physicians, hospitals, and the medical school—in aiding the city's physical and economic development, and even as a key employer.

By the early twentieth century, the growing trade with Latin America—primarily for agricultural products like bananas and coffee—and tourism had become key drivers of the New Orleans economy. Boosters sought to develop business associations, steamship companies that sailed directly from New Orleans to Latin American ports, and foreign trade organizations to make New Orleans the "Gateway to Latin America." By 1914, over 75 percent of imports by value to New Orleans came from Latin America.[13] In 1913, the Association of Commerce formed. The organization created a tourism and convention bureau and launched a nationwide tourism media campaign to attract visitors and professional conventions.[14]

Starting in 1910, to further boost the image of the city, New Orleans civic leaders began a several-year push for the 1915 Panama–Pacific Exposition; they also hoped to be designated the official port of entry when the canal opened. New Orleans competed with San Francisco for the exposition, with extensive business and political lobbying. As part of its effort to win the event, San Francisco underwent a significant municipal improvement and beautification process. Both sides also engaged in smear campaigns. San Francisco pamphlets criticized New Orleans on several fronts: inadequate number of hotels, a less developed commercial sector, lack of "fit drinking water," "unsanitary conditions," and a "big negro population." San Franciscans proudly proclaimed their city as 98 percent white.[15] Ultimately, Congress awarded the exposition to San Francisco. The loss demonstrated a continuing problem in the minds of white elites in New Orleans. To attract both visitors and trading partners, the city had to eliminate public health issues and project an image of good health and sanitation. Many outside New Orleans still viewed the city as unsanitary and unhealthy due to the city's high mortality rate—21.35 per 1,000 in 1910, far above San Francisco's rate of 15.1 and the overall national rate of 14.7 per 1,000.[16] Additionally, many whites viewed the large Black population, the second biggest of any American city, as another stigma. In the first three decades of the twentieth century, white leaders of the city sought to combat these issues, first tackling public health, then turning toward segregation.

Through the dawn of the century, New Orleans remained significantly behind other major American cities because it had no sewer or drainage system, no garbage collection, refuse and open trash containers throughout the city, no street cleaning, wooden plank sidewalks, and unregulated ownership of domestic animals and storage of foodstuffs. These issues favored the estimated 1 million rats in the city. Open pools of water like cisterns served as breeding grounds for mosquitos that served as vectors for yellow fever and malaria; New Orleans had a malaria rate of 104 per 100,000 in 1900. The use of privies rather than a sewer system led to the mixing of human waste and drinking water, which facilitated outbreaks of typhoid and cholera; the typhoid rate was 38 per 100,000 in 1900.[17]

The municipal government, with the backing of the medical system, initiated efforts from 1900 to 1940 to deal with the scourges that continued to afflict the city, notably malaria, tuberculosis, typhoid, and yellow fever. The city focused on improving public health knowledge, eliminating sources of contagion by closing open pools of water like cisterns and privies, initiating mosquito control, paving roads, the raising of buildings, creating modern sewer, drainage, and sanitation systems, and providing better treatment through public health clinics. Of the public health problems, tuberculosis received perhaps the most attention as it remained one of the highest causes of death with a mortality rate of 326 per 100,000 residents from 1900 to 1904, one of the nation's highest rates.[18] In 1906, activist Kate Gordon organized the New Orleans Tuberculosis League, which partnered with the Louisiana Anti-Tuberculosis League to provide free tuberculosis clinics and pushed for the opening of the Orleans Anti-Tuberculosis Hospital in 1926 in the Gentilly neighborhood and the John Dibert Tuberculosis Hospital, also opened in 1926 as part of the growing Charity Hospital complex.

Tulane University became actively involved in both public health and hygiene issues. In 1912, Dr. Creighton Wellman founded the New Orleans School of Tropical Medicine and Hygiene as part of Tulane University. Samuel Zemurray, who owned Cuyamel Fruit, which shipped fruit from Honduras to New Orleans, funded the school, further demonstrating the ties between the commercial trade industry and public health measures. In October 1912, Wellman published "The New Orleans School of Tropical Medicine and Hygiene," a lecture he originally delivered before the OPMS in March 1912. In his paper, Wellman highlighted the international shift toward "preventative medicine" and made the case for New Orleans as an important center in this new approach. Wellman argued that with the creation of the school, New Orleans would be the center of a "great movement for the study and conquest of disease, and particularly tropical disease." New Orleans and Tulane, he posited, were "marked for a great and manifest destiny of educating the Western Hemisphere in the vital questions of ridding ourselves of the disease scourges which have too long hindered the commercial, social, and moral growth of the many."

In his view, and those of other trade boosters, New Orleans, as a major trading port for Central and South America, made a natural choice to be the central location for studying the eradication of tropical disease like yellow fever, malaria, and typhoid. Tulane would train the "future custodians of health," providing education along the "broadest possible scientific lines" based on the recent advances in bacteriology, pathology, and laboratory science. Wellman also pledged to work with the Board of Health, other government and civic officials, educators, and the general public to educate about and confront the city's public health problems.[19]

By 1920, New Orleans had undergone a radical shift in its approach to public health. The city employed what were considered to be "progressive" and "scientific" approaches to shift away from reaction to prevention of epidemics through education; civic improvements, including drainage, water, and sewage lines; sanitation and hygiene initiatives; and new clinics and hospitals to not only tackle public health problems, but to also boost the city's trade and tourism image, which would make New Orleans again a leading center of medicine.

A White Medical District

Buoyed by municipal leaders, economic boosters, and increasing federal medical research funding, the city's largest medical institutions—Charity Hospital and Tulane University—underwent significant expansion in the early twentieth century by acquiring numerous blocks in the Medical District. Charity built the Richard Milliken Memorial Children's Hospital in 1899, the Delgado Hospital in 1909, and the John Dibert Tuberculosis Hospital in 1926 as part of its complex, in addition to an ambulatory building, nurses' residences, and support units. Tulane moved its medical program into the nearby Richardson Building in 1893 on Canal Avenue, renovated and expanded in 1902 and renamed it the Josephine Hutchinson Memorial Building. In 1922, the city council granted Tulane's initial request to construct its own hospital on their campus.[20] Ultimately, the Board of Administrators decided not to go forward with their hospital plan, and instead built the new Hutchinson Memorial Building on Tulane Avenue, which contained a clinic with hospital beds, next to Charity Hospital in 1930.[21] A second medical school joined Tulane in the Medical District. In 1931, the Louisiana State University (LSU) School of Medicine opened. Pushed by Governor Long, who wanted to create a medical school for residents of the state—most of Tulane's students came from outside of Louisiana—the school constructed a building on Tulane Avenue, across from Charity, on land owned by the hospital. Despite initial opposition from Tulane, the school enrolled 171 students for its first full year of operation in 1932, with a faculty largely raided from Tulane—further drawing its ire. The two schools agreed to have an equal number of beds at Charity, partially mollifying the private school.[22]

As the hospital and medical schools expanded, the institutions and white city leaders began removing the Black presence in the Medical District, which was part of a larger push for segregation and spatial concentration of African Americans. Throughout the early twentieth century, New Orleans had relatively low levels of segregation, primarily due to African Americans living close to white residences where they labored as domestics.[23] This changed in the early twentieth century. With the expansion of municipal services like drainage, water, sewage, and roads, neighborhoods on the urban periphery previously considered undesirable and flood-prone—and thus having higher concentrations of Black residents due to low property values—became appealing for white residents.[24]

Following the lead of other Southern cities starting with Baltimore in 1910, New Orleans adopted a residential segregation ordinance in 1924; they did so despite the Supreme Court declaring such ordinances illegal in *Buchanan v. Warley* (1917). City leaders justified the ordinance as a defense of white property values, arguing that Black residents in neighborhoods would decrease the values. They also stated they adopted the ordinance to prevent racial animosity and violence, and as a public health measure because African Americans had higher disease rates and would spread disease to whites.[25] In the following three years, white residents used the ordinance, backed by police threats of arrest and acts of violence including a series of bombings of Black homes and businesses, to prevent African Americans from moving not only into predominantly white blocks, but also into many racially mixed neighborhoods, or spaces that whites hoped to claim as their own after city improvements made those areas desirable. Thousands of African Americans were directly affected, charged with violating the law, prevented from moving into homes they had legally purchased or rented, and made to sell property they owned to whites at losses—even though the city's improvements had significantly increased their property value. In addition, Black residents who should have received the health benefits that accompanied the extension of municipal services into their neighborhoods found themselves forced out and again living in areas with flooding and other health hazards.

Although lawsuits by Black residents, supported by the local chapter of the NAACP, led to the Supreme Court declaring the ordinance unconstitutional in *Harmon v. Tyler* in 1927, efforts to expand segregation continued into the following decades. White residents and police officers continued to harass and attack African Americans that attempted to live in or even access areas considered to be "white spaces." Developers and homeowners instituted racially restrictive covenants to prevent the renting or selling of homes to African Americans.

Most significantly, in 1929, the city instituted its first comprehensive zoning plan. Drafted by nationally renowned planner Harland Bartholomew, the document employed racial zoning practices to propagate segregation. As seen in figure 4.1, the plan designated mostly white neighborhoods like the Garden District and Uptown areas around Tulane University (marked numbers 1, 14–17) as "Residential A," permitting only single- or double-family homes, as well as spaces like parks, churches, and golf courses. With this designation, whites

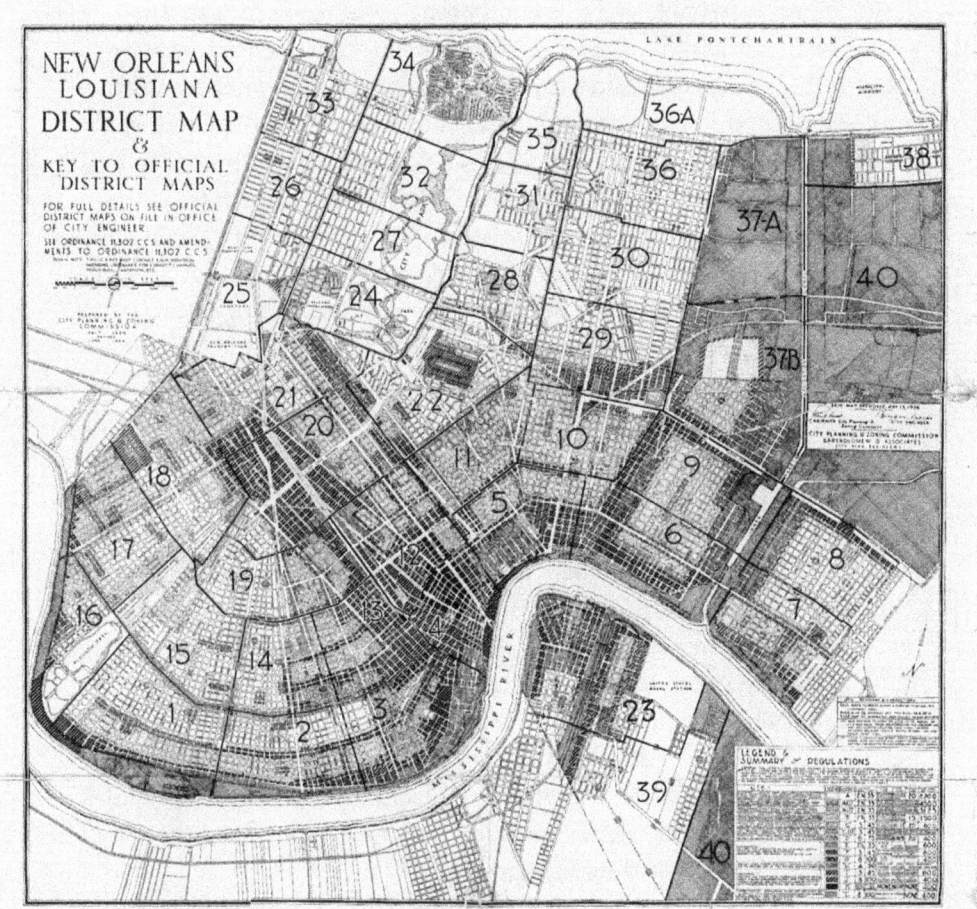

FIGURE 4.1 The 1929 New Orleans Comprehensive Plan (City Planning Commission Records, City Archives, New Orleans Public Library).

could build homes with racially restrictive covenants and prevent the building of apartment buildings, which African Americans may have been able to afford, a practice known as exclusionary zoning. The plan designated Black neighborhoods like Central City and B. W. Cooper (marked numbers 13 and 4) as "Multiple Dwelling," which permitted apartment buildings; "Unrestricted," which allowed any building type; or "Industrial." The "Unrestricted" and "Industrial" designations allowed the building of factories, oil refineries, municipal dumps, and the municipal incinerator on blocks with Black residences. Even before the 1929 plan, African Americans were significantly more likely to live near potential pollutants. Unable to pay the higher real estate prices of more desirable and less flood-prone areas, many African Americans often could only afford to live in areas that already contained industry, like the Central Business District and the Warehouse District; and along the urban periphery, neighborhoods like the Ninth Ward where the city placed wharves and warehouses. The comprehensive plan codified Black exposure to health hazards, particularly air and water pollution from industrial plants.

In its narrative report for the comprehensive plan, the City Zoning Commission celebrated its "scientific" and "progressive" approach. Zoning, it argued, "must relate to the public health, safety, convenience, or general welfare." Zoning helped individual property owners by preventing the "depreciation of property values . . . and in most cases adds to its value by giving it a character of stability and permanence." Zoning helped improve health by mandating standards for single- and double-family dwellings and separating "Residential A" districts from industrial; after all, they stated, "it is a well-known fact that poor health conditions go hand in hand with poor housing facilities." Commission members made no mention of the poor housing facilities and poor health conditions of Black residents. Like their public health efforts and other measures carried out under the mantle of "progressivism," zoning benefited whites and further hurt Black health.[26]

By 1930, New Orleans had redefined urban space. The laws, discriminatory real estate practices, police intimidation, violence, and zoning had increasingly concentrated African Americans in neighborhoods viewed as undesirable. The city coupled these practices with new ordinances passed after World War I that ordered racial segregation of public spaces and entertainment venues like parks, museums, bars, restaurants, and sporting events, designed to attract white tourists from the North.

White leaders subjected the Medical District to these segregation efforts, using their powers to remove the growing Black medical system in the neighborhood. By the 1910s, in addition to Flint Medical College, Flint Goodridge Hospital, and J. T. Newman's Provident Sanitarium, Black physicians' offices and pharmacies dotted the area (see map A.1). The Black-owned Pythian Temple, on Loyola Avenue, contained the offices of several doctors, dentists, and life insurance companies. Thus, the Tulane Gravier neighborhood served as the primary medical district for African Americans in the early twentieth century, as it did for whites.

Flint Medical College was the first institution removed. In 1910, Flint Medical College officials planned a $50,000 enlargement of the building by 50 percent in the hopes of allowing more students and to meet new standards established by the American Medical Association. In 1904, the American

Medical Association created the Council on Medical Education to study and standardize medical education. The council asked the Carnegie Foundation to fund a study, led by Abraham Flexner, of all medical colleges in the United States. The 1910 Flexner Report faulted Flint Medical College for having "scant equipment in anatomy, chemistry, pathology, and bacteriology" and described the rooms as "in poor condition." The report concluded that "Flint College is a hopeless affair, on which money and energy alike are wasted," and recommended closing the school and redirecting all of Flint's students and resources to Meharry College in Nashville, which it opined should be the only school for Black physicians in the South. While having no official authority to close schools, the report warded off needed donors from the schools criticized in the document, mostly Black medical colleges, and the AMA instituted new accreditation guidelines based on the report. Unable to secure funding to changes mandated by the AMA to maintain accreditation, Flint Medical College closed in 1913, one of five Black medical colleges that closed due to the Flexner Report, leaving only two programs open, Meharry and Howard. All Flint students transferred to Meharry, although periodic efforts to reopen the school continued for several years afterward.

During its existence, Flint Medical College produced a total of 102 doctors and sixty-two pharmacists. The loss of the medical school would have a devastating impact on Black health care not just in New Orleans, but throughout the South. Flint graduates practiced in larger cities like Dallas but also in thirty smaller towns in Louisiana and in towns in Mississippi, Texas, Arkansas, Oklahoma, and Georgia. The closure of Flint severed the pipeline of Black physicians to these rural Black communities. New Orleans experienced an almost immediate drop in Black physicians. In 1910, forty-two Black physicians practiced in the city, double the number from 1900, with most either graduates of or instructors at Flint. By 1920, seven years after Flint's closure, the number of Black physicians declined to twenty-nine, dropping New Orleans from the fourth highest total of Black physicians to twelfth; the beginning of the Great Migration may have also partially accounted for the attrition.[27] Regardless, for the first time since the early nineteenth century, New Orleans experienced loss, not gain, of Black physicians (see Table A.2). That loss would especially be felt when the graduates of Flint began to retire or die in midcentury, without the medical school producing the next generation of Black doctors to replace them. Additionally, the closure of the medical college hurt Flint Goodridge Hospital, depriving the institution of most of its residents, and making the hospital ineligible for many of the research grants the federal government began to distribute to university-affiliated hospitals.[28]

Flint Goodridge Hospital almost suffered the same fate as the medical college when city officials used municipal powers to shutter the space in 1912. An inspection by the city Board of Health found the structure to be "unsafe," and after administrators were unable to raise money to make improvements, they closed the facility. Hospital leaders eventually secured additional financial support from the MEC, Caroline Mudge, and the descendants of John Flint, and converted the empty medical college building into a new sixty-bed hospital, renamed Flint Goodridge Hospital, which opened in January 1916. Black and white community leaders including Mayor Martin Behrman attended the dedication ceremony. Reporters described the new space as "modern, convenient, and well equipped." However, the new building lasted less than fifteen years.[29]

In 1926, Charity Hospital sought to further erase the Black presence in the Medical District by making Black patients less visible. Since 1877, the hospital had segregated patients by using a smaller building on Gravier Street, behind the main building on Tulane Avenue, as the "colored ward." In 1926, the hospital announced a change in policy, now requiring Black patients to use a separate entrance on Gravier Street, rather than the main one on Tulane Avenue. Black leaders immediately condemned the action, with board members of the NAACP local branch—led by Flint graduates Dr. George Lucas and Dr. Joseph Hardin—presenting a petition of protest signed by hundreds of residents. Black leaders framed their opposition in several ways. First, they presented an economic argument, highlighting the unfairness of the policy due to the financial contributions to the institution and the city as whole, as laborers, taxpayers, and donors to hospital fundraising drives. Second, they argued the unfairness of the policy in light of decades of medical students, residents, and interns learning by practicing on Black patients. The NAACP's petition stated that African Americans had "contributed more than his share of subjects for studious consideration of the white novice. He has been a veritable storehouse of knowledge to the embryo pathologist." The *Louisiana Weekly* was even more critical, writing of "the living sacrifices they have made in their bodies and their very lives for the sake of making physicians—white physicians, if you please."[30]

Black leaders also noted the connection between the policy and the city's residential segregation ordinance, at that time still awaiting a ruling by the Supreme Court. The NAACP told the Board of Administrators that it had "inadvertently permitted its policy to be shaped so as to put the institution in the same category with certain persons . . . who not only advocate public segregation but whose teachings and doctrines tend to the most injurious form of racial oppression." Both the *Weekly* and the NAACP highlighted their opposition to all forms of "public segregation," describing it as "unjust," "unnecessary," and "embarrassing." The NAACP noted that whites cited avoiding racial conflict as a reason for segregation, but Charity's policy would have the opposite effect, planting "deep in the heart of every self-respecting Negro the seeds of discontent, dissatisfaction, and unrest—yea even rancor." Charity's Board of Management responded that they did not intend the "result of racial discrimination" with the policy, but rather "to facilitate the movement of the crowd," and refused to accede.[31]

While Black leaders spoke of their opposition to "all forms of public segregation," their petitions were limited in scope. They did not call for the end of segregated treatment at Charity. Instead, they pushed for the enforcement of the "equal" part of the court's "separate but equal" provision. The local NAACP chapter—dominated by upper-class medical professionals in six of the eight executive board positions—and the Federation of Civic Leagues favored an "accommodationist" over an integrationist approach in the period. They propagated Booker T. Washington's model of "racial uplift," with the "better class" leading the effort to improve the standing of African Americans and gaining acceptance by whites.[32] They sought smaller concessions over radical changes like integration, instead pushing for better funding for separate Black spaces like schools, parks, and playgrounds, and municipal services for Black neighborhoods. Similarly, at Charity, they requested not integration, but instead equal funding for the Black ward and equality through using the same entrance.[33]

White leaders ignored these petitions and the racialized medical system grew, and it was increasingly fueled by federal funding. Passed in 1933 in response to the Great Depression, the National Industrial Recovery Act created the Public Works Administration (PWA), which funded public works including schools, bridges, and hospitals. In 1933, Charity applied for Public Works Administration funding to build a larger hospital, a move opposed by the OPMS, who viewed the expansion as detrimental to other private hospitals and argued Charity had too many beds. With opposition from the OPMS as well as a frosty relationship between President Franklin Roosevelt and Governor Huey Long, the PWA delayed approval. Despite the OPMS's claims, Charity was overcrowded and underfunded, as it had been through much of its existence. In 1936, the hospital served an average of 2,781 patients daily in a space that contained 1,814 beds.[34] This problem particularly afflicted the Black ward, with many patients forced to sleep two or three to a bed, or on cots and wooden pallets in the halls.[35] When Morris Fishbein, the editor of the *Journal of the American Medical Association*, inspected Charity in 1936, he publicized his findings, drawing national attention to the "horrible conditions" of hygiene and sanitation he found in the Black ward.[36] This report and coverage in *Time* magazine led to further calls for improvement, and the federal government approved funding in 1936—after the assassination of Governor Long.

The new Charity, the second largest hospital complex in the country with 2,860 beds in the main structure and an additional 850 beds in affiliated buildings, took three years to construct. Through the PWA, the federal government paid 45 percent of the costs—Charity was the most expensive PWA-sponsored hospital project—including "slum clearance" measures to clear out the surrounding blocks. This action—physically carried out largely by Black WPA laborers—displaced hundreds of Black residents and businesses—including Black pharmacists, the last remnants of the Black part of the Medical District—and churches, as well as the Chinese business district on Tulane Avenue (see figures A.1 and A.2 in Appendix).[37] African Americans remained the majority of residents of the neighborhood. In 1939, the Home Owners' Loan Corporation noted that Tulane Avenue, which housed Charity, was 100 percent white and contained "the best properties in the area"; overall, though, the association gave the surrounding Black neighborhood its lowest rating, as "hazardous." The characteristics contributed to redlining, the practice in which the Federal Housing Administration refused to grant insurance to loans and mortgages for homes in areas identified by the Home Owners' Loan Corporation maps as "declining" or "hazardous." Private lenders including local banks in New Orleans too used the maps as guidance. Because almost all Black neighborhoods were designated as "declining" or "hazardous," Black residents in Tulane Gravier and other Black-majority neighborhoods faced extreme difficulty in securing necessary loans or mortgages to become homeowners.[38] Charity, Tulane, and LSU would all expand in the following decades, pushing more African Americans outside of the neighborhood and further away from medical care. Like Charity, federal funding also funded the growth of Tulane and LSU—and indirectly the displacement of more Black residents. Both schools benefited from federal grants that helped them expand their programs, student numbers, and physical presences.

New Orleans as a "Medical Center"

In 1929, physician C. C. Bass gave a speech to OPMS entitled "New Orleans as a Medical Center," which celebrated the Crescent City as the leading medical center of the South and highlighted the importance of the medical field to the city's economic prosperity. Bass held up the city's hospital facilities as "unequalled in the South" and New Orleans as the "leading center for the entire South for almost one hundred years." Bass noted the significance of the medical field in sustaining trade with Latin America. In fact, he argued, New Orleans had become the place to which the surrounding Southern territory and "tropical countries" turned for research on tropical disease. Thus, in Bass's opinion, New Orleans was not just a key site for medical care, but also a leading medical research center. The "researches and contributions of the medical profession of New Orleans," he stated, "have commanded attention and high esteem in every civilized country in the world." As such, it attracted medical students from every state in the United States and internationally, especially increasingly from Latin America due to the "tropical disease research" and the "rapidly increasing number of patients." The color line that rejected African Americans as doctors and medical students did not apply to individuals from Latin America, who could attend the city's two medical schools, join the OPMS, and work in hospitals. The benefits of this tropical research to Latin American countries and the training of medical students from there, in his view, greatly improved the relationships between New Orleans and Latin America, leading to "increasing friendliness in matters of business and commerce." Bass opined that the future of New Orleans, the "Queen of the South," depended on this trade relationship and its broader role as a major port city, which relied heavily upon the medical field: "As a city's health is a city's wealth, so shall this phase of our civic development keep pace with our commercial advancement."

With these growing institutions fueled by federal funding and support from economic boosters, by the 1930s New Orleans had returned to its pre–Civil War status as one of the leading medical centers of the South. In addition to being home to the nation's second largest public hospital, a boom in hospital construction in the 1910s and 1920s expanded the capacities of the French Hospital, Presbyterian Hospital, the Ear, Eye, Nose, and Throat Hospital, Hotel Dieu, and the U.S. Marine Hospital; two medical schools, with hundreds of students; and hundreds of practicing physicians. The city also offered nursing programs at Charity Hospital (started in 1895), Touro Infirmary (1896), Flint Medical College (1896), Hotel Dieu (1899), and the New Orleans Hospital and Dispensary for Women (1908). Thousands worked directly or indirectly in the city's health care sector and by 1930 the hospital industry became the fifth-largest enterprise in the country.[39]

Bass noted "With the worthy record as a medical center for the past and present that New Orleans has, the future can hold only increasingly glowing prospects." He identified Tulane University—where he taught—as the heart of the burgeoning medical center. Bass praised Tulane as a "center for medical knowledge" and argued that the school's continued development "will greatly increase the importance of New Orleans as a medical center."[40]

Bass was not the only physician to hold these views. In his 1931 inaugural address, incoming OPMS president Emmet Lee Irwin held up New Orleans as "one of the nation's leading centers for the dissemination of medical knowledge." Irwin used his speech to call for increased funding for medical research, of vital importance to the city: "When the dividends are declared through extermination of disease, relief of suffering, better health, prolongation of life, and a more desirable community in which to live, the investment is quite small." Greater federal aid and other forms of funding would allow New Orleans, as a "famous Medical Center," to "take the lead in vast research problems and claim her just position in the medical world."[41]

In many ways, Bass's and Irwin's assessments were correct. The growth in the number of hospitals and the larger health care economy and improvements in medical research had greatly aided the city's economic development and improved the health and lives of many. However, the health efforts mostly benefited white residents and excluded African Americans. Tulane became integral in New Orleans's success as a medical center, as it produced many of the city's leading physicians and surgeons and served as the main center for the city's research in tropical medicine, largely funded by federal grants. But African Americans could not attend Tulane or LSU, or any medical school in the Deep South; nor could they join the OPMS or work as a nurse or physician at any hospital in the city except Flint Goodridge. All private hospitals supported Jim Crow by refusing to admit Black patients. Black patients in the "leading medical center of the South" could only use Flint Goodridge or Charity, the latter of which also upheld Jim Crow in its new hospital. When the federal government approved PWA funding to construct a new Charity, many in the African American community hoped the complex would provide better care for Black patients. "With this announcement," reported the *Louisiana Weekly*, "comes hope on the part of Negroes of Louisiana that adequate provision will be made for them."[42] This hope did not materialize.

During the three years it took to construct the new building, the hospital temporarily transferred Black patients to the Pythian Temple. Because the Knights of Pythias chapter owed several years of back tax payments, the state forced the organization to rent the space, which contained the offices of Black physicians, two Black-owned insurance companies, and the *Louisiana Weekly*. Some businesses stayed on the ground floor, while others, including the physicians, were forced to relocate.[43] African Americans looked on the move with suspicion. One newspaper columnist saw the action as a "subtle movement to remove Negro property owners from the immediate location of proposed new City Hall." The state attempted to force the Knights of Pythias to sell the space by auction (with white ownership likely). However, an attorney for the Knights of Pythias successfully blocked the move at the U.S. Circuit Court of Appeals in 1937 and maintained the Knights as the owners.[44] Local Black business and civic leaders then "banded together for the common good" to help the Knights secure a loan, saving "the most valuable real estate owned by Negroes in Louisiana."[45] During its three-year occupation, hospital administrators made some repairs to the building, but the same problems of overcrowding and poor funding in regards to Black patients continued. Morris Fishbein of the AMA reported "terrible conditions" after visiting in November 1937, noting that he found twenty-seven patients in ten beds and infected tuberculosis patients being held next to children.[46]

Black New Orleanians were most affected by the temporary closure of Charity between 1936 and 1939. Beyond the limited space in the Pythian Temple, which contained fewer beds than the Black ward at Charity, Black patients' only other choice was Flint Goodridge. Whites could turn to over twenty other hospitals. When the new Charity building opened in 1939, the same discriminatory treatment continued. State hospital laws required segregation in all aspects of medical treatment. The hospital had separate entrances, blood banks, and a "colored wing." White and Black patients shared a waiting room, with separate seats for each race. However, fewer seats existed for Black patients. Even if all the Black seats were full and white seats were unoccupied, security guards prevented Black patients from using those seats; Black patients often had to stand for hours waiting to be seen.[47]

Charity physicians continued the legacy of experimentation on Black patients from the antebellum period. Former Charity chief of staff John Salvaggio told a 1994 congressional inquiry, "The whole population of the hospital was used for guinea pigs ... You could pick anyone you wanted and do any tests you wanted."[48] In the 1950s, the Atomic Energy Commission sponsored fifteen different radiation studies at Charity, which were carried out by doctors affiliated with Tulane University. These tests on 300 Black patients included having them swallow radioactive mercury without their consent or knowledge of the dangers. This was part of a larger series of studies carried out by the Atomic Energy Commission on Black hospital patients nationwide.[49]

Segregation and exclusion persisted in other health care institutions and endeavors, including the city's celebrated public health measures. Kate

Gordon spearheaded many of these efforts and embodied many of the contradictions and hypocrisies of the Progressive Era. In some ways, Gordon was a radical who pushed for equality. Born in New Orleans in 1861, Gordon was a leader of the women's suffrage and women's rights movement in Louisiana, including successfully pushing Tulane to admit its first women as medical students in 1915. She campaigned for the end of child labor and the creation of a juvenile court to try youth offenders. She helped push through the creation of the city's Sewage and Water Board in 1899, street improvements, and food inspections.

However, Gordon was also an avowed white supremacist. In a 1901 interview, Gordon espoused her views on the importance of enfranchising white, educated, tax-paying women: "The question of white supremacy is one that will only be decided by giving the right of the ballot to the educated, intelligent white woman of the South ... Their vote will eliminate the question of the negro vote in politics, and it will be a glad free day for the South when the ballot is placed in the hands of its intelligent, cultured, pure and noble womanhood."[50] Kate and her sister Jean Gordon were also leading eugenicists who felt the state's anti-miscegenation laws did not go far enough in preventing mixed-race children. The Gordon sisters campaigned for state laws to forcibly sterilize individuals considered "degenerates" and prevent interracial children. Speaking before the legislature on behalf of the bill in 1924, Jean warned of the dangers if the state did not enact the law: "If something of this sort is not done soon, our nordic civilization is gone and race preservation is the highest form of patriotism." The state medical society endorsed these policies, and Jean read letters of support to the state legislature from New Orleans physicians and Tulane University professors; echoing Jean's racist warning, Tulane professor of gynecology and obstetrics S. D. M. Clark argued that the "scientific" perspective demanded eugenics "for maintaining the purity of the white race in Louisiana."[51] To the frustration of the Gordons and their allies, the state legislature narrowly voted down the four eugenics bills between 1924 and 1930, primarily due to opposition from the Catholic Church. Undeterred, Jean carried out her own personal eugenics campaign. Jean took children from the Milne Home for Destitute Girls, which she founded and directed from 1919 to 1932, to doctors Sara Mayo and Ada Kiblinger at Presbyterian Hospital, where they performed sterilizations of 125 children for free.[52]

Kate Gordon brought these principles of white supremacy, and contempt for Black lives, to her public health work. Gordon advocated for segregation and exclusion of African Americans from her tuberculosis campaigns. In addition to organizing the New Orleans Tuberculosis League, she led the campaigns to establish the organization's tuberculosis clinics and their Camp Hygeia, a retreat for tuberculosis patients on the other side of Lake Pontchartrain; as well as the Orleans Tuberculosis Hospital, which she managed. Camp Hygeia—and all the nearby tuberculosis sanitariums and retreats—refused to admit Black patients. The tuberculosis clinics and Orleans Tuberculosis Hospital only treated African Americans as outpatients in separate, smaller, and underfunded clinics. Only Flint Goodridge and Charity accepted Black tuberculosis sufferers as inpatients, and the latter only in a small, segregated space in the old hospital, reserving the entire newly opened John Dibert Tuberculosis Hospital building for whites. The city's focus on whites and refusal to address the root causes of tuberculosis that disproportionately affected African Americans—like poverty, low-quality and overcrowded housing, and unequal access to health care—kept the Black tuberculosis rate three times the rate for whites through the 1930s, and the overall death rate for African Americans double that of whites.[53]

To compound this exclusion, white officials and physicians blamed African Americans for their public health problems like tuberculosis—caused by the factors listed above, all stemming from Jim Crow segregation and discrimination—and used these castigations to support their segregation efforts. One example was Rudolph Matas, a professor at Tulane, doctor at Charity, and one of the nation's leading surgeons. In his 1896 paper "The Surgical Peculiarities of the Negro," Matas argued that whites were physiologically "the superior race," and that "mulattos" were "liable to disease" like tuberculosis which they could spread to whites. Matas used these claims to advocate against "miscegenation," much as half a century earlier Samuel Cartwright and others used the same arguments to support slavery.[54] In their 1906–1907 biennial report, the Louisiana Board of Health stated that "improvement in the colored death rate has been retarded by the reckless and improvident ways of the race and their utter disregard of all hygienic and sanitary laws"; they recommended separating death rates by race so as to avoid negative views of whites by outsiders.[55] These calls for separation of health statistics transformed into the demands in the 1910s and 1920s for residential segregation and spatial containment previously detailed.

New Orleans experienced significant advances in municipal services and public health in the Progressive Era. Yet, the gains did not extend to all residents; indeed, white leaders purposely excluded Black New Orleanians and used the resulting racial health disparities to justify the larger system of Jim Crow. In July 1917, the editors of the *Times Picayune* wrote a piece titled

"A Gilt-Edged Investment," which lauded the public health improvements and accompanying decline in the white death rate, and also perfectly captured the relationship between the "Progressive" measures and white supremacy: "A city without care is bound to be a city without character. Fortunately, New Orleans has never stood in that contemptible class. She cared for white supremacy and shed some of her noblest blood to overthrow the carpetbag regime; she cared for her people's poorer health and spent thirty million, out of relatively slender resources, to assure it; she cared for her commerce and devoted millions to its upbuilding."[56]

Despite the self-congratulating of whites, New Orleans in the early twentieth century, and throughout its history, was "in that contemptible class" as a "city without care." New Orleans cared to improve public health and promote commerce, two goals closely aligned. However, the city did not extend this care to African Americans. Instead, as the editors celebrated, "she cared for white supremacy."

Excluded from the public health measures and the historically white medical system in general, and blamed for their own health problems, African Americans in the first decades of the twentieth century turned to their own health care system. Black civic organizations initiated public health measures, and Black medical professionals created their own alternate medical district in Central City; chapter 5 explores these efforts.

CHAPTER FIVE

Jim Crow Black Health Care, 1927–1950

On October 30, 1931, over 15,000 people came for the dedication of the cornerstone for the new Flint Goodridge Hospital in Central City. Grand Marshall Joseph Geddes led a parade of thousands of members of fraternal organizations, civic associations, and marching bands. The Tonic Triad military band and a chorus of 150 singers led the crowd in a rendition of the "Negro National Anthem," followed by a series of speeches by Bishop R. E. Jones, Dillard University board vice president Dr. Emile LaBranche, master of ceremonies Edgar Stern, U.S. Veterans Affairs hospital superintendent Colonel E. H. Ward, and Southern University president Joseph Clark. The speakers all lauded the success of the fundraising efforts for the building, with contributions from both white and Black citizens and organizations. "The problem of one group is the problem of another," Stern told the crowd. Clark echoed this theme: "the unselfish cooperation of the white people of New Orleans and the state to safeguard the health of the colored people is one of the best evidences of their faith in cooperation." He also urged further contribution from Black residents through their wills and donations, "leaving to the outstanding credit of the race a glorious heritage."

Clark furthermore summarized the importance of the growing health care system, which had helped decrease rates of disease and mortality nationwide. The expanded Flint Goodridge would address these problems and provide training for many Black medical professionals, providing invaluable service to the community:

> Disease, poverty, and crime have linked themselves together and stared civilization in the face as a mighty monster, waging war against prosperity, peace, and happiness, but fairness and justice are demanding that these monsters surrender their claim, and to that end thousands of hospitals have been erected, making it possible for the sick to be cured, and the lame to walk, the blind to see, and the deaf to hear . . . This is a unit of the great Dillard University where nurses will be trained and sent forth to the bedside of the suffering with a balm of comfort; where doctors will come and get their interne practice, and go forth to cure; where patients will be brought and their lives extended by the treatment of operation.[1]

Builders completed the hospital, one of the largest Black hospitals in the country, the following year. Hundreds of thousands of dollars in donations from Black and white residents as well as philanthropic groups made possible its construction. However, as this chapter demonstrates, it was hardly an example of benevolent interracial cooperation that guided the giving by whites, as the speakers in 1931 led the crowd to believe. The same desires for racial segregation and spatial concentration that led to Flint Goodridge's removal from the white Medical District served as the main impetus for most whites' support. Nevertheless, Clark's assessment of the significance of the hospital proved correct. Over the next five decades, Flint Goodridge spearheaded the effort to tackle Black public health issues. The hospital trained generations of nurses and physicians. And Flint Goodridge anchored a new Black medical district.

This chapter explores the efforts of Black New Orleanians to create an alternate medical district in the Central City neighborhood. It details the initial attempts to create two hospitals, the unsuccessful Colored Hospital and the new Flint Goodridge Hospital. The chapter examines the initial challenges of the hospital—like fundraising and staffing—and the vision of Flint Goodridge as not just a hospital but a health center focused on three main goals: expanding hospital care for African Americans throughout the region, addressing Black public health issues, and serving as a training center for Black medical professionals. Finally, the chapter explores two significant issues for the hospital: the deliberate effort of the municipal government to prevent the growth of the hospital with WPA-sponsored "slum clearance" and building of public housing units around the institution, and the post–World War II exodus of Black physicians from the Jim Crow city.

Creating a Black Medical District

Excluded from official public health initiatives and blamed for their high disease rate, African Americans attempted to address these problems through grassroots efforts. Black churches and civic organizations participated in public health campaigns and neighborhood cleanups as part of the National Negro Health Week, started by Booker T. Washington's Tuskegee Institute in 1915. In 1927, Dr. Joseph Hardin formed the Seventh Ward Civic League, an organization that followed the self-help and accommodationist model promoted by Hardin and other leaders of the local NAACP chapter. Led primarily by upper-income Black business and civic leaders, the Seventh Ward Civic League—and other leagues that formed in other Black-majority wards—

carried out neighborhood cleanups, pressured the city for more funding for Black schools, lobbied for the creation of Black parks and playgrounds, and self-funded street lighting, paved roads, and other improvements the municipal government refused to fund in Black neighborhoods.[2]

Flint Goodridge Hospital too became involved in these endeavors. The hospital extended its reach by offering outpatient clinics in schools, charities, and churches. However, the hospital's clinics and the grassroots efforts could not overcome the impact of systemic racism, particularly the exclusion from the larger medical establishment, to adequately meet the needs of the city's 99,000 Black residents, or the 1.5 million African Americans who lived within a 200-mile radius of New Orleans. Black leaders still favored the accommodationist approach of pushing for gradual change and enforcement of the equal provision of "separate but equal" over pushing for integration of white hospitals. Angered by the requirement of using the separate entrance and facing continued discrimination and lower quality of care at Charity, Black leaders focused on three different approaches: the creation of a separate Black public hospital; the creation of a second private Black hospital; or the expansion of Flint Goodridge. Although proposed as an option in the *Louisiana Weekly*, no existing historical records indicate that African American leaders approached the city or the state for the creation of a municipal or state-administered and financed separate Black hospital. Instead, they focused on the latter two options, in the process creating a division within the Black community.

By the late 1920s, many African Americans had lost confidence in Flint Goodridge Hospital's leadership. An all-white board appointed by the Methodist Episcopal Church ran the institution and selected the hospital's superintendent—who was always white—which rankled many members of the Black community. This model of white leadership existed in many of the Black hospitals funded by institutions like the MEC and philanthropic groups like the Rockefeller Foundation.[3] Frustration with this situation, especially over allegations of prejudice by white doctors at the hospital, including Superintendent T. Restin Heath, boiled over in the late 1920s. In 1925, Black nursing students went on strike over "unbearable conditions," alleging that Heath was "overbearing" and refused to call them by their surname, only by their first name, a practice of disrespect dating back to slavery in which many enslavers renamed enslaved individuals and often gave no surname, in the process stripping them of their identity and status as equals. Physicians claimed that Heath bore "anti-Negro feeling," favored white physicians, acted "discourteous" to Black physicians, and only hired whites for his personal office staff. A Black patient made a formal complaint against a white doctor at the hospital, alleging that the physician beat him, prompting investigations by the NAACP. Although Heath promised to give Black physicians a voice in administration, Black doctors and nurses continued to feel ignored. In March 1926, officials from the MEC visited the hospital and Heath offered his resignation; the MEC refused and told Black leaders who requested a Black physician take his place that it was an "idle dream for anyone to figure that a colored man would be made head of the institution as long as the white people, through the church agencies, supplied the money for the hospital."[4] In August 1926, Heath reorganized the staff and he purposely omitted Dr. Rivers Frederick, his most vocal critic. Outraged, Black medical and civic leaders demanded the restoration of Frederick to the hospital staff and the MEC's immediate removal of Heath, which the MEC again refused to do.[5]

With the African American community angry at both Flint Goodridge and Charity Hospital, a third hospital for Black patients nearly came to fruition. In 1926, several of the board members of the Colored Hospital Association, which had halted their efforts to build a Black hospital in Central City in 1921, resumed their quest. The *Louisiana Weekly* heartily endorsed the project, stating in September 1926 that the one good thing that emerged from the "disgusting and muddled situation" at Flint Goodridge was that it "impressed upon the people of New Orleans the need of another hospital in the city."[6] Similarly, they wrote of the "Uncharitable Hospital": "We are not wanted at Charity Hospital . . . Give Negroes a separate hospital where they won't feel as though they are not fit subjects . . . If we must sacrifice our bodies for the making of physicians, permit us to make a few Black physicians."[7] Noting that it did "not mean to discard the existing hospital," the newspaper urged Black residents to support this second Black hospital "that serves without being circumscribed by denominational lines"—taking a direct shot at the MEC—and "which can appeal to and serve the whole people.[8]

By September 1926, the Colored Hospital Association announced plans for a $300,000, 200-bed institution—with half the beds allocated for free service for indigent patients—on the same lot purchased by James Newman in Central City, far exceeding the hospital they had hoped to build five years earlier and the sixty-four beds at Flint Goodridge. Additionally, the hospital would feature a nurse training corps. Many of the city's leading Black business and civic leaders led the project. Almost all served in leadership roles for the NAACP, the Federation of Civic Leagues, or both. Almost all participated in exclusive Creole social and pleasure organizations. Almost all sat on boards of Black life insurance companies. And almost all favored accommodation, in the form of a separate Black institution, rather than integration. "Help Yourself," urged advertisements for the hospital in the *Louisiana Weekly*. Writing in support of the hospital in October 1926, the newspaper urged all Black citizens to aid the project, following a model of self-help: "Let us evidence the spirit of independence. We should let the whole world see that we are determined to help ourselves in our affairs as far as human endeavor is possible."[9]

Initially, it appeared the Colored Hospital Association would succeed this time. A fundraising drive commenced in October netted $40,000 in its first week. All the local white newspapers gave "favorable editorial comments upon the movement," noted the *Weekly*, which also reported in September 1926 that "assurances have been given by leading white citizens that they will support the project with funds."[10] Mayor O'Keefe endorsed the project and promised to pave the roads—most of Central City still had dirt roads—as soon as they constructed the hospital.[11] "The sentiment in favor with New Orleans Colored Hospital is indeed strong among both races," reported the *Weekly*, including white physicians who supported the Black hospital "as one in the interest of scientific advancement."[12]

Despite this enthusiasm and seeming progress, the hospital encountered the same problems as the earlier attempts. Most significantly, the "assured" financial support from whites never materialized. Without this contribution or the support of a large philanthropic organization that helped finance many Black hospitals—including Flint Goodridge—the effort collapsed, and in 1928 the Colored Hospital Association ceased to exist.

The leaders of the Colored Hospital Association pledged the raised money to expand Flint Goodridge instead. Administrators initially sought to buy property adjacent or elsewhere in the Medical District. However, like the opposition faced by Newman as part of the effort to evict African Americans from the Medical District, white landowners refused to sell the land for the Black hospital. Faced with this obstacle, hospital leaders looked elsewhere, but again found their efforts limited. White property owners throughout the city refused to sell property. Additionally, administrators had to obtain permission from the all-white city council to build a hospital in any section of the city under the 1894 municipal ordinance.[13]

The heads of Flint Goodridge announced plans to construct a new building in October 1927. Having been unable to purchase property from adjacent white landowners and facing a constant threat of closure by city inspectors, Flint Goodridge became part of a larger transformation of racial space in the city. With the backing of both school's administrators, the AMA and MEC jointly announced a merger of Straight College and New Orleans University into a single school named Dillard University. Leaders hoped the union would create a leading and financially stable—both colleges had been losing money for years—higher education institution for African Americans. The institutions would move as well. New Orleans University—still downtown on Canal Street—and Straight—located uptown on St. Charles—would consolidate onto the proposed site of Dillard in the Gentilly neighborhood. As part of the merger, Flint Goodridge affiliated with Dillard. Flint would relocate from the Medical District to Central City, one block from the site of the proposed location of the Colored Hospital. By that period, Central City had the largest concentration of Black residents and had become the hub for the Black working class. Central City contained asphalt, gravel, and timber industries mixed with dairies like the Woodside Dairy—which occupied the land that administrators later purchased for Flint Goodridge Hospital—and Black residences. The area lagged behind other neighborhoods, as the city refused to pave roads or extend water or sewage lines in the early twentieth century.

White New Orleanians favored the hospital moving to the Black-majority neighborhood, and the city council granted permission and amended the residential zoning ordinance for the desired property on Louisiana Avenue.[14] White leaders viewed the less desirable property in Central City as the perfect location for Black residents, meeting their desired goal of Black spatial containment. To facilitate this process, the city built the first Black school and only Black playground there in the early twentieth century and steered Flint Goodridge there in the late 1920s. The city council also approved this measure to continue the removal of the Black medical profession from the main medical district in the Tulane Gravier neighborhood. Flint Goodridge left that area in 1932, following the earlier closing of Flint Medical College and Provident Sanitarium.

Although Flint Goodridge left the Medical District and the proposed Colored Hospital never came to fruition, the relocation of Flint Goodridge fostered the creation of an alternate Black medical district in Central City. A cluster of medical practitioners already operated on Dryades Street, about a mile from the site of Flint. This grouping included two dentists, eight physicians, and the Unity Industrial Life and the Eagle Life Insurance Company. Starting in the 1920s, Unity Industrial hired Dr. Raleigh Coker to run a clinic at its headquarters to provide free services—primarily infant and maternal care, vaccinations, and care for minor health problems—for any member of the Black community, hoping to attract more subscribers.[15] Six other doctors had offices in other parts of Central City, in addition to four more pharmacies. Central City was already functioning as an alternate Black medical district by the 1920s; the relocation of Flint Goodridge solidified this status.

Flint Goodridge's Many Initial Challenges

Finding a location for a new hospital proved to be only one obstacle for Flint Goodridge's leaders. Most pressingly, the hospital needed to raise hundreds of thousands of dollars. This was a monumental task for an institution that had relied primarily on several thousand dollars a year from the MEC to supplement patient fees and one that struggled throughout its first decades to remain financially solvent. Hospital leaders worked with the Community Chest to form a fundraising campaign to raise a total of $2 million, with $1.5 million going toward Dillard and $500,000 for the hospital. Volunteers solicited the money from 1929 to 1930. The MEC and the AMA each pledged $500,000, and leaders secured an additional $500,000 from the Rockefeller Foundation and $250,000 from the Rosenwald Fund, which had recently decided to expand its philanthropy beyond education to Black health care. The latter two groups stipulated that they would only donate the money if locals raised an additional $250,000. Fundraising leaders set a target goal of $200,000 for whites and $50,000 for Black residents. More than 1,200 Black residents donated, but campaign workers struggled to meet the $50,000 goal due to the poor economic situation of most Black New Orleanians.[16] On the other hand, white New Orleanians surpassed their quota of $250,000, with 3,000 residents giving a total of $328,000. For some whites, an altruistic desire to support public health efforts and a general interest in equality may have motivated giving. White and Black leaders of the hospital publicly expressed this sentiment. Flint superintendent H. W. Knight wrote that with the funding "the white men of the city have expressed themselves as understanding the colored man and liking him." Head of the Rosenwald Fund, Edwin Embree stated that "a new record was set for any southern city both in the sums involved and in the spirit of partnership between the races working for a common civic purpose." The NAACP's *Crisis* stated the "genius" of the hospital "is not that of doing something for Negroes, out of the white man's wisdom and abundance. Instead, it is that of pooling the resources and the intelligence of both groups in a great community enterprise for the advantage of both—a policy that evidences a breadth of mind, of sympathy, and of cooperation that would be a credit to any community."[17]

Yet, despite these celebrations of interracial cooperation, three less altruistic concerns appear to have been the primary causes of white support: fear of disease, a desire to have healthy workers, and the push for residential segregation and spatial concentration of African Americans in Central City. Fundraising leaders repeatedly emphasized the first concern in their quest to garner white support. Fundraising material prominently featured the phrase "The Microbe Knows No Color Line!" A 1929 report put out by the hospital to support fundraising emphasized the "proximity" of Black health hazards to whites due to the "constant contact of both races, by reasons of locality, employment, transportation, and recreation." Speaking at a dedication of the hospital's new site in October 1929, Dillard University president Dr. W. W. Alexander told the assembled crowd: "The two races cannot be considered apart from each other in their problems, whether health or economics. If there is an epidemic among negroes, there will be an epidemic among the whites." This fear prompted white support of the new Black hospital. To protect themselves while still maintaining segregation, they donated to the separate Black hospital.[18]

Connected to this idea was the need to have a healthy Black labor force. The namesake of the university, Dr. James Hardy Dillard, argued: "In improving the health of the negro, the white people are protecting themselves since negroes are necessary to the community and must be taken care of properly if local industries are to prosper."[19]

White leaders encouraged white donations to facilitate the relocation of the Black hospital and the affiliated Black schools out of the neighborhoods deemed "white spaces." Speaking to a crowd in 1930, Mayor T. Semmes Walmsley told the white audience that "it was worth the entire amount asked to get the race schools off the sites they occupy." City councilmen too pushed for the plan, including attempts to assuage white residents of the Gentilly neighborhood who protested at a December 1930 city council meeting that locating Dillard University nearby would depreciate their property values and that the school would "form the nucleus of a Negro colony."[20] Whatever the motivation, white residents responded by giving $328,000.[21]

In October 1931, over 20,000 people attended an opening ceremony for the hospital (figure 5.1). Designed by modernist architect Moise Goldstein, the four-story brick and stone hospital "combined permanence and utility with exceptional beauty and good taste," noted the *Crisis*. The total cost for the property, building, and equipment came to $435,000, less than the projected $500,000, in sharp contrast to Charity's final cost of $12.5 million, over $4.5 million above the original approved cost.[22]

Advocates of Flint Goodridge saw the hospital as a significant milestone not only for Black New Orleanians, but for African Americans throughout the Deep South. This modern institution, now Black owned and operated, was still the only hospital in the region with Black physicians. Philanthropist Julius Rosenwald described the venture as "one of the most epoch-making

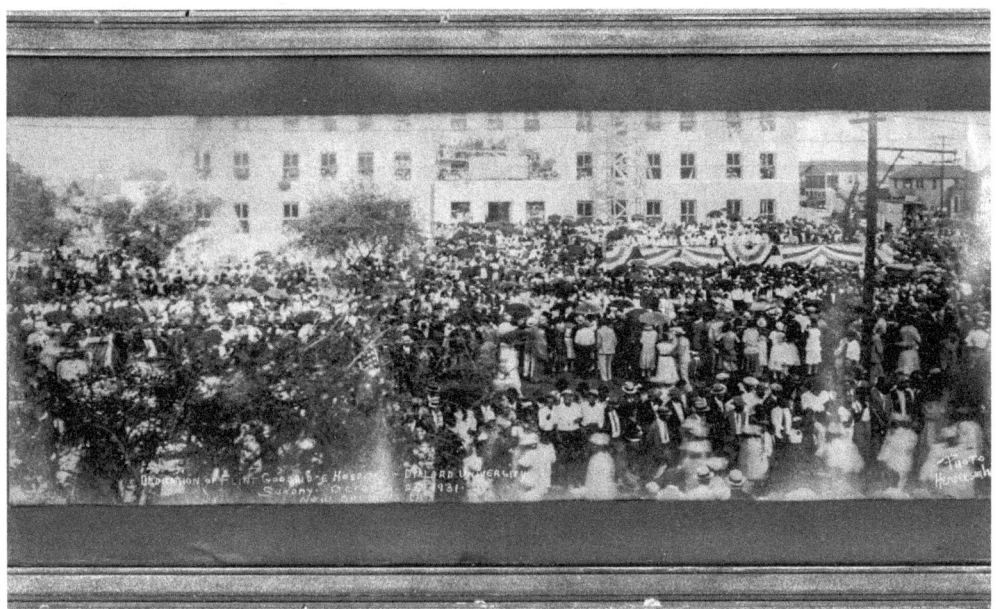

FIGURE 5.1 Dedication of Flint Goodridge Hospital in October 1931 (Flint Goodridge Hospital Collection, Dillard University Archives).

steps on behalf of the Negro since Lincoln's Emancipation." Edwin Embree spoke of the institution becoming one of the "Big Four" of Black hospitals in the country, joining Provident Hospital in Chicago (founded 1891), Provident Hospital in Baltimore (1894), and Frederick Douglass Memorial Hospital in Philadelphia (1895).[23]

The three hospitals that Embree cited shared many similarities with Flint Goodridge. All had been founded in the 1890s. All three included in their mission statements three primary goals: care for Black patients, providing hospital opportunities for Black physicians, and offering training for Black nurses. All three started as small, private hospitals in buildings in Black neighborhoods, relied primarily in their early years on donations from the Black community, used women's auxiliaries to lead fundraising drives, turned to white civic and business leaders in support of fundraising, treated a small number of white patients, struggled financially due to providing reduced or free care to the low-income Black patients that were the majority of admissions, and repeatedly sought to expand and moved into a succession of buildings in their early decades. Two of the three entered into partnerships with white medical schools: Provident Hospital in Chicago with the University of Chicago, and Provident Hospital in Baltimore with Johns Hopkins University and the University of

Maryland. By the 1920s, these partnerships and financial support from philanthropic groups like the Rosenwald Fund and the Rockefeller Foundation brought financial stability to the hospitals. In contrast, Frederick Douglass Hospital refused to establish ties to the University of Pennsylvania. In response, the state legislature ended annual appropriations to the hospital. Out of the three, Frederick Douglass Memorial Hospital was the most financially unstable due to its lack of wealthy benefactors, and repeatedly lost accreditation in the 1920s. Flint Goodridge followed the path of the Provident Hospitals in securing financial support from philanthropic groups.[24]

With a location found and money raised, the administration turned to the controversial task of staffing the hospital. With previous protests centered on having only white administrators and allegations of discrimination against those administrators still fresh, the new board of directors—headed by Dillard University president W. W. Alexander and Edgar Stern of the Rosenwald Fund—chose Albert Dent to become the new hospital's first Black head. Dent previously worked in accounting and fundraising in life insurance and higher education, and he was considered a brilliant administrative mind even at the age of twenty-seven. Alexander successfully recruited Dent, who was also considering a similar position with a Black hospital in Chicago and a posting with the Public Works Administration's new housing program.[25] Dent and others on the board then focused on hiring the physician staff. The administrators quickly realized the dearth of Black physicians in the city. In 1930, forty-two Black doctors practiced in New Orleans, for a ratio of 1 physician to every 2,758 Black residents, and only thirty-five were fully licensed to work at a hospital; in contrast, 708 white doctors practiced, for a ratio of 1 physician for every 465 whites. The closure of Flint Medical College, the lack of professional opportunities, and exclusion from the OPMS prevented Black doctors from enrolling in postgraduate training or even using the medical library. Only two of the physicians in the city had completed internships; overall, just forty internships existed nationwide for Black physicians—Charity alone had 124 internships for white doctors. The hospital hired thirty-three of the Black physicians in New Orleans, but they needed more to fully staff the institution—Charity's combined staff of regular, visiting, and interning doctors exceeded 600. Due to the small number of available Black doctors, Flint Goodridge's administrators made the controversial decision to name white doctors as heads of six of the seven departments, with Black physicians as associate heads. Dr. Rivers Frederick led the surgery department. The board also continued the practice of allowing white doctors to treat their Black patients at the hospital.[26]

Some praised the use of an interracial staff. The *Crisis* described the program as a "notable example of interracial cooperation." Other Black hospitals—including Provident Hospital in Chicago and Provident Hospital in Baltimore—also used interracial staffs. Yet some assailed the lack of Black leadership positions. The *Chicago Defender* criticized the move and contrasted it with the Colored Hospital Association's earlier plan to only have Black doctors on the full-time staff, with white doctors as consultants. "To the layman," the newspaper wrote, "it is easily apparent if Race men are excluded from serving as chiefs, one of the prime needs of the hospital is nullified." The article continued, "the biggest function of the Race in the new hospital would be to supply patients to the Race institution, heralded at the time of the drive for funds for it as the salvation of the Race physicians in this section of the South." The newspaper further speculated that the lack of Black leadership at the hospital may have led to Black residents declining to contribute to the fundraising drive.[27] The criticism of white supervisors also came from groups like the NAACP, which expanded its condemnation to creating a separate Black hospital in the first place. In 1931, the board of directors of the national NAACP passed a resolution condemning the actions of the Rosenwald Fund—especially the creation of separate Black hospitals like Flint Goodridge—as propagating segregation. In response, Embree argued the necessity of institutions like Flint Goodridge, and he pointed to the fact that only ten Black hospitals in the entire country were approved by the American Medical Association and American College of Surgeons to have Black patients and train Black physicians and nurses.[28] While proponents held up Flint Goodridge and other Black-operated hospitals as vital to the African American community, debate about and criticism of separate Black hospitals like Flint continued until the 1960s.

A Black Health Center

Dent and the other leaders of Flint Goodridge envisioned a new role for the hospital, one that matched the ideals first imagined when New Orleans University attempted to establish New Orleans as a medical hub centered around their planned medical school in the late nineteenth century. In 1929, the same year that C. C. Bass gave his speech predicting New Orleans as a "Medical Center" with Tulane's medical school as the key institution, Flint Goodridge released a booklet to support the fundraising effort that proclaimed its dream of New Orleans as "one of the five great health and education centers for colored people in the United States."[29] Under Dent, Flint Goodridge embraced this expanded role and joined other Black hospital movement leaders who saw improved health as an important part of the larger "racial uplift" principle popular in the era.[30]

The 1929 booklet addressed the major health issues that Flint Goodridge and Black health activists needed to address in New Orleans, where African Americans had a death rate more than twice as high as whites (28.1 per 1,000 compared to 13.7 per 1,000, respectively). The number of Black deaths in 1929 exceeded the number of births, meaning that if not for migration from outside the city, the Black population would have declined. The researchers found the Black mortality rate was the highest among the eleven cities with the largest Black populations. The report identified several major causes: maternal/infant death rate, with 76.7 stillbirths for every 1,000 births, 16.5 maternal deaths per 1,000 births, and an infant mortality rate of 12 percent (compared to white rates of 44.5 and 11 per 1,000, and 5.9 percent respectively); heart disease (762 per 100,000 vs. 382 for whites); tuberculosis (310 vs. 101); pneumonia (288 vs. 46); and cancer.[31]

Hospital administrators focused on what they identified as the "three main health liabilities of the Negro": tuberculosis, maternal/infant health, and syphilis.[32] To address these issues, Dent secured outside funding to create outpatient clinics specializing in all three problems by 1936. For the tuberculosis clinic, the hospital partnered with the Tuberculosis and Public Health Association of Louisiana, the Tuberculosis Committee of New Orleans, the Rosenwald Fund, and later the state Department of Health. The clinic conducted studies on incidences of tuberculosis and tested all babies seen at the hospital, all Black schoolchildren, and all patients at any of the hospital's clinics. This resulted in the testing of nearly 6,000 people in 1936 alone. They were also able to give free treatment for the indigent and free biweekly lectures and demonstrations for any Black doctor within a 150-mile radius, in addition to free testing and treatment consultation. The tuberculosis clinic was the first in the city to offer the cutting-edge pneumothorax treatment. The hospital operated a syphilis clinic with the same setup.[33]

With the infant and maternal health clinic, Dent hoped to reduce the number of women who used midwives instead of delivering babies in hospitals—21.7 percent of Black New Orleanians and 89.9 percent of Black Louisianans living in rural areas outside of the city. Dent hired a social worker to form mothers' clubs and teach prenatal and infant care and advise about "the inadvisability of trafficking with midwives." After determining that most of women used midwives because they were cheaper than hospital services, Dent determined a $10 flat fee for having a birth at Flint Goodridge. As a result, births at the hospital increased 400 percent between 1932 and 1938, and by 1939 more whites used midwives than African Americans. The hospital also started "well-baby" clinics—with 1,242 visits in 1932 and 4,385 in 1938—and pediatrics clinics, as well as providing periodic free diphtheria immunization and whooping cough clinics.[34]

Clinics provided much needed treatment not only in addressing the major public health issues like tuberculosis, but also in more standard care that most Black residents could not typically afford. For example, hospital clinics held a "Sight Saving Week" during October 1936, offering free services for low-income residents. Of 700 patients that came for exams, doctors found eye defects and diseased tonsils in half, and diseased teeth in a quarter. By 1939, the hospital added clinics for gynecology; urology; ear, nose, and throat; diabetes; and dental care.[35]

Through the clinics and other services, the hospital found its original mission shifting. The founders in the 1890s created the hospital primarily to provide care for patients who could afford to pay for services, and thus were ineligible for treatment at Charity Hospital, with 20 percent of Flint Goodridge's beds set aside for free services for the indigent. However, the health needs of low-income Black residents pushed the hospital to expand these services; by the late 1920s, one out of every three patients received free care.

When administrators envisioned the new hospital in 1929, they planned to reduce the amount of free care back to the original 20 percent level. However, the hospital opened as the Great Depression gripped the country, with African Americans disproportionately impacted, with higher rates of unemployment and poverty than whites. While African Americans made up fewer than 31 percent of households in New Orleans in 1935, they comprised 50 percent of all the unemployed and 65 percent of the families on federal relief. In New Orleans, as in many Southern locations, whites received preferential treatment for relief and reemployment programs, especially in the early 1930s; as domestic or unskilled laborers, many African Americans were exempted from the National Recovery Administration and minimum wage regulations. They also often did not meet the minimum income for public housing. These conditions severely impacted the hospital in two ways: the Great Depression increased the number of patients in general and made the public health initiatives more difficult and more needed; and these conditions pushed more Black New Orleanians into poverty, adding to the number of free patients.[36]

In its first year in the newly opened building, nearly 46 percent of patients received free care. By 1935, that number climbed to nearly 59 percent, and 11 percent of patients received reduced fee treatment. While the hospital served more patients overall, seeing an increase from 2,098 patients in 1932 to 5,719 in 1936, the high percentage of partial-pay and free patients kept income low. The outpatient clinics experienced a similar pattern. In 1932, 7,790 patients used the clinics, with 41.4 percent receiving free care. By 1935, the number reached 21,084, with 81 percent receiving free care. Additionally, many Black patients chose to transfer their services to Flint Goodridge from Charity due to poor treatment, which further expanded the free care.[37]

In 1935, Dent started a penny-a-day hospital insurance program to increase working-class access. It allowed patients up to twenty-one days a year in the hospital for $3.65 a year. By 1938, over 3,200 people had enrolled. The American Medical Association endorsed the plan and identified it as the cheapest in the nation. In September 1939, *Life* magazine ran a feature story on the program, citing it as the best hospital insurance plan in the country and praising it as needed inspiration during the Great Depression: "Frankly this is a success story; one that makes a heartening comment on democracy, in these dark days of race hatred and persecution. It is one of those things, we think, that makes you genuinely happy to belong to the human race."[38] The *Louisiana Weekly* described the penny-a-day insurance plan and other programs as strengthening the hospital's "position in the community where its desire to operate as a Health Center and not merely as a hospital has long been recognized."[39]

However, even with the income from the penny-a-day program, the hospital struggled to remain financially solvent due to the high number of nonpaying patients, and they were forced to rely on fundraisers by the hospital's women's auxiliary and sources like the Community Chest and the Rosenwald Fund to pay for the indigent services. Donations to the Community Chest remained low due to the Great Depression, and the organization distributed money to numerous other causes; funding from the chest—raised throughout the 1930s primarily from whites using the repeated slogan "the microbe knows no color line"—stayed at $12,000 a year.[40] The Rosenwald Fund proved a much more reliable source throughout the decade. Son-in-law to Julius Rosenwald, Edgar Stern proved a valuable ally, serving on Flint's board of management and continually approving increased funding. However, the fund ran out of money in 1943 and other ways to support the hospital needed to emerge. Although the city appropriated money to private, all-white hospitals, they regularly turned down Flint's requests. For example, in 1936, the city gave $30,000 to five white health institutions, but denied Flint's request for $3,000 "on the grounds that it was not possible to add any new appropriations to the City Budget this year."[41]

Patient numbers, and corresponding fees, increased steadily nearly every year. However, more patients led to the need for more personnel. Additionally, equipment replacement proved continuous and costly and was exacerbated by uncollected patient debts and threatened loss of accreditation. These problems plagued the hospital throughout its existence. Despite these difficulties, Dent and the hospital leaders sought to increase the hospital's impact, including efforts to improve Black medical education. Dent planned to restart Flint's medical school, although that never occurred. Dent began an internship program to help address the lack of internships available nationwide to new Black doctors and created a postgraduate training program. Dent started the latter program in response to the exclusion of Black physicians from local American Medical Association chapters, which meant that not only were they not allowed to work in white hospitals, but they were also denied postgraduate opportunities provided by the AMA. To counter this, Dent opened an annual two-week postgraduate program, featuring leading Black and white medical educators (primarily from Tulane University and LSU) and physicians from throughout the city, and offered it free for any Black physician in the country. From 1936 to 1940, the course had 207 participants from ten states. Over 33 percent of the Black physicians in Louisiana and 20 percent of Black physicians in adjoining states attended. The Rosenwald Fund also gave funding to support Black physicians at Flint doing postgraduate fellowships at hospitals throughout the country and internationally to further their training.[42]

While these programs significantly helped the Black medical profession, attracting Black staff proved a persistent problem. With Howard and Meharry still the only Black medical schools in operation and the impact of the Great Depression further limiting the financial abilities of African Americans to afford to attend medical school, the number of Black physicians had declined nationwide by the 1930s. Despite the opening of Flint Goodridge and their educational programs like the postgraduate seminar, New Orleans experienced this decline in Black physicians. In 1930, forty-seven Black physicians practiced in the city; this number dropped to thirty-nine in 1940 even as New Orleans's Black population grew by nearly 15 percent. The ratio of Black physicians per Black residents fell from 1 per 2,758 in 1930 to 1 per 3,821 in 1940; in comparison, the number of white physicians increased from 708 in 1930 to 855 in 1940, improving the ratio of white physicians from 1 per 465 to 1 per 404 white residents (see table A.2). This forced Flint Goodridge to continue to rely heavily on white physicians.

Additionally, the hospital's nurse training program, the only one for Black nurses in the state, was not producing enough graduates to meet the expanded hospital's needs. In 1932, representatives from the Louisiana Board of Nurse Examiners, the National League of Nursing Education, and the National Organization for Public Health Nursing reviewed Flint Goodridge's nursing program on Dent's request as he sought accreditation. The representatives reported that the number of instructors, the hospital's facilities, and number of patients were inadequate for accreditation, and in 1934 the nurse training program ceased, ending the program's twenty-eight-year run in similar fashion to the forced shuttering of Flint Medical College. Dent pushed unsuccessfully for eight years to reopen the program. Instead, the hospital hired Black graduate nurses from existing programs outside of Louisiana like Spelman College, but nursing numbers remained persistently low.[43]

Slum Clearance in Central City

Guided by Dent's vision of Flint Goodridge as the focal point for a health center for African Americans in the region, administrators early on planned to expand the hospital as its patients and services increased. However, federally funded municipal action forever altered this vision and hampered not just the growth of Flint Goodridge but the Black medical district also. In 1937, the year state and local officials began displacing hundreds of Black residents to build the new Charity Hospital through PWA funding, the city applied for additional PWA funding to build separate Black and white public housing units. When Congress passed the National Industrial Recovery Act in 1933, which created the Public Works Administration, advocates of public housing—inspired by state-sponsored housing in Europe—successfully pushed to include housing as one of the PWA's authorized goals. Initially, the PWA built communitarian-modeled units like the Carl Mackley Houses in Philadelphia (1935), which included a kindergarten and cultural center. However, conservative legislators used amendments to the Housing Act of 1937 to limit the nature of government-subsidized housing. The Housing Act provisions required slum clearance to precede the building of housing, limited the amount that could be spent on construction (lowering the building quality), set caps on tenant incomes, and gave greater control to local governments over the projects.[44]

When New Orleans applied to build a Black public housing complex (officially titled the C. J. Peete Public Housing Development but colloquially known as the Magnolia Projects) under the PWA, initially Black leaders, including Flint's administrators, supported the proposal. The *Louisiana Weekly* reported that African Americans "joyfully received the news." The newspaper connected the issue of housing to health, noting that poor housing conditions contributed to the "disease epidemics," with the "homes of the wealthy whites being no forbidden grounds" due to their reliance on Black domestic workers. The paper sought through "slum clearance" the eradication of "dilapidated, unsanitary, 'revenue' houses" and replacement with public housing.[45]

However, only months later Black leaders changed their position when the city announced that it intended to use the PWA funding to clear the blocks surrounding Flint Goodridge Hospital as the intended site for the Black public housing. In an editorial titled "Not the Proper Location," critics decried the location: "If there was ever territory which needed slum clearance less than that adjoining Louisiana Avenue," the article argued, "we have yet to discover it in this city." Opponents noted that the city relied on a study conducted in the early 1930s by white Tulane University students—"we can think of no group more ill-suited to the task"—with no updates or input from Black leaders. Working-class Black residents largely comprised the Central City neighborhood around the hospital. Over the objection of Black leaders, the clearance went forward.[46] The city repeated this process for the other Housing Act–funded projects, using "slum clearance" to remove hundreds of Black residents in the adjacent B. W. Cooper neighborhood for Calliope; in Tremé for Lafitte; and near Dillard University for St. Bernard. All units were Black housing projects. Additionally, the city displaced hundreds of more Black residents to build two white housing projects, Iberville in Tremé and St. Thomas in the lower Garden District. The *Weekly* prophetically lamented the fate of the displaced working-class families, who would be pushed "to the farther reaches of the city, beyond the care of agencies which know and now meet their needs." For these residents forced to move from Central City and B. W. Cooper, the agencies included Flint Goodridge; many would have practically no access to health care until integration.[47]

The building of the housing projects had several other negative consequences. First, the Magnolia Projects, finished in 1941 and expanded by an additional six blocks in 1955, boxed in Flint Goodridge, curtailing future expansion. Second, while many envisioned public housing as helping improve the lives of lower-income individuals, due to the Wagner Act provisions the government used cheap, low-quality material to build the units. Rather than living in improved housing conditions, residents often found themselves trapped in quickly deteriorating units, isolated, and exposed to health issues— including lead poisoning and problems caused by exposure to toxins. The city placed the Calliope Projects and the first Black public high school near the municipal incinerator and on top of the recently closed Silver City Dump. This placement explicitly demonstrated the direct relationship between Jim Crow and negative Black health. Unbeknownst to Black residents, the soil on top of the dump—WPA workers filled in the dump and covered it with a layer of soil—contained high levels of carcinogenic toxins. The 1929 Comprehensive Plan designated B. W. Cooper as "Unrestricted" and thus permitted hazards like the incinerator, which exposed residents to carcinogenic byproduct blown into the air from the burning of trash; the incinerator operated until 1986.[48] These hazards caused severe health problems for residents of Calliope and Magnolia, and they primarily used nearby Flint Goodridge. In turn, this raised the number of free-care patients, which financially hurt the hospital and also stigmatized the institution for its association with the projects and the neighborhood, which increasingly acquired a reputation for crime and drugs.

The use of federal funding for projects in the 1930s in the two medical districts, the white one in the Tulane Gravier neighborhood and the Black one in Central City, demonstrated the power of federal laws and money in supporting local racialized health care systems. Starting in the 1910s, the federal government, primarily through the public health services and later with the National Institutes of Health (created in 1930), began awarding research grants to universities and university-affiliated hospitals for research on public health issues and new treatments. Under New Deal programs like the PWA and WPA, the federal government started in the 1930s to fund the expansion of hospitals nationwide. Both sources helped lay the groundwork for the postwar period of growth of the medical–industrial complex, with an increasing number of hospitals and physicians, supported by increasing federal government funding. Tulane's and LSU's medical schools received federal research grants that supported their growth in the pre–World War II period. Similar to the PWA-sponsored "slum" clearance and building of the new Charity in the 1930s, federal funding helped support their physical expansions in the Tulane Gravier neighborhood, and their student bodies by increasing the schools' revenue. With an expanded Charity Hospital, Tulane and LSU—which each ran one of the wings in the hospitals—had increased opportunities for conducting research and more spots for students to train. The physical presence of the three institutions in the form of Charity Hospital and Tulane University's medical school—housed in the Hutchinson Memorial Building adjacent to Charity and connected to the hospital by an underground tunnel completed with WPA funding in 1937—and the LSU School of

Medicine—located next to Charity—on blocks that used to contain Black homes and businesses attested to the power of federal government funding for historically white medical institutions.

In contrast, Flint Goodridge did not receive federal research grants. Due to the forced closure of Flint Medical College, the inability of Dillard University to start its own medical program, and the refusal of Tulane and LSU to affiliate with the hospital, the hospital was not a university hospital, and thus was largely ineligible for federal research grants. Additionally, the municipal government used PWA money to prevent Flint Goodridge's expansion through its displacement of Black residents to build segregated public housing units. The use of federal funding to support the racialized health care system continued throughout the century.

World War II and Postwar Problems

World War II and the postwar period brought new obstacles for Flint Goodridge. In 1941, Albert Dent left his position as the hospital's chief administrator to become the president of Dillard University. He continued to play an active role with the hospital through his position as president and board member, but his direct daily running of the institution ceased. The hospital faced labor shortages during the war as many nurses and physicians joined the military. Dent helped address the dearth of nurses by successfully lobbying for financial support from the General Education Board, the Julius Rosenwald Fund, and the United States Public Health Service to start the state's first collegiate-level nursing program at Dillard in 1942, the third baccalaureate program in the country, and the first at an HBCU. By 1948, the program produced twenty graduates, but only seven worked at Flint Goodridge, hardly solving the nursing shortage, which became exacerbated as many nurses left Flint Goodridge for paying work at Charity—which began using Black nurses due to its own shortages caused by the war—and hospitals outside of New Orleans.[49]

The double bind of racism and sexism also kept down the number of nurses. By this period, nursing had been gendered as women's work, and Black women in particular faced difficulties in becoming nurses. High levels of poverty, low levels of education, and gender-role expectations that women focus on the home sphere not only undermined Black women's ability to become physicians, but also decreased chances of admittance to the few nursing programs like Dillard that admitted African Americans. Additionally, Southern states like Louisiana made Black women take separate nursing exams from whites, refused to permit needed training in hospitals, and denied them membership in professional organizations.[50]

Lacking nurses, in late 1945 Flint Goodridge closed twenty-three beds. The hospital hoped this would be temporary. To counter the loss, the hospital required employees to work longer hours and offered slightly higher wages to attract more nurses after the war ended, but the beds remained closed for over two years.[51]

The loss in beds led to a sharp decline in the hospital's revenue, exacerbating the continuing financial problems. In 1943, the Rosenwald Fund ceased. Fortunately, under Dent, Dillard assumed a large financial responsibility for the hospital, regularly paying off yearly deficits. The ending of the Rosenwald Fund forced the hospital to rely primarily on patient fees. In 1932, 53 percent of the hospital's total income came from patient fees; by 1944, this figure had climbed to 88 percent of the budget.[52] An increase in patient numbers and slight decline in free care occurred, reflecting the gradually improving economic condition of African Americans in the postwar period. However, the racist hierarchy limited these gains, as whites continued to discriminate against Black residents in hiring, promotions, and pay, leading to the perpetuation of higher Black rates of unemployment, underemployment, and poverty. Thus, Flint Goodridge's patient base never offered the stable support of the clientele at the private, all-white hospitals. Additionally, patient usage led to the need for more supplies, larger staff, and greater taxing of the building and equipment. In his 1944 annual report, new superintendent C. C. Weil noted the building and much of its equipment already needed costly renovations and replacement, a blood bank, and expanded laboratory facilities. The report also detailed that patients owed thousands in uncollected debt. The collection issue remained a continual problem for a hospital with a large majority of low-income patients. As a result, the hospital depended on fundraising by the Community Chest—which refused to raise annual allocations above $17,000—and individual donors, not just of money but everyday supplies like linen and cutlery. This reliance on an unstable funding base made the hospital's finances perpetually precarious. Inspecting the hospital in 1947, Dr. Basil MacLean—former superintendent of Touro Infirmary and an original Flint Goodridge board member—warned administrators they needed to broaden their financial support to "ensure survival."[53] Even with increased use of the hospital and a return to the target of 80 percent paying patients and 20 percent free patients with the postwar improved economy, financial instability (the hospital estimated that it spent $11.40 per patient-day in 1949 and income per patient-day only averaged $9.05 for the year) made annual survival challenging.

Board member Edgar Stern estimated the costs for free patients exceeded funding from their donation bases by over $31,000 in 1952, and the hospital needed $60,000 for renovations and new equipment.[54]

The need for equipment replacement and building renovation also reflected concerns over accreditation. Regular inspections by historically white organizations including the Joint Commission of Hospital Accreditation, the American Medical Association, the American College of Surgeons, and state and local bodies like the Board of Health forced the hospital to make improvements or face the loss of accreditation and forced closure, as occurred in 1914. In July 1954, the Joint Commission of Hospital Accreditation briefly stripped the hospital of accreditation. Although quickly restored after complying with the recommendations on improved policies and equipment, the threat hung over the hospital for decades to come.[55]

Another problem arose over hospital insurance, which white-owned companies refused to provide Flint Goodridge. As president of the Louisiana Life Insurance Company, Chief Surgeon Rivers Frederick directed his company in 1952 to draft a policy, but insurance coverage became an ongoing concern and an increasingly costly expenditure.[56]

Attracting Black physicians remained an issue as well, following a nationwide decline in Black doctors in the 1930s and 1940s due to the closure of Black medical schools and increasing poverty during the Great Depression. The inability to attend medical school in Louisiana and the poor treatment of Black doctors in the Jim Crow city also lowered the number of available Black physicians for Flint Goodridge. Testifying before a House Committee on Interstate Commerce hearing on the Hospital Construction Act in 1958, Flint Goodridge's Dr. William Adams informed the group of the exodus of Black physicians from the Crescent City in the postwar years, pushed out by segregation—including the refusal of the OPMS to admit Black physicians and LSU and Tulane's excluding them from seminars and lectures—and pulled by greater professional opportunities and better treatment in the North and West. Adams told the committee: "Our younger persons have left the city and the state primarily to California and other places because of their refusal to stay in an atmosphere where their further study is hindered by discriminatory laws." From a peak of forty-seven Black physicians in the mid-1930s, only fifteen Black doctors practiced in New Orleans by the mid-1950s. This loss of physicians hurt Flint Goodridge's ability to maintain an adequate full-time staff.[57]

As a result, the hospital increasingly granted attending privileges to more white physicians who brought their paying Black patients to the hospital but did not work full time for Flint. Hospital administrators argued that the interracial makeup of the staff served as a valuable counter to segregation, and Basil MacLean told the *Times Picayune* in 1947 that Flint's plan "has served as model" for other hospitals elsewhere. Regardless, the number of Black doctors working at the hospital and in New Orleans in general declined significantly after the war, rather than increasing as the hospital hoped.[58]

Beyond Flint, the decline in the number of physicians hurt the Black community in two main ways. First, with only fifteen physicians for over 200,000 Black residents, visiting a doctor's office or having them visit a patient at home became even more difficult. Second, New Orleans lost many civic leaders.

For 100 years, New Orleans had been a Black health center and the home of several generations of leading Black physician-activists. The first generation were the antebellum Creoles of color who followed in the wake of James Durham, the first Black physician. This group included Louis Charles Roudanez and Joseph Chaumette, individuals who, in a country that equated Blackness with slavery, in the words of historian Gretchen Long, used their positions of relative privilege to "doctor freedom." Barred from attending medical school in the United States, they obtained medical degrees in Europe and then returned home to provide care for other free people of color—predominantly the wealthy Black Creoles—and advocate for Black rights. A second generation of Creoles of color followed. Like their predecessors, these individuals, including James Newman and L. B. Landry, could not obtain medical degrees in their home city of New Orleans and gained medical education abroad or in newly formed Black medical schools. They too returned to the Crescent City to establish and lead that city's own Black medical college and hospital in a new world of supposed freedom that revealed itself to be Jim Crow. This second generation pushed against the boundaries of racialized health care and trained the third generation at Flint Medical College and in Flint Goodridge Hospital. Unlike their predecessors, the third generation did not have to travel to Europe or Canada or even Washington, D.C. or Nashville. Locals like Raleigh Coker and Ruby Vining and transplants like Joseph Hardin and George Lucas earned medical degrees in New Orleans, the leading Black medical center of the Deep South. They also carried on the tradition of Black physician activism, leading organizations like Black fraternal associations, ward civic leagues, and the NAACP. The shuttering of Flint Medical College in 1913 ruptured this legacy. Once again Black New Orleanians wanting to become doctors had to look elsewhere, if they were fortunate enough to even have that opportunity. And when they obtained their medical degrees at Meharry and Howard, most did not return, lured by the promise of the Great Migration that brought them instead to Chicago, New York, and California. Missing too from this generation were the Black medical students who would have come to New Orleans for medical school and stayed to provide care in the Black medical district, or individuals like Rivers Frederick who came to teach and lead. When the third generation retired or passed—both Hardin and Frederick died in 1954—fewer Black physicians existed in New Orleans to take their mantle. Flint Goodridge carried on its mission in the postwar decades, and doctors like William Adams provided leadership at the institution and in the larger Black freedom struggle. But the decreasing number of Black physicians foreshadowed that institution's own decline and the diminished role of Black physician-activists in New Orleans.

Even with these physician losses, Flint Goodridge's administrators increasingly recognized the need to expand the hospital as the Black population continued to grow, reaching over 181,775 in 1950. Thousands visited the crowded clinics each year, reaching a peak of 32,274 in 1944, over four times the number of the hospital's first year in 1932. Births increased tenfold, from 63 in 1932 to 631 in 1944. In the wake of criticism of the quality of care at the hospital due to the above-described problems, Superintendent Weil launched a publicity campaign in 1950 to highlight some of the hospital's improvements, including new equipment, a blood bank, cubicles in the wards to create privacy, and higher nurse salaries. Remarkable given its limitations and the poor health conditions of Black residents, Flint Goodridge had the lowest death rate of any hospital in the city. The hospital's maternity clinics and flat-rate birth plan achieved a dramatic drop in infant mortality, from a rate of 119 per 1,000 in 1932 to 34.5 in 1952. This improvement and other health measures spearheaded by Flint Goodridge and Black physicians and health activists led the overall mortality rate to drop from 23.53 per 1,000 for Black residents in 1930 to 12.13 in 1950; in comparison, the white mortality rate improved from 11.32 per 1,000 in 1930 to 10.04 in 1950. While still higher, the gap between Black and white residents, which had consistently stayed at 200 percent since the Civil War, had closed to 20 percent higher, with the biggest gains made since Flint Goodridge had opened its new space. In those first twenty years of existence, the hospital had treated 142,198 different individuals, about 80 percent of the Black population in 1950, over the course of 550,148 separate hospital visits, and oversaw the birth of 6,740 Black babies. While the hospital struggled financially for its initial decades, its accomplishments for the Black community were undeniable. The hospital increased Black health care access, created hundreds of Black jobs, and addressed many of the Black public health issues.[59]

Despite these results, Flint Goodridge alone could not overcome the limitations imposed by racialized health care. By midcentury, New Orleans had returned to its pre–Civil War status as a "Medical Center." Nine hundred and fifty-three students studied medicine in Louisiana in 1947–1948, with the majority at Tulane and LSU, representing 3.46 percent of all medical students in the United States. Every person studying medicine in New Orleans, and Louisiana, was white. Nationwide, 588 Black students—2.14 percent of all medical students, despite being 10 percent of the total U.S. population—studied medicine, with more than 84 percent at Meharry and Howard. Only fifteen Black physicians practiced in a city with population that was 31.87 percent Black, compared to nearly 1,000 white physicians who operated out of private practices and staffed the two medical schools, Charity Hospital, the private hospitals, and the other historically white medical institutions. Flint Goodridge remained the sole Black medical institution.[60]

Change was coming, though, not just for Flint but for all health care institutions. In the 1950s, Black New Orleanians increasingly pushed for the integration of health care. Chapter 6 explores the Civil Rights struggle for equal access to health care.

CHAPTER SIX

Health Care in the Era of Civil Rights and Resistance, 1950–1968

In January 1953, Jessie Frohm took her son, aged two and afflicted with cerebral palsy, to Charity Hospital. A social worker at Charity referred Frohm to the state-funded Cerebral Palsy Center in New Orleans and they promised to schedule an appointment. Frohm waited for weeks to hear back and called repeatedly to find out when they would see her son. She finally secured an appointment in March. However, when she showed up for the visit, the administrator informed her that "they didn't have any provisions for Colored." The woman told Frohm that possibly in the future the center would offer one day a month for treating African Americans, but she did not know if or when that would happen. Frohm informed the social worker at Charity, who noted that the center repeatedly called her asking her to send over white children from Charity as the center had few patients. With few options, Frohm wrote to the local branch of the NAACP. Frohm pressed the organization to take on the issue and "see that facilities are provided for Negro children the same as for whites."[1]

Jessie Frohm's fight for her son was part of the decades-long struggle to desegregate the historically white health care system, explored in this chapter. Starting in the late 1940s, African Americans dropped the push for enforcement of the "equal" part of "separate but equal," and increasingly pushed for the end of Jim Crow, including integration of the health care system. Sadly, Frohm's son would be a teenager by the time health services like the cerebral palsy center opened for African Americans in the 1960s. But the actions of his mother and others like her led to significant change in health care in New Orleans.

This chapter explores the period of health care civil rights activism. It examines a seemingly paradoxical problem with Flint Goodridge: the desire to expand the Black hospital—thwarted for years by the state's denial of federal Hill-Burton funding—occurring as Black leaders pushed for access to all hospitals. This chapter details the new strategies employed by civil rights leaders like A. P. Tureaud, who turned to litigation to integrate medical schools, and the impact of federal court decisions and legislation like the Civil Rights Act of 1964, Medicaid, and Medicare. This chapter also details the concentrated efforts of Charity and private hospitals to defy integration and the creation of "white flight" suburban hospitals. As this chapter demonstrates, the late 1960s were another potential "crucial turning point," and white municipal and health care leaders fought to preserve the racialized health care system.

Flint Goodridge Hospital and Health Care Desegregation

Flint Goodridge was both a vestige of earlier efforts to create separate Black spaces and at the forefront of the health care civil rights struggle. Hospital leaders pushed for desegregation of health care, even as they sought to maintain their growing institution. In the postwar period, patient numbers at Flint Goodridge continued to climb—more than 20 percent between 1949 and 1954—even as the number of Black physicians in the city declined. The additional patients drove up income, allowing the hospital to withstand rising insurance costs, a burgeoning payroll for the 344 affiliated physicians and the 200 other employees by 1959, as well as needed improvements. In 1932, the hospital's budget was less than $50,000 per year; by 1959, the budget topped $750,000.[2]

With more income, and a growing number of patients, expansion seemed logical, but first the hospital needed to secure a funding base. In 1954, the newly formed Flint Goodridge Board of Management—which replaced a board of Dillard University administrators and gave more direct control to the hospital—applied for funding through the 1946 Hospital Survey and Construction Act, commonly known as the Hill-Burton Act. The legislation made federal funding available—with the federal government providing two-thirds of the cost—for the expansion of existing hospitals and the construction of new ones, with the goal that each state would reach a quota of 4.5 beds per 1,000 residents. From 1947 to 1971, the bill provided $3.7 billion in federal funding on 10,748 projects nationwide, creating nearly 500,000 new beds. Like other Black hospitals, Flint Goodridge faced difficulty in securing Hill-Burton funding. The legislation was supposed to determine funding based on which areas needed beds. However, the bill allowed hospital funding to be used for all-white or segregated hospitals as long as some area facilities treated African Americans and the number of beds for African Americans in the area matched the number of beds for whites. Additionally, the individual states, not the federal government, would administer the funding. In the New Orleans area, Hill-Burton funding aided the construction of nearly every new hospital as well as the expansion of existing institutions over the following twenty-five years. Administrators disregarded the needs-based formula and the requirement that an equal number of beds existed for Black residents as for whites.[3]

In 1954, and for the following four years, the state Board of Hospitals denied Flint Goodridge's request for Hill-Burton funding, stating they had already filled their bed quota for New Orleans. Instead, the board allocated the funding for expansion of the all-white Touro Infirmary and the Children's Hospital, and it funded construction of the whites-only, 250-bed Ochsner Foundation Hospital. The state legislature denied Flint's requests throughout the decade, even though African Americans accounted for 97.6 percent of New Orleans's population growth between 1950 and 1958.[4]

The state finally approved Flint Goodridge's funding in 1959. Flint Goodridge board president Rosa Keller—a white socialite, civil rights activist, and heiress to the Coca-Cola fortune—played a leading role. Edgar Stern asked her to serve as the chair of the hospital board of management and Keller used her political connections to seek support. After the state repeatedly turned down Flint's Hill-Burton request, Keller and chief administrator C. C. Weil traveled to Washington to seek federal support from HEW officials. When the state still refused Flint's requests despite support from HEW, Keller arranged a personal meeting with Governor Earl Long—he would only meet with Keller, not Weil who was Black—and he agreed to support the spending.[5] With $500,000 secured through Hill-Burton, the hospital launched a drive in 1958, headed by Keller, to raise an additional $450,000 from New Orleanians. Similar to the 1929–1930 campaign, prominent white citizens like Mayor deLesseps Morrison encouraged white residents to support the drive. Keller sought his aid, and the mayor served on the campaign's committee of sponsors. Morrison and his aides directly contacted business leaders to solicit donations and allowed the campaign to use utilize payroll deductions for city workers.[6]

Akin to the campaign to build the new Flint Goodridge in the 1920s, desire to maintain Jim Crow motivated Morrison's support. The civil rights struggle in New Orleans had intensified throughout the 1950s, achieving significant victories including desegregated transit in 1958 and successful boycotts of businesses that forced them to hire Black employees. In response, Morrison and other white leaders fought to maintain Jim Crow, especially after the Supreme Court's 1954 *Brown v. Board of Education* ruling led to a federal district court order to desegregate the Orleans Parish school system. White citizens' councils formed, including a chapter that started in 1955 in New Orleans, to oppose integration through boycotts, protests, threats, and violence. This push for equality and violent backlash created the context for Morrison's support of the hospital's campaign. Morrison strongly endorsed segregation, and it was his desire to keep the city's hospitals segregated that led to his involvement in Flint's fundraising. Earlier actions foreshadowed this role. For example, Morrison bowed to pressure from Black leaders to support the creation of the Pontchartrain Park golf course after the NAACP sued to desegregate City Park and Audubon Park golf courses. Morrison told white opponents of the proposed Black park in May 1950: "We have got to just make up our minds that if we are going to preserve traditions and habits of our city that we are going to have to provide facilities to meet the demands of the Negro people." Morrison continued to support the funding of separate Black facilities like recreation places, schools, and Flint Goodridge to prevent integration through the end of his term.[7]

In addition to the specter of integration, the fear of the spread of disease again played a significant role in garnering white contributions. Using the same kind of rhetoric as the earlier drive, the official campaign pamphlet warned that "civilization has progressed to the point where a city the size of New Orleans can be saved from disease by one inoculation, or blown into oblivion by one explosion." The document also emphasized the economic benefits of Black health. The pamphlet described the hospital as having "helped thousands of those employed by local industries to a healthier and more secure life, and therefore added to the economic wellbeing of the city."[8]

These strategies worked, as residents gave over $450,000. In total, the campaign, federal funding, and philanthropic giving netted $1.36 million, which the hospital used to build a four-story addition in 1960. With the new wing, the hospital expanded its number of available beds from 88 to 128.[9] The following year, despite the addition of the new beds, the hospital reported a waiting list for patients.[10] Thus, the hospital's new wing not only seemed prudent, but also was a harbinger of further expansion. With increased patients and income, the financial troubles of the past appeared to be behind it, and the 1960s looked to be the hospital's most promising decade. Flint Goodridge flourished in the early 1960s. With 350 affiliated physicians and 220 full-time workers, Flint served as the largest Black employer in Louisiana. Continuing its mission of improving health care access and addressing public health issues, Flint helped reduce the Black mortality in the late 1960s to 10.06 per 1,000, nearly equal to the white rate of 9.15, a remarkable achievement.[11]

Despite these accomplishments, Flint Goodridge found itself in a conundrum. Flint Goodridge had accomplished much in previous decades for the Black community, although some Black leaders continued to criticize its very existence as propagating health care segregation. Yet, even as they faced this criticism and continued to advocate for their institution's expansion, many associated with the hospital pushed for the end of segregated health care, most visibly Keller, who used her social position to seek out other white allies. Keller was part of a group from Flint Goodridge that met with members of the OPMS about integrating the organization in 1954. The contingent argued that the denial of membership to Black physicians had helped drive Black doctors away from New Orleans and jeopardized the hospital's future. OPMS Hospital Committee chairman Dr. C. Walter Mattingly told the Flint Goodridge representatives that the OPMS would not integrate, and that Flint's real problems were inadequate facilities and "poor hospital administration." Mattingly also argued that part of the reason that Black doctors left was because "the colored man wants a white doctor. How are you going to change this?" Mattingly informed the Flint contingent that integration "was not the solution to Flint Goodridge's immediate difficulties" and refused to support the idea.[12]

Undeterred, that same year Keller met with Ochsner Hospital president Dr. Alton Ochsner to seek his support on integration and ask him to both serve on Flint Goodridge's board and hopefully form a partnership between Flint and Ochsner Hospital. Ochsner refused, and Keller noted that his "racist" behavior and hostility to Black medical professionals left her "terribly frightened." Similarly, when she met in 1959 with the heads of LSU's medical school about allowing Black physicians to use LSU's library and attend medical meetings, they rejected her requests and replied "I can't understand this [training Black doctors]. Why would a n—— want a n—— doctor anyway?"[13]

This exclusion from professional opportunities, combined with everyday discrimination, was in large part responsible for the exodus of Black doctors from New Orleans. Dr. George Thomas recalled in a 1985 interview that he inherited his practice in New Orleans in 1947 after a fellow Black physician was arrested while driving home from a medical conference in Mississippi for "indecent behavior"—his crime was stopping by the side of the road to eat his lunch. Upon his release, he left the city because he was no longer willing to put up with the treatment.[14] This episode demonstrated the synchronicity between the racialized health care system and the larger system of Jim Crow. The medical system and the larger system of Jim Crow excluded Black physicians and patients, drove away Black doctors, and prevented the growth of Black medical institutions.

In turn, white medical professionals used the health disparity caused by inadequate access to health care and the negative social determinants that resulted from discrimination to continue to justify Jim Crow, particularly as the civil rights movement intensified. White proponents especially used higher Black disease rates as a main argument against integrating the school system. In November 1955, the Board of Directors of the OPMS adopted the following resolution: "Whereas, the statistics of the Louisiana State Department of Health for the years 1950–54 for the Parish of Orleans and the State of Louisiana as a whole, indicate a tremendously greater incidence of venereal diseases and illegitimacy of births among the Negro race than the white race of school age; therefore be it, Resolved, that the Orleans Parish Medical Society go on record as being of the opinion that it would be a distinct health hazard to integrate the races in the schools of Orleans Parish, as well as other Parishes." The board planned to have its resolution read as part of the school board's legal fight to prevent desegregation. At an OPMS general meeting, over 150 members voted on the resolution; OPMS bylaws required a unanimous vote on the measure as it had been introduced without an announcement at the previous meeting. With exactly one member—not identified in the meeting minutes—voting in opposition, the resolution failed.[15] Although the OPMS general body never formally adopted the resolution, in December 1955 the Orleans school board filed affidavits in its federal case from eight white doctors stating that integration of the schools would "present a danger to the health of white children" and would "lead to an increase in the incidence of venereal diseases." Three psychiatrists also attested that integration would cause "psychiatric damage," and noted the threat of Black children who "harbored tremendous hostile feelings to the predominate culture."[16]

One of the doctors who signed the affidavits attesting to the "health menace" of integration was Emmett Lee Irwin. Born in 1893 in Clinton, Louisiana, Irwin attended Tulane's School of Medicine and became a professor at the school and a surgeon at Charity, Baptist Hospital, and Touro Infirmary. He served as the first director of LSU medical school's surgery department and on the LSU Board of Supervisors. In 1931, the OPMS elected him president, and in 1942 he became the president of the Louisiana State Medical Society. By the 1950s, Irwin was one of the most venerated figures in the city's white medical profession. Irwin was also one of the leading advocates of white supremacy. In 1955, he was the founding member of the Citizens' Council of New Orleans; he personally registered the organization with the state. He served as chairman of the group from 1956 until his death in 1965, and led its opposition to integration of schools, buses, and other institutions.

Irwin epitomized the legacy of white supremacy and scientific racism in the white medical field. He learned from and joined a lineage of teachers at

Tulane who all promoted ideas of scientific racism. In his numerous speeches, television appearances, newspaper editorials, court affidavits, and letters to officials, Irwin offered a mix of his predecessors' ideas. Like Samuel Cartwright 100 years earlier, he proffered the idea that God had created different races, with whites as superior. He cited earlier advocates of scientific racism, including extensively quoting Thomas Jefferson's ideas of the "natural inferiority" of African Americans in the Citizens' Council resolution he authored in opposition to integration of the city's buses.[17] He frequently espoused the language of the proslavery advocates who decried the abolitionists in the nineteenth century as creating racial tension. In a Citizens' Council statement written by Irwin in 1958, he labeled the NAACP "part of the Communist conspiracy" and argued the group was "fomenting strife and discord between the white and Negro races in the South and is disrupting relations between these races which heretofore have been—and at present are—harmonious and friendly in every respect."[18]

He also repeatedly cited higher rates of Black disease, particularly sexually transmitted infections, in his opposition to integration, and combined it with the threat of Black sexual violence. In 1958, he told a television audience—he regularly used the Citizens' Council's funds to sponsor pro-segregation programs on local television—that all women's organizations should be active in pro-segregation efforts as "you white women are the ultimate goal of the integrationists."[19] While he was espousing these racist views, he was still an active surgeon at Charity, where he operated on Black patients.

Irwin's position as the leader of the Citizens' Council hardly hurt his social standing in the medical field. In a 1957 letter to the editor of the *New Orleans Item*, a resident praised Irwin's leading of the Citizens' Council, which he described as "such a fine group of American citizens," and lauded Irwin as a "credit to the profession which he represents—because the health and moral welfare of the white people are his greatest concern."[20] Many other prominent white physicians shared these same "concerns." The medical director of the Orleans public schools and the president of the Louisiana Board of Health joined Irwin in signing the affidavit submitted to the federal court in opposition to school integration. Alton Ochsner was perhaps the most prominent physician who actively opposed integration, although often less publicly than Irwin. In addition to his hostility toward integrating the OPMS, detailed earlier, Ochsner used his social standing to lobby politicians to oppose integration and civil rights legislation.[21] Other doctors were open members and leaders of the Citizens' Council and other white supremacist organizations, just as a century earlier doctors led the White League and other paramilitary groups in their reign of terror. These individuals lent the guise of intellectualism and professional stature to the pro-segregation and white supremacist cause.

White civic and political leaders like Leander Perez—one of the leaders of the Citizens' Council with Irwin—used the rhetoric of scientific racism and disease threat promoted by doctors in their own advocacy of segregation. Senator Allen Ellender told a Black reporter in support of his opposition to school desegregation in February 1955: "I do not particularly like to quote venereal disease statistics about any group, or to cite crime rates, but these are things we must recognize."[22] That same year, in the immediate aftermath of *Brown v. Board*, the state legislature passed a bill that required segregated schools under the state's "police power" to maintain "public health, morals, better education, peace, and good order."[23] In many ways, proponents justified this legislation by citing the threat of African Americans spreading disease exactly as the generation before did in its defense of residential segregation ordinances.

While proponents of segregation continued to use the rhetoric of poor Black health—often discussed as a sign of physical inferiority and moral ineptitude—and the disease risk posed by integration, they refused to discuss the root causes of the higher Black disease and mortality rates. They also remained unwilling to use the historically white health care system to improve Black health. The Jim Crow system was largely responsible for the health disparity. The segregation of Charity and denial of admittance at private hospitals combined with many of the issues that civil rights organizations fought against—white violence; false arrests of African Americans in "white spaces" for disturbing the peace, vagrancy, and loitering; police brutality; employment discrimination; school segregation; and environmental racism—which had so severely damaged Black health. For instance, the rate of tuberculosis—caused by factors like low-quality housing conditions—was 107 per 100,000 for Black residents in 1947 compared to 53 per 100,000 whites.[24] Thus, Jim Crow helped create a self-perpetuating cycle. Segregation caused higher Black disease and mortality rates, and whites used higher Black disease and mortality rates to justify segregation. Black New Orleanians recognized the hypocrisy of this cycle. In a July 30, 1963, editorial in the *Louisiana Weekly* entitled "A Pattern of Gross Indifference," the newspaper criticized the city's neglect of Black health and its use as justification for Jim Crow: "Arguing against desegregation of schools, public and private institutions, attorneys for the City of New Orleans have not hesitated to haul out morbidity reports to substantiate their claim that Negroes are the chief sufferers of various infectious and contagious diseases. Yet, the city itself is guilty of contributing to such a condition."[25]

Civil Rights and Health Care

After World War II, Black New Orleanians began shifting their approach to problems like access to health care and those "patterns of gross indifference" the *Louisiana Weekly* noted. In earlier years, leaders favored the accommodationist model of pushing the city not to integrate but rather to uphold the "equal" part of "separate but equal." However, whites in no way made any pretense to maintain the "equal" part of "separate but equal" health care. The awarding of Hill-Burton funding to all-white hospitals over Flint Goodridge, despite the already higher number of beds for white residents, was just one example. In medical education, although the state supported Southern University to maintain segregation in higher education—with LSU for white students and Southern for Black students—the state never appropriated enough funding to start a promised medical school for African Americans. Similarly, while Charity admitted African Americans into a short-staffed and underfunded segregated ward, the state failed to provide other needed medical services. In response, Black residents like Jessie Frohm pushed for access to health care, as patients and as workers. In April 1951, three women—Katherine London, Marie Williams, and Marguirite Brown—attempted to enroll in Charity Hospital's nursing program. Told that the program was "not offered to the Colored because of the lack of sufficient facilities and housing," the women, like Frohm, brought the issue to the NAACP.[26]

Through this activism, health care became part of the civil rights struggle. Although it never received as much focus as issues like housing, employment, or voting, these efforts led to complaints filed by the NAACP, and then litigation pushing for integration as new NAACP leadership increasingly adopted more direct challenges to Jim Crow. In 1941, George Lucas, Joseph Hardin, and other members of the city's Black economic elite that favored a more accommodationist approach lost power to a cadre called "the Group," led by A. P. Tureaud and Reverend A. L. Davis. The Group favored direct challenges of segregation, particularly with litigation.[27]

The Group included one physician, William Adams. In many ways, Adams was the mirror opposite of Emmett Lee Irwin, the white physician who led the Citizens' Council. Born in 1900, Adams grew up in New Orleans. Unlike Irwin, who attended Tulane, Adams could not attend the city's whites-only medical school, and the Flexner Report closed Flint Medical College a decade prior to his pursuit of a medical degree. Instead, Adams attended Meharry Medical College and returned to New Orleans, joining Flint Goodridge in 1929 and later serving as chief of staff. Adams was also a civil rights leader.

Adams served on the NAACP's executive committee in the early 1950s, and in 1957 Adams became the leader of the New Orleans Improvement Association (NOIA), an underground organization formed after the Louisiana legislature passed a bill forcing the NAACP and other organizations to turn over membership lists. When the NAACP refused, the state declared the group illegal and forbid it to operate in the state. Adams led the NOIA's voter registration drives and successful lawsuits for the desegregation of buses in 1958, Audubon Park in 1959, and airport facilities in 1963.[28] In these efforts, Adams repeatedly opposed Irwin; Adams described Irwin's tactics as head of the Citizens' Council as similar to "those used in Fascist Germany under Adolph Hitler" in a 1956 speech.[29]

A. P. Tureaud served as the lawyer for the NOIA and NAACP lawsuits, and as part of his efforts to desegregate education he filed lawsuits for Black access to historically white nursing and medical schools. In 1946, Tureaud sued LSU on behalf of Viola Davis, a Louisianan who had completed her first year as a medical student at Meharry but wanted to transfer to LSU.[30] Although Tureaud lost in the Davis case, he won three lawsuits against LSU between 1950 and 1952, which forced the school to admit Black students, including Flint Goodridge's head nurse Dayle Foster, who enrolled in LSU's nursing program. With Foster's legal victory in 1952, the judge imposed a permanent injunction against LSU barring Black applicants to its School of Medicine. However, despite this victory and a similar fifteen-month court battle that forced Tulane to drop its whites-only policy in 1963, administrators continued to deny every Black applicant at both schools as subjectively "unqualified." LSU did not admit its first Black medical student until 1965, and Tulane not until 1967.[31]

Activists also used litigation to desegregate all-white hospitals, although these institutions too delayed integration for years. The NAACP and the National Medical Association—formed by Black physicians excluded from the American Medical Association in 1895—filed lawsuits nationwide to integrate historically white health care institutions.[32] In 1956, the two groups filed suits to end the separate but equal provision of the Hill-Burton Act. Although they lost their first cases, the organizations continued to file suits in different states. In 1962, the NAACP filed suit in North Carolina in *Simkins v. Moses H. Cone Memorial Hospital*. After losing at the district court level, they appealed, with the Supreme Court upholding a federal appeals court ruling striking down the separate but equal provision as unconstitutional in March 1964.[33]

While activists pursued these cases elsewhere, through early 1964, civil rights leaders in New Orleans continued to focus on other issues, eschewing hospital integration. Local groups filed lawsuits to integrate schools, the municipal auditorium, parks, and recreation facilities, but not hospitals. In February 1963, Flint Goodridge's Board of Management discussed suing Charity to force it to hire Black physicians, despite this potentially further draining Flint Goodridge's own already limited doctor pool; ultimately, it did not pursue the lawsuit.[34] In September 1963, over 10,000 New Orleanians participated in a freedom march from Shakespeare Park in Central City to City Hall. The leaders of the event, the Citizens' Committee of New Orleans, attempted to give Mayor Victor Schiro a "Petition to the Greater New Orleans Community." Schiro refused; instead, the group presented the document a week later to the city council. An initial draft of the petition demanded desegregation of hospitals in the city as point nine. However, the final version only included the first seven points that addressed hiring of Black employees, repeal of city segregation ordinances, and integration of city properties; they dropped the request for hospital integration.[35]

It was not until the Supreme Court's ruling in 1964 that struck down the separate but equal provision of the Hill-Burton Act and the HEW's subsequent announcement that all hospitals receiving funding must desegregate or lose Hill-Burton funding that hospital desegregation efforts in New Orleans started. The week of the Supreme Court ruling, two Baton Rouge hospitals—Our Lady of the Lake and the Baton Rouge General Hospital—announced they would allow Black physicians to treat their Black patients in the hospitals. However, New Orleans hospitals that had received Hill-Burton funding ignored the court ruling and the HEW order. In response, New Orleans NAACP branch president Ernest Morial stated the organization had been "studying" litigation "for some time" and he anticipated that the branch "will take action in the future toward the full implementation of the supreme court's ruling."[36]

Despite Morial's statement, litigation did not immediately occur. Again, this may have reflected the NAACP's focus on other issues deemed more pressing. It also may have been the result of the decline in influence of Black physicians within the NAACP and other civil rights groups. With the loss of power of the physician elites to the Group and the exodus of Black physicians in the postwar period, few Black physicians outside of Adams played an active role in the leadership of civil rights organizations. Few Black doctors in New Orleans even publicly called for hospital integration. At its annual meeting in February 1963, National Medical Association president John A. Kennedy urged all members as "social engineers" to personally advocate for the desegregation of hospitals; this did not occur in New Orleans.[37]

An April 5, 1964, editorial in the *Weekly* noted that Black physicians led the push to integrate the Baton Rouge hospitals, and chastised the public silence of Black doctors in New Orleans: "it is indeed surprising to say the least that even at this late date there has been no voluntary public expression on the issue by Negro members of the local medical profession who have been hampered by racial discrimination even more-so than Negro patients . . . It is now discouraging that Negro doctors have given absolutely no public indication that they too will seek to implement the Simkins-Cone decision in the local hospitals which are now receiving or which have received Hill-Burton and other federal funds."[38] Instead, individual citizens, with support from the NAACP, pressed for hospital integration, an issue that was aided significantly by federal legislation, particularly the 1964 Civil Rights Act. Passed after years of Black advocacy—and over the opposition of all of Louisiana's white federal representatives—the act contained Title VI, which mandated that all hospitals desegregate and no longer discriminate or be subject to the denial of all federal financial assistance.

The same month that President Johnson signed the Civil Rights Act of 1964 into law, Callie Castle, the grandmother of civil rights leader Oretha Castle Haley, became the lead plaintiff in a class action lawsuit filed in federal court to desegregate Charity, claiming the continued segregation violated the equal protection clause, the due process clause, and the 1964 Civil Rights Act.[39] Facing the lawsuit, Charity slowly started to integrate. In October 1964, the hospital board voted to integrate the tuberculosis wards. That same month, Dr. Gilbert Tomsky, the chairman of the hospital's medical committee, said that Charity was 80 percent integrated and that the integration of the tuberculosis wards represented "one more step towards a gradual elimination of physical segregation in the hospital."[40] In January 1965, Charity announced that the "colored" and white signs had been completely removed.[41]

Louisiana continued to maintain segregation in other state-administered hospitals, including those in the Charity system. In June 1965, the Louisiana Civil Liberties Union filed a lawsuit to desegregate the Washington–St. Tammany Hospital in Bogalusa, which was followed by an NAACP lawsuit against the Charity hospital in Alexandria. In December 1965, District Court Judge Gordon West ordered the desegregation of all state hospitals. State Hospital Director R. B. Walden stated that all hospitals would comply by the end of the year and pledged that all personnel for state hospitals would be hired without racial discrimination. The ruling did not apply to Charity Hospital in New Orleans and Confederate Memorial Hospital in Shreveport, as they had their own boards; however, Walden falsely claimed that both hospitals had already completely desegregated.[42]

At the municipal level, the New Orleans Board of Health considered openly rejecting the federal nondiscrimination order and accepting the loss of federal funding. Director of Health Rodney C. Jung wrote to Mayor Schiro in February 1965 to ask if the board should sign a required document pledging nondiscrimination or decline all further federal funding. Schiro ultimately decided to order the document signed so as not to lose the needed revenue source.[43]

Despite these public announcements of compliance with desegregation, most medical institutions privately refused to integrate. In the following years, civil rights leaders in New Orleans and throughout the South filed repeated suits for noncompliance. Patients complained about being denied admission or the continuation of segregation to the NAACP, which in turn forwarded the complaints to HEW. After HEW refused to enforce compliance, the NAACP Legal Defense and Education Fund filed federal lawsuits. Starting in February 1965, the NAACP sued dozens of hospitals, including New Orleans's Sara Mayo Hospital, which only treated Black patients in separate facilities and continued to refuse to hire Black doctors.[44]

Sara Mayo's administrators defended their hiring decisions by arguing that official hospital policy was to only hire physicians that were members of the OPMS, which maintained its whites-only member requirement. By the mid-1950s, most county medical societies nationwide and all state medical societies except for Louisiana and Mississippi admitted Black members.[45] OPMS members brought up integration in the 1950s. In November 1956, two members introduced a measure to drop the "white" requirement. The organization held a vote at their December 10th meeting. With a 107–88 vote in favor of dropping the white requirement, the measure failed the required two-thirds threshold.[46] After this failed vote, the OPMS became more entrenched against integration, especially during the school desegregation battle. In 1958, William Adams testified before the House Committee on Interstate Commerce and informed them of the problem Black doctors faced due to exclusion from the medical society: "In New Orleans, no Negro appointments are allowed on the hospital staffs either as interns, residents, or staffmen . . . We have considered the proposition of getting on the [hospital] staffs and participating in the work, we are always told that in order to become eligible for the staff you will have to join the parish society. Of course, the society has a lockdown against Negroes. Thus, you can't get into the society because you are a Negro and you can't get on the staff because you can't get into the society." Because the state medical society and all the local societies maintained their whites-only membership clauses through the 1960s, before 1965 Black doctors in Louisiana could only serve on the staff of Flint Goodridge. Adams informed the members of the committee that he and other physicians and civil rights activists were planning to sue the OPMS and other parish medical societies that denied Black membership. Adams told the committee that some doctors in northern Louisiana had initially opposed the effort because they feared retaliation, particularly from the state, as the state had already denied reimbursement for providing care for indigent patients. Adams asked the committee for guidance on whether they should initiate litigation; congressional records do not document any response by committee members to this question, and no court records of such a lawsuit against medical societies in Louisiana have yet been found by this researcher.[47] As the mother organization, the American Medical Association could have mandated that all state- and county-level AMA affiliates drop whites-only clauses. Despite more than a dozen proposals introduced from 1944 to 1965 by state-level AMA chapters and continuous requests from the National Medical Association, it was not until 1966 that the AMA amended its bylaws to investigate discrimination by local chapters and potentially strip them of affiliation.[48] The AMA's intransigence gave medical societies in Louisiana carte blanche to continue discrimination. Both the OPMS and the Louisiana State Medical Association refused to integrate until 1965, making the state the last one in the nation to integrate. Following the April 1965 lawsuit against Sara Mayo, which highlighted its OPMS membership stipulation, at its May meeting, the OPMS finally voted to eliminate the word "white" from its bylaws, and in June admitted four Black physicians.[49]

In July 1965, President Johnson signed into law Medicare and Medicaid. Implemented in Louisiana in 1966, Medicare and Medicaid offered a stream of federal revenue to hospitals, provided they meet the requirements of the Civil Rights Act of 1964 and served as a further integration push.

In private practices, many white physicians continued to refuse to treat Black patients or desegregate waiting rooms. In September 1965, State Board of Public Welfare Commissioner Garland Bonin sent a letter to all doctors and dentists stating the maintenance of segregated waiting rooms would prevent them from participating in the federal medical vendor program, a state program that provided funding for treating some low-income residents prior to Medicare and Medicaid's implementation. Those that wished to participate would have to sign a nondiscrimination document; doctors who wished to keep segregated waiting rooms could opt out of the program. Bonin noted his personal reluctance to enforce the provision, writing in his letter that he was "only passing on federal government's interpretation of the Civil Rights Act."[50]

Both the OPMS and state medical society opposed the requirement. In anticipation of the requirement, in August 1965 the newly integrated OPMS passed a resolution—over the objection of the new Black members—to not "violate the freedom of physicians" by requiring them to sign the nondiscrimination form. The state medical society also voted to advise physicians to refuse to sign nondiscrimination documents. Society president Charles Odom argued that opposition was not based on racism or in opposition to the Civil Rights Act, but instead about principles of freedom: "any demand that a physician sign a written agreement that he will abide by a law is contrary to our American way of life." Bodin and Odom went to Washington to meet with HEW and got the department to drop the signing. Instead, bills for payment to the physicians from the federal government for services rendered through the vendor program included a nondiscrimination statement as a reminder. After they secured this change, the state medical society issued a statement supporting the right of white physicians to not treat Black patients: "All persons concerned agreed that the patient has free choice of physicians and the physician has a right to accept or not accept any individual as a patient."[51]

Integration at Charity

Despite this initial resistance, many African Americans remained hopeful in the late 1960s that lawsuits and federal laws would lead to the end of the racialized health care. The most significant integration occurred at Charity, which witnessed an immediate increase in the number of Black patients from under 50 percent prior to the integration orders to 77 percent in July 1965, three months after the directors announced the end of segregated wards and nearly a year after the Civil Rights Act of 1964 forbade the practice. However, official integration did not lead to the end of discrimination. Many at the hospital defied the court and federal mandates to end discrimination, leading to years of confrontation between Black patients and the white employees and administrators. In the face of this continued discrimination, Black patients pushed for better treatment. In 1966, Black residents formed a "Committee for Better Health Services." In April, they sent a letter to the administrators asking to speak with them. When they received no reply, they created a petition and sent it, along with documented complaints of poor treatment and racial discrimination compiled by the NAACP, to the hospital. They also asked the Office of Economic Opportunity to help them distribute the petition citywide, and the *Times Picayune* printed it in June 1966. The petition read:

> Whereas, we the poor are unemployed, and underemployed, forced into Slum Housing, having no money, are subjected daily to conditions which contribute to disease, poor health, chronic illnesses, high infant deaths and many other unhealthy atrocities. Having already requested an audience with the heads of Charity Hospital by our committee, and having not yet heard from Charity, and being concerned with poor communications between Charity Hospital and the consumers of medical services, who are for the most part, "poor people," and, having documented statements from citizens at Charity Hospital. We the undersigned request an open hearing to air documented complaints against you; and, to work to eliminate the cause of the many problems that affect the health of the poor.[52]

The most documented complaint was delay in treatment, with white patients given higher priority than Black patients in waiting rooms. Lois Jones detailed how she had waited in the intake office for seven hours with a rheumatic fever of 104 degrees before her husband drove her to a friend of her father's home; he made a call to a contact who worked at the hospital and finally got her admitted. Others without these types of connections were not as fortunate. The NAACP conducted interviews with workers at Charity and found that administrators regularly required Black patients to undergo lengthy eligibility checks prior to treatment. Patients had to provide proof of residency in Louisiana for at least six months and steady employment. Charity set an income limit of $225 monthly for an individual person, with an additional twenty-five dollars allowed monthly per child. Patients who met the requirements received an eligibility card for hospital services. However, many individuals seeking treatment in Charity's emergency room did not have eligibility cards or did not bring with them the necessary proof to obtain one. In the emergency room, administrators often required Black patients to first prove they were eligible before they offered treatment, while white patients received care before their status was determined. As detailed by Myrtle Perron, "They don't care if you're dying or what; you have to wait until they find out if you are eligible." Hubert Alvin described how after he was attacked and severely wounded by a gang, Charity caseworkers refused to treat him, even though he was a full-time student at Southern University of New Orleans and thus was automatically eligible for care. Alvin presented his student identification card, but the caseworker demanded he present documents detailing his financial situation. While Alvin used the bathroom, a white supervisor, seeing that Alvin had previously served in the military, called the military police to have him arrested, even though he had been honorably discharged. Elsie Brazile-Brown, a Black worker at Charity, reported to the NAACP in January 1966 that she witnessed a Black woman come in with severe burns. The white supervisor insisted the Black caseworker take her out in the hallway and determine her eligibility before they treated her. Mystis Keelen described her problems getting an eligibility card from the hospital. Keelen, a mother of six, earned twenty-four dollars a week, far below the eligibility threshold, but the hospital refused to give her the card, accusing her of being dishonest: "They said I was lying because nobody could get along on 24 dollars a week with six children." When they rejected her, the caseworker told her to instead "find the father of my children and make him support them." Brenda Soublet told the NAACP in March 1966 that her son Louis was attacked and beaten unconscious. She brought him to the hospital, but before he could be treated a white supervisor administered ammonia to wake him and question him about his eligibility.[53]

The process of proving eligibility often proved arduous and humiliating. In 1969, the Human Relations Council—an interracial group of civic leaders— detailed the complex task of trying to receive care at Charity. In two articles written by physicians, "Are You Strong Enough to Be Sick?" by Dr. Jeff Gordon and "Poor People's Panacea" by Dr. Dan Bloomenthal, the two physicians detailed the problems at the hospital and called for needed improvements. Bloomenthal described the process of using Charity as such: "For the person who cannot afford a personal physician and entry into the regular medical care system, adequate health care may be an impossibility; degradation and dehumanization are certainties."[54] Patients first had to prove their financial eligibility, as detailed above. Individuals could have the income requirement waived by physicians working for LSU or Tulane. Additionally, many whites wrote to the mayor, asking him to help get the income requirement waived, a task Mayor Schiro repeatedly did in the 1960s; Schiro wrote over 100 such letters in 1963 alone for white constituents. With no representation at the hospital, among the physicians at LSU or Tulane, or in the city council and mayoral administration, African Americans who exceeded the income requirement but still lived in poverty and thus could not afford a private hospital had no means to seek treatment at Charity and could not receive hospital care.[55]

For those who qualified, Charity recommended patients bring with them to the hospital—even when seeking emergency treatment—contact information for their employer and a letter from their employer or other proof of employment like a paycheck. Patients were expected to provide a copy of their 1040 tax return, their welfare card, insurance policies, proof of residency like utility bills, and copies of previous hospital bills and time payment plans. Granting of eligibility for nonacute cases usually took weeks or months. If patients needed medicine that they could not afford, they had to go through a separate process. First, they had to visit the Social Services Department. From there, they would then have to visit the State Welfare Department. Then they were directed to Charity to have a physician fill out a form saying they needed the medicine. If they completed these steps, they would be granted a card that entitled them to a prescription, but not refills; to obtain a refill, they had to go through an additional process. If patients wanted immunization shots, they had to visit a neighborhood center. For birth control, they had to go to a family planning center. For other medicine, they had to go to city hall. Patients receiving medical treatment rarely saw the same physician at Charity twice, even if they were undergoing long-term treatment. Patients primarily received treatment in open wards with no privacy. There was virtually no hospital follow-up and no real options for preventive measures. Overall, Bloomenthal found the system to be confusing, degrading, and extremely difficult to navigate, perhaps purposely so to discourage use and to punish the poor. He reflected, "One finds that he has been fed into a huge depersonalizing machine that strips him completely of human dignity."[56]

Beyond this byzantine process, Black patients continued to face other indignities at Charity. In its 1966 petition, the "Committee for Better Health Services" noted that the hospital continued to require Black patients to sit on a separate side of the emergency waiting room from whites, a practice forbidden under the 1964 Civil Rights Act.[57] This was not the only documented cases of segregation at Charity in the late 1960s. The NAACP reported that the hospital continued an unofficial policy of separate water fountains, waiting rooms benches, and even telephones.[58] The hospital's school for children of patients segregated the children by race for lessons, and the hospital refused to admit Black babies to the nursery.[59]

Black patients also suffered from physical and sexual assaults by white doctors. Victoria Jones reported one such incident in October 1966. A caseworker gave Jones a referral slip to see a physician at Charity's clinic for her hemorrhoids. When she visited the clinic, she gave the slip to the nurse, who attached the paper to the doctor's clipboard, which also contained her chart and a description of her ailment. However, when she saw the doctor he claimed not to have her slip nor to know what was wrong with her. She tried to explain her problem, but the doctor interrupted her and told her "I'm not interested in that" and refused to treat her. She tried again to explain her ailment, but the doctor again cut her off and began cursing her, telling her "you don't have as much brains as a jackass or a monkey." She finally got the doctor to examine her, but as he did so he punched her in the back and told the woman to "get your bitch self out of my room." Upon leaving, Jones reported the incident to the hospital's chief administrator, Dr. Charles Mary. Jones informed Mary that this was the second time a white physician at Charity had physically assaulted her. She also reported the incident to the NAACP, which in turn pressed Mary to investigate. Mary promised to do so but promptly dropped the matter, and neither Jones nor the NAACP heard back from Mary about the matter.[60]

Charity also continued to play a controversial role with its decades-old relationship with the police and the Orleans Parish jail. Officers would take African Americans they assaulted to Charity for quick treatment before bringing them to the jail. In her complaint filed with the NAACP in September 1968, Eliza Reynolds detailed how police falsely arrested her twenty-five-year-old son Joseph and accused him of burglary. The police came to her home, dragged Joseph off the swing he was sitting on, and severely beat him. They took him to Charity Hospital where a doctor hurriedly treated him for six broken ribs and an eye out of the socket, then immediately brought him to jail, where they beat him again.[61]

Black workers also made complaints over discrimination in hiring, promotion, and treatment by white supervisors. The NAACP sent these complaints to Charity but received no response. They launched their own investigation and determined in March 1966 that white supervisors continued to deny Black workers promotions, good assignments, and leaves of absence. The organization also documented that Charity had no Black supervisors in most departments. The hospital placed no Black nurses or physicians in the nursery and grouped all Black nurses, aides, and maids on the twelfth floor. When the NAACP conducted its investigation, it reported that white supervisors placed "much pressure" on Black workers to not cooperate with the NAACP and threatened to fire anyone who did.[62] In his report filed with the NAACP in June 1968, James Sanders, an orderly at Charity, detailed how his supervisor called the police and had him arrested that April. On his break, Sanders went to speak with a receptionist, who then left to talk with a patient. Sanders sat at her desk while he awaited her return. Two guards came and told him he could not be there. The guards then called his supervisor and accused Sanders of cursing at them. The supervisor had him arrested. When the head nurse asked the supervisor if an apology would suffice rather than Sanders being taken to jail, the supervisor, a Mr. Davis, replied: "I've got to show these people something." When another nurse approached and asked if she could help, Mr. Davis told her to "shut up" or he would have her arrested too. Sanders noted in his statement to the NAACP that it was a "definite racial incident because of the timing of when it happened"—the day after the assassination of Martin Luther King Jr. Sanders was one of many who filed reports for wrongful termination of employment or for being unjustly kicked out of the hospital's nursing program, which continually dismissed Black students with no cause.[63]

Private Hospitals Defy Integration

While African Americans continued to face discrimination at Charity, few ended up at the historically white private hospitals, many of which even more overtly defied integration. Despite issuances of assurances of nondiscrimination, segregation continued. For example, at the Home for the Incurables, a facility for those suffering from long-term or terminal health problems, the institution's board passed a resolution to integrate in June 1965 in accordance with the Civil Rights Act. For decades, they had provided care for Black patients at one building and whites in another. Although they pledged to desegregate in 1965, the hospital continued to house Black and white patients in separate buildings until 1970.[64] Many hospitals refused to hire Black doctors, nurses, and other workers. Those that found employment faced harassment from white coworkers and supervisors. In April 1966, Ellis Hull Jr. sent a letter to the Department of Justice documenting his experience of racial discrimination. In the late 1950s and early 1960s, Hull worked as a porter at Charity before leaving to work in another field. Hull returned to the hospital in early 1966 in the same position, but the hospital fired him after three months with no cause. He then got a job at Touro Infirmary. Although the hospital hired him as a porter, it proceeded to use him as a janitor. At first, Hull did not complain as he needed the work. However, his supervisors made his work exceptionally difficult, assigning him to changing shifts, constantly giving him new tasks, and issuing contradictory orders. For several weeks, one white supervisor stood behind Hull and followed him around, watching him do his work. Hull noted in his letter to the Department of Justice that he believed this harassment stemmed from white opposition to integration. Hull wrote: "I think these people just wanted to see me as a CORE or NAACP worker, rather than a citizen looking for a job." For these white workers, Hull represented the civil rights groups that pushed for integration and they trained their animosity on him.[65]

Others experienced similar treatment. The only five Black nurses employed at the Ear, Eye, Nose, and Throat Hospital filed a complaint with the NAACP in April 1968 that the hospital remained segregated in nearly every way: a separate ward for Black adult patients; Black babies were not placed in the nursery ward but rather in the Black adult ward; every Black nurse, except for a very light-skinned woman, worked in the Black ward; doctors and administrators addressed white nurses with their title in front of their name, but only addressed Black nurses by their first name; the hospital paid Black workers less; Black nurses had to congregate and punch their time cards in the basement, unlike white nurses who did so on the first floor; and the hospital even used separate thermometers for Black and white patients.[66] Black nurses at the Veterans Affairs hospital filed a list of grievances in June 1968, documenting "bias throughout the hospital." The women descried "constant harassing treatment" and "mental cruelties" intended to "force nurses to quit an already understaffed Nursing Service." Their list of included unfair requirements for promotion to administrative positions—including mandating degrees for Black but not white nurses and filling positions in secrecy rather than on a competitive basis—to prevent African Americans from applying for them, and the dismissal of Black nurses for unfavorable criticism by white supervisors.[67]

Although the NAACP brought these complaints to HEW, the federal agency took little action in the late 1960s. In March 1967, the regional program director of HEW's Office of Equal Health Opportunity wrote to the administrators at the historically white private hospitals asking them for data on admissions by race to determine their compliance with the Civil Rights Act. The hospitals—some of which still identified patients' blood to segregate by race and carried out other practices of discrimination based on the patient's race identified on the admission form—refused the federal government's request to count patients by race, arguing doing so would violate freedom of the hospitals and patient confidentiality. In April 1967, the OPMS voted to endorse this decision. HEW ultimately refused to press the matter, and thus had no data to show hospital violations.[68]

White Flight Hospitals

In addition to the federal government's failure to enforce compliance in the city's hospitals, it played another role in the perpetuation of racialized health care: providing funding for "white flight" hospitals. Like other Southern cities, white migration to New Orleans's suburbs began in the immediate postwar period, with the lure of cheaper housing, lower taxes, and larger lots. Government policies aided suburban growth, with highway expansion projects, subsidies for oil that kept gas prices low, and federally backed mortgages. In the New Orleans area, as in many metropolitan regions, whites primarily benefited and made up most of the movers. White New Orleanians had higher incomes that allowed them to purchase homes and afford mortgages from banks or programs like the G.I. Bill, which were often denied to African Americans. Real estate agents played an active role in the creation of white suburbs by refusing to show or sell African Americans homes.

Government funds also aided the construction of hospitals, another driving factor in suburban growth. Hill-Burton money and municipal bonds funded the construction of hospitals, with nearly all private hospitals built prior to 1964 refusing to admit Black patients and public hospitals only treating them in segregated wards. Municipal bonds and Hill-Burton aid helped fund the building of Metairie Hospital, which opened in 1947; St. Tammany Parish Hospital (1954); Chalmette General Hospital (1954); St. Bernard General Hospital (1959); Slidell Memorial Hospital (1959); West Jefferson General Hospital (1960); Methodist Hospital (1963); Lakeside Hospital for Women (1964); East Jefferson General Hospital (1971); and Lakeview Regional Medical Center (1977), all constructed in the suburbs of New Orleans. The extension of federal highways and gas subsidies also helped bring in patients, and it expanded municipal services that provided them needed gas, water, and electricity. Clinics and private practices followed these hospitals to suburbs as well.

In Jefferson Parish, the expansion of Ochsner Hospital served as one of the largest pulls. The hospital became the leading employer, not just in the parish, but in the state. However, the hospital started as a whites-only institution and fiercely resisted integration. The aforementioned Alton Ochsner founded the hospital and guided much of the hospital's growth. In the 1920s, Ochsner served as the chief of surgery at Charity and gained national renown as the first physician to link smoking to lung cancer. While a professor at Tulane, Ochsner pushed the school to break its ties with Charity and instead create its own private hospital, as well as a clinic which Ochsner would head. When the school demurred, Ochsner and four other physicians established the Ochsner Clinic, the first group medical practice in the Deep South, in 1942. In 1944, the group created the Ochsner Medical Foundation and sought support to create their own hospital. In 1946, the foundation purchased

Camp Plauche in Jefferson Parish from the federal War Assets Administration and converted it to a whites-only, 200-bed hospital. The former army site contained fifty-three wooden-frame buildings, though, and the foundation looked for a more modern structure. In 1952, with money from a fundraising campaign and Hill-Burton funding secured from the state, it built a five-story, whites-only, 250-bed building on twenty-two acres in Jefferson, just outside of New Orleans boundaries. In the following decade, it built the Brent House Hotel, used for long-term patients and physicians' offices, a residence building for nurses and physicians, a helicopter landing pad, a research building, and the relocated Ochsner Clinic. By the 1960s, the hospital was a leading center for research and cutting-edge medical procedures. Over the next half-century, Ochsner acquired other hospitals and became both the largest employer in the state and the biggest private health care system in the region.[69]

The all-white institution was aided by several factors unavailable to Flint Goodridge Hospital. The founding partners of the clinic were all professors at the whites-only Tulane University and doctors at the segregated Charity Hospital. Through the wealth acquired in working in the racialized health care system, the founding partners gained the capital necessary to start their own practice. The partners solicited patients from their work at Charity and Tulane to create a financially secure, white clientele. The partners also used their connections to secure the hospital's first location, purchased from the military; to solicit money during their fundraising campaign; and to gain Hill-Burton funding in the same period the state repeatedly rejected Flint Goodridge's requests for expansion, even though the number of white beds already far outnumbered beds for Black patients, a violation of the legislation.

The role of hospitals in facilitating white flight can most explicitly be seen in the creation of the Methodist Hospital in New Orleans East. New Orleans East first developed in the early twentieth century as the Gentilly neighborhood expanded. In 1923, the Industrial Canal opened, followed by the Intercoastal Waterway in 1944, which physically separated the East from the rest of the city and effectively slowed its growth. Development picked up again in the late 1950s through the 1970s with white flight to new suburban subdivisions. Mayor Schiro personally championed the growth of New Orleans East, as he hoped to encourage movement to the area, within official city bounds, in lieu of migration to suburbs in other parishes. Industry—primarily shipping, warehouses, and manufacturing—helped pull development, with the Intracoastal Mississippi River–Gulf Outlet Canal, completed in 1965, aiding the placement of inner harbor wharves along the Industrial Canal. The National Aeronautics and Space Administration (NASA) took over the Michoud

Assembly Facility, constructed during World War II as part of the Higgins Industries' war production efforts, in 1961. The area benefited from a strengthened levee system after severe flooding during Hurricane Betsy and the building of Interstate 10, started in 1957.[70]

The construction of Methodist Hospital, opened in 1968, also helped the East's growth. The idea for the hospital originated with members of the Gentilly Methodist Church in 1959, who were concerned about the lack of medical care available to area residents. In 1961, the Methodist Hospital Association incorporated. Church member Kenneth Schor and Reverend John Koelemay led the $3.5 million fundraising campaign, with contributions from other Methodist congregations and business and civic leaders, and government funding. Serving as president of the Methodist Hospital Association, Schor solicited the support of Mayor Schiro and the OPMS, the latter primarily for its application for Hill-Burton funding. The hospital association sent both the OPMS and the mayor a document entitled "Memorandum Supporting Methodist Hospital" with several arguments in favor of the hospital.

First, the association noted a significant drop in the patient base for existing hospitals in New Orleans with a 9.9 percent decline in population from 1950 to 1959 due to white flight. In contrast, they highlighted the "exploding population" in the area of the proposed hospital, which witnessed a 67 percent increase in population. Methodist Hospital would meet the medical needs of the East's burgeoning population. In addition to providing treatment for the acutely ill, the hospital planned to offer long-term care, psychiatric care, and services for the growing elderly population.

Second, the boosters hailed the proposed hospital as "essential in attracting new industry to any community." Schor argued that a medical center would help lure commercial and industrial businesses to locate in New Orleans East as the hospital would service their employees. Mayor Schiro, who became a vocal advocate for the hospital, fully embraced the hospital board's vision, personally sending out letters to business and civic leaders asking for donations. Speaking at the hospital's first anniversary in 1969, Schiro stressed the role of the hospital in helping the East develop, which he argued was of vital importance to the city's overall success. The East, Schiro stated, possessed the largest land area for growth. Without this space, he warned, the city "would soon be strangled with a glut of population and buildings, unable to reach the destiny predicted for us." The destiny he spoke of was for the city to become a "manufacturing center" based primarily out of the East. Schiro predicted that half a million people would end up in New Orleans East (nearly the city's entire population at the time). "With this anticipated growth staring us in the face," he told the crowd, "we cannot afford to think of less than realizing the full goal" of an additional $500,000 for hospital expansion. Thus, in Schiro's proffered vision, Methodist Hospital was linked to the city's future. The hospital, he stated, "fills a need felt by every person living and working in this part of our city, both present and future."[71]

Third, beyond attracting industry, both the hospital leaders and the mayor celebrated the hospital itself as a significant employer. In his fundraising letter, Schiro called the hospital "a new industry"; similarly, Koelemay, who served as the hospital's promotional director, spoke of "what the hospital means to the community as an industry."[72] Schiro and Koelemay were hardly alone in their assessment of the hospital as an industry. By the late 1960s, medical costs nationwide had soared, buoyed by health insurance and growing incomes, and hospitals had become profitable, with companies increasingly interested as investment opportunities.[73] Methodist Hospital planned to operate as an independent hospital, with no backing from a hospital corporation. However, the hospital benefited from support from powerful companies. Members of the hospital's building fund advisory board included executives from Merrill Lynch, Hibernia National Bank, Southern Bell Telephone, and Coca-Cola. The hospital's leaders projected its annual income to continually increase—nationwide, income at private hospitals nearly doubled in the second half of the 1960s—as New Orleans East's population grew.[74] The increasing population would fuel the hospital's growth, and they projected it would be one of the East's two largest employers, along with the Michoud plant, and employ hundreds.[75]

Fourth, the hospital's founders and promoters appealed directly to racism. In its memorandum, the hospital association stated it decided to locate the institution in its proposed site, in the northern section of the East, so that it would serve a majority-white population. The Black population, which they noted was concentrated in the southern section, would be "outside of the expected service area." The memorandum highlighted the recent increase in the Black population in the southern section and argued that the hospital could help counter this by facilitating the growth of the northern part, which would see an "accelerated increase in the white residents." The hospital association made its desire to serve white patients and help the white population grow explicit, and used it as a main selling point of the hospital to the mayor, the OPMS, and other supporters.

The fundraising campaign proved successful, bringing in $1.9 million from the community, in addition to the $2.6 million from Hill-Burton aid and a $3 million mortgage loan. The hospital opened in 1968 and immediately began expanding, reaching 181 beds by 1971. New Orleans East saw steady growth in population in the 1960s and 1970s, although never reaching Mayor Schiro's vision of half a million people. Up until the 1980s, the vast majority of residents were white, proving the hospital association's predictions correct. The hospital, the Michoud plant, and the city's improvement efforts turned New Orleans East into a white suburb within city bounds. Despite opening after the passage of the Civil Rights Act of 1964, the hospital, by design of its location and purpose, served a mostly white patient base and hired mostly white workers. So much so that Methodist Hospital was one of the city hospitals sued by Black residents and charged with racial discrimination by HEW.

CHAPTER SEVEN

Two-Tiered Health Care, 1965–1974

Attorney John Dowling was adamant that residents of the Tulane Gravier neighborhood opposed the proposed expansion of the Medical District being debated at a December 1970 city council meeting. Dowling argued the plan would mean forced relocation for hundreds of mostly Black residents. "There is no doubt in my mind that the majority of the people in this area don't want their homes taken away from them by a blue-ribbon board or some unthinking politician," Dowling stated. Created in 1968, the state agency the Health Education Authority of Louisiana (HEAL) planned to expand Charity and Tulane's and LSU's medical schools, as well as build a new hospital for Tulane, parking garage, medical offices, and housing for thousands of employees and medical students (see figure A.3 in Appendix). HEAL hoped to secure funding from the U.S. Department of Housing and Urban Development (HUD) to pay two-thirds of the $30 million project. The money would also help fund urban renewal of the surrounding area, replacing over 800 residences and businesses deemed "substandard," "deficient," or "blighted." Hundreds of mostly Black residents and business owners would potentially be displaced despite their opposition, as the state granted HEAL the power of eminent domain. Speaking to the city council on behalf of the Owners and Tenants Association of Greater New Orleans (OTAGNO), Dowling was blunt: "When they confiscate our property, they will relocate us. I haven't heard this term (relocation) since the days of Hitler."[1]

This chapter explores the post–Civil Rights period when the promise of an integrated health care system evaporated and the racialized health care system became re-entrenched, similar to what occurred in New Orleans a century earlier. This chapter starts with juxtaposed stories: the simultaneous attempts to expand the white Medical District, including the successful creation of Tulane's new hospital, and the stymied work to expand Flint Goodridge, which entered into decline. It explores the creation of HEAL and its efforts to displace Black residents and businesses. This chapter also explores continued Black health activism, which took several forms. First, Black residents of Tulane Gravier organized against the expansion of the Medical District. Second, Black residents and the NAACP initiated litigation against the historically white hospitals that continued to discriminate, leading to federal investigations, efforts undermined by the failure of the federal government to enforce integration. Third, Black residents pushed for Health Department and federally funded Model Cities health clinics in the public housing units and Black neighborhoods, and the Black Panther Party (BPP) created its own People's Clinic in the Desire neighborhood; all the clinics proved short lived. Finally, the chapter examines the transition of Charity Hospital to a "de facto" Black hospital, and the accompanying decrease in state funding and quality of care.

A Modern Medical Center

While white flight hospitals like Ochsner and Methodist grew, the two hospitals that served the majority the city's Black residents, Flint Goodridge and Charity, began a steady phase of decline. Initially, the leaders of Flint Goodridge expected the desegregation of health care to aid the hospital and result in it being a leading part of the growing health care sector. The Board of Management looked upon the passage of Medicare and Medicaid as a potential boon. While patient numbers had increased through the early 1960s, the hospital still faced concerns that made the projected steady stream of Medicaid and Medicare patients—and more importantly, government compensation— attractive. The hospital lacked a steady funding base beyond Dillard University. The hospital's average length of stay for adults of nine days significantly exceeded the national average of seven days, due primarily to its reliance on visiting physicians who earned income based on patient length of stay, not on a set salary. This induced physicians to admit patients in the hospital for longer than necessary, financially benefiting the physician but hurting the hospital. Because the hospital's patient base was primarily low income and many lacked health insurance, the hospital continually struggled to collect unpaid bills. Finally, the hospital's expansion in the 1950s and increased services led to higher salary and operating costs.[2]

Almost immediately into the hospital desegregation period, Flint Goodridge experienced some negative effects. Although many historically white hospitals continued to discriminate against Black health care workers, Flint's administrators noted in 1965 a "high turnover rate" as some nurses left for better salaries at other hospitals or with the government. This loss of workers forced the hospital to raise nursing salaries to retain employees, which cut into revenue. Hurricane Betsy compounded this financial hit by causing wind damage. In response, the hospital temporarily closed several areas for years, which resulted in the hospital's first decline in patients in over fifteen years and a drop in much-needed patient payments. Even worse, administrators discovered the hospital's insurance policy did not cover wind damage, so the hospital had to pay for the repairs out of its revenue.[3] That November, the hospital raised rates to make up for losses.[4] However, administrators looked at the patient drop as an irregularity caused primarily by the storm and continued to express optimism for the hospital's future. Administrators believed patient numbers would increase again when Medicare and Medicaid went into effect in July 1966. As such, the hospital attempted further expansion by offering to purchase public housing property from the Housing Authority of New Orleans (HANO) in 1966. Writing on behalf of the Board of Management in February 1966, Vice President Charles Kohlmeyer Jr. noted the apprehension of board members over displacing HANO tenants on the property they hoped to buy, but stated that they believed "that the Community need for the expansion of the Hospital facilities outweighed the need for relatively few apartments which would be lost in the move." HANO officials initially appeared willing to accept Flint Goodridge's offer of $370,000. However, HANO then reneged and demanded more money, which led to negotiations that dragged on for several years. Kohlmeyer raised the offer to $425,000, but HANO stated it would not sell for less than $525,000, and it would not turn over the property until all the tenants had relocated.[5] With Flint Goodridge unable to raise that amount, HANO ended the negotiations. Other local officials further curtailed the hospital's growth. In 1964, the hospital applied to the City Property Office to close Toledano Street between Freret and LaSalle Streets, fill in the street, and use it for a new building. The department rejected the claim; after a series of appeals that lasted three years, the city again denied the move, ending the struggle in 1967.[6] While the city had pledged to end discrimination in health care, little seemed to have changed in the municipal government's attitudes toward the Black hospital.

Administrators still had hopes for expansion though, pinned primarily to the enactment of Medicare and Medicaid. Flint Goodridge's leaders strongly believed these two programs would increase Black usage of health services, and that Medicare and Medicaid would provide a stable source of income. Unable to foresee the future problems of under-compensation from Medicare and Medicaid, the hospital again applied for Hill-Burton funding. In November 1965, the state Department of Hospitals announced the further availability of Hill-Burton funding for New Orleans's hospitals. The department anticipated that when Medicare when into effect in 1966, the resulting increase in patients in the New Orleans area would lead to a projected need of

295 more hospital beds. Flint Goodridge's administrators requested to add onto the hospital to create 100 of these beds. They noted that in a reversal of the slight decline the hospital experienced in late 1965, patient use had increased in early 1966, leading to a shortage of beds.[7] Hospital representatives noted their occupancy rate of 103.5 percent compared to the citywide average of 75.3 percent demonstrated the need for more beds for Black residents. With this over-occupancy in mind, they urged the state to award Hill-Burton funding to allow the hospital to have a 260-bed capacity. Administrators contacted Congressman Hale Boggs in hopes of his assistance in securing the funding.[8] Under the 40 percent compensation formula available at the time through Hill-Burton, the hospital anticipated federal funds to cover $1.192 million of the $2.98 million estimated cost, leaving the hospital to raise $1.788 million through a fundraising campaign.[9]

Leaders envisioned hospital building space more than doubling from 69,451 to 160,000 square feet. Even after this growth, the administrators believed the hospital would operate at "near capacity" and be a "financially sounder operation." Additionally, the board wanted to build a new ninety-three-bed, five-story nursing home on adjoining property for $685,000, financed through Fair Housing Administration funding.[10]

Flint Goodridge's vision for an expanded hospital in some ways rested on complex and perhaps even contradictory ideas. Black civic leaders fought hard for desegregation of the city's institutions. However, some worried about the fate of the city's Black institutions like Flint Goodridge. Would integration lead to a massive decline in Black usage of the hospital? Would whites enter as patients? The hospital made a concerted effort to attract white clientele. Consultant Jesse Bankston told board members in February 1967 that the extent of integration "will determine the future success of this hospital." While the historically white hospitals resisted integration, Flint Goodridge pushed for integration to survive, based on the belief they needed white patients and doctors to remain viable. Their vision proved prophetic, as a lack of white patients helped doom the institution in following years.[11] At the same time, the hospital's board members emphasized to state and federal officials that the health care needs of African Americans would continue to be best filled at Flint. Administrators wrote of their expectation that "there will be a tendency for Negroes to indicate a preference for admission to Flint Goodridge."[12] This expectation proved only partially correct, as many upper-income Black patients left the hospital in the following years, taking away needed fees.

Ironically, doctors affiliated with Flint Goodridge greatly precipitated this exodus. In 1966, the hospital announced a new policy that doctors who continued to only treat their Black patients at Flint Goodridge and their white patients at the historically white hospitals would lose admitting privileges. Administrators did so to encourage white doctors to treat their white patients at Flint Goodridge. In response, nearly all the white affiliated doctors resigned, and they transferred their higher-income Black patients to other hospitals. By May 1967, 236 of 350 total physicians dropped their affiliation with the hospital.[13] The removal of their patients proved particularly devastating because they made up most of the paying patients. In the wake of this move, Flint Goodridge reverted to its Great Depression role as the Black version of Charity, with an even greater percentage of indigent patients than in the 1930s.

Flint Goodridge's last year in the black was 1967. Between 1965 and 1968, patient use dropped 36.2 percent; births dropped 47.5 percent; and clinic visits declined 56.2 percent. In 1967, Dillard University recommended formally cutting ties with Flint Goodridge as they considered the hospital to be a "liability" due to "financial difficulties."[14] That year the hospital reported losses of $72,000.[15] To counter, the board raised rates again in 1967 for the third straight year.[16] Thus began a desperate gamble. By raising prices, administrators hoped to bring in additional revenue from the remaining patients. Yet, by doing so they also risked driving away those that could not afford the new rates.

In late 1968, the hospital experienced another temporary increase in patients, which it hoped was the sign that the earlier idea of Flint Goodridge taking on a large percentage of the new Medicare and Medicaid patients was happening. Optimistic about the future, that May the hospital released a new "expansion report." The bold plan, which called for an additional 150 inpatient beds (for a total of 278); a health clinic; childcare center; educational center; a 160-bed long-term care facility; and separate Desire Housing Project and Lower Ninth Clinic Ward clinics, would create a massive institution that would serve an estimated 70,000 patients a year. Administrators still expected most of the city's Black, and many white, Medicare and Medicaid recipients to use Flint Goodridge, and not Charity, especially in light of poor treatment at the latter. They wrote in the expansion report: "The experience the poor, particularly the poor Blacks, have endured at Charity Hospital, have often been anything but pleasant. For these reasons, it can, I believe, be safely assumed that once the Medicare and Medicaid programs are fully enacted, that most, if not all of the indigents of our community, will look away from Charity Hospital for their health needs." Administrators also believed that Flint could apply for funding through the federal Model Cities program. Started in 1966 as part of President Lyndon Johnson's war on poverty, the program offered funding for antipoverty programs, including clinics and public health initiatives.

The hospital they envisioned meant both a significant leap forward toward serving as a modern health center and a return to the hospital's original mission of increasing access, addressing public health issues, and training and employing Black medical workers. The report described the need for services in the Lower Ninth Ward, which had "practically non-existent" health services, and as a result had high infant mortality and tuberculosis rates. The Lower Ninth clinic would also be "community controlled" through a partnership with residents and offer vocational rehabilitation in addition to health services. The mental health facility would offer special programs for treatment of alcoholism and narcotics addiction. The education center would offer a three-year associate's degree in conjunction with Dillard and other universities, with second- and third-year students working at the hospital, and with a noted outcome of "upward mobility" as the ultimate goal; a two-year work study program in physical therapy; a program in inhalation therapy; and training in radiology. Finally, the plan envisioned a strengthened connection with the community. The hospital, the report urged, should take a holistic approach and partner with community leaders to "involve itself in the full range of urban ills besetting our communities," which it identified as crime, education, urban development, zoning, housing, land use, and transportation.[17]

The plan never materialized. The state refused to give further Hill-Burton funding, which doomed the expansion. Furthermore, the municipal government carried out more measures to halt the hospital's growth. Already hemmed in by HANO, the city council passed a zoning ordinance, redesignating areas near the hospital as commercial, despite the protestation of the hospital; the commercial zoning made the hospital ineligible to buy that property.[18] The 1960s initially appeared to be the most promising decade in the hospital's history and also offered the seeming end of racialized health care. However, both of these dreams evaporated by 1970. Racialized health care remained, and Flint Goodridge struggled through the next decade and a half, before closing in 1985.

Health Education Authority of Louisiana

While government officials used their powers to limit Flint Goodridge, they simultaneously aided the growth of the historically white health care institutions. Introduced originally in 1968, HEAL's proposal initiated what would become a fifty-year effort to expand the white Medical District. By the mid-1960s, both LSU and Tulane wanted modern university hospitals, with the former hoping to replace Charity or establish a partnership with another hospital, and the latter planning to create its own hospital. Tulane operated a clinic in the Hutchinson Building since the mid-1960s, with more than 66,000 patients annually and an annual budget of $12 million, with two-thirds of costs coming from federal funding. However, federal funding had decreased in recent years and operating costs increased, leading to a deficit. The university still had a large endowment—over $51 million—but hoped to find a consistent revenue source.[19]

In a 1969 paper titled "The Future of Medicine in Society is Tulane's Future," Tulane vice president John Walsh argued that "the feeling of the American people, whether we agree or disagree with it, is that they are entitled to quality health care." This supposed change in viewing health care, coupled with rising incomes and insurance, resulted in more health care spending and use of hospitals. Walsh urged Tulane to build its own hospital to benefit from these changes. Tulane's administrators believed that creating their own private hospital would generate significant revenue.[20]

Tulane's push for a hospital received great aid from the formation of HEAL, with the explicit mission to help Charity, LSU, and Tulane acquire more property in the Medical District. Leaders of LSU and Tulane worked for several years to introduce and win support for HEAL. In a 1968 lobbying pamphlet, proponents argued the Medical District was "once renowned as a great concentration of medical education and care," but had now been surpassed by centers in other cities, including Houston and Birmingham. They noted concerns over patient loss, modernization, and changes with new policies like Medicare. They also warned if LSU and Tulane could not build new facilities—with government aid—they would "vacate" the Medical District and "Charity's demise would only become a matter of time." "Downtown blight," they predicted, "would spread" as a result. In contrast, if the institutions expanded, "an area destined for decay would become one of the community's bright spots, a vibrant area producing opportunities and new wealth, as well as better health for the community, the state, and even the nation."[21]

The 1968 HEAL legislation authorized the creation of a board of directors composed of business leaders, lawyers, heads of insurance companies, and members of the chamber of commerce, and led by hospital management executive Jack Aron and Dr. J. Jefferson Bennett, who previously helped develop and direct the planning for the University of Alabama's Medical Center Complex, which took over sixteen blocks in downtown Birmingham. The legislation also created twelve representatives to the board: two from Tulane, two from Charity, two from LSU, two from the executive board of the Louisiana State Medical Society, one from the Louisiana Dental Association, one appointment by the governor, and one selected by the New Orleans mayor. HEAL could initiate voter-approved bonds for the eligible institutions to buy property and build new structures and parking lots, use eminent domain to acquire lots that refused to sell, and offer expert advice and networking for securing additional funding, including applying for federal grants and technical expertise from planners and architects. Finally, HEAL sought to erect training centers and housing for the medical professionals and students the district would attract as it expanded.

The creation of HEAL reflected several important threads in New Orleans's medical history. HEAL's vision of—in the words of Tulane representative Darwin S. Fenner—"a medical complex second to none in the nation," matched the rhetoric of Fenner's ancestor E. D. Fenner in the 1850s, C. C. Bass in the 1930s, and other historical proponents of New Orleans as a leading medical center. As was the case in these earlier promotions of New Orleans as a medical center, advocates held up the economic benefits of a strong health care system. In the past, proponents promoted health care to protect and expand the city's leading industries—the slave trade and slave-based economy in the antebellum period, and the commercial trade with Latin America and tourism in the early twentieth century. By the 1960s, the health care economy itself had become a booming industry, employing thousands of New Orleanians. HEAL would further the growth of this burgeoning field by adding an estimated 2,500 jobs and thus boost the city.

Proponents also wrapped their arguments for HEAL in the language of urban renewal that marked a deeply ironic switch of many white leaders on federal involvement. After the federal government ordered desegregation of schools following the Supreme Court's *Brown v. Board of Education* decision, the Louisiana state legislature passed laws that banned the state and municipal government from participating in federal programs or receiving federal funding; this included urban renewal grants. The state maintained these stipulations until the late 1960s, over the objections of Black proponents who advocated for participation in President Lyndon Johnson's Great Society programs. The ban on urban renewal funding protected New Orleans from large-scale scourges of urban renewal that decimated Black neighborhoods in cities throughout the country. When Louisiana finally lifted the ban on urban renewal, New Orleans belatedly carried out several projects, including the building of the I-10 overpass on Claiborne Avenue, a new city hall complex and jail in the Tulane Gravier neighborhood, and the Theatre for Performing Arts and Louis Armstrong Park in Tremé, all of which displaced hundreds of Black residents and businesses. The proposed medical complex was part of this push for urban renewal. In April 1970, HEAL signed a contract to work with the city's Community Improvement Agency (CIA), which administered the city's urban renewal project. This occurred after a three-to-two vote of approval by the CIA, with the two Black members of the executive board voting in opposition. With this partnership, HEAL and the CIA would carry out urban renewal for a proposed 289 acres, with thirty acres for the medical complex, and the rest redeveloped for housing and other facilities (see figure A.3).[22]

HEAL reflected the continuing power of the racialized health care system. No African Americans served on the appointed board of directors. The potential beneficiaries of HEAL were all historically white health care institutions. In addition to Charity, LSU, and Tulane, the legislature designated the Veterans Affairs Hospital, Hotel Dieu, and the Ear, Eye, Nose, and Throat Hospitals as potential recipients, all located in the Medical District. Forced out of the neighborhood decades earlier, Flint Goodridge was ineligible to receive the badly needed funds. The legislation authorizing HEAL stated that the authors intended it to "promote the health and welfare of its citizens." However, the participants in HEAL continued to face complaints, lawsuits, and federal investigations for racial discrimination.

With the adoption of the HEAL legislation and the creation of the board, the organization turned to acquiring property. In an effort designed to cause the same displacement of Black families that justified "slum clearance" in the 1930s in Central City and in the Medical District, the state again turned to federal funding in the 1970s, this time in the form of HUD grants. To apply for these grants, HEAL had to secure approval by the city council before submitting its applications. HEAL's representatives and its proponents made several arguments. They highlighted several economic benefits, including the direct gain creating the projected 2,500 new jobs, and the indirect benefit of using the medical complex to attract large companies. They noted that Louisiana had a shortage of physicians, which could be addressed with expanding the medical schools. Finally, they touted the health benefits for all residents and the opportunity to "improve" the Tulane Gravier neighborhood with urban renewal. J. Jefferson Bennett also stated that residents would not be displaced, as opponents claimed. He argued the medical complex and the urban renewal project would have a "beneficial impact on the residential areas" and have no "detriment to the families and businesses occupying the area."

A powerful coalition backed Bennett and HEAL, including Mayor Moon Landrieu, who called the project a "fantastic opportunity for the city"; the executive director of the CIA; the chancellor of LSU; the president of the Greater New Orleans American Federation of Labor and Congress of Industrial Organizations (AFL-CIO); the president of the chamber of commerce; and the bishop of the Roman Catholic Archdiocese of New Orleans all spoke in favor of HEAL's proposal at the December 1970 city council meeting.

Dwarfed in terms of civic and political clout, members of OTAGNO spoke against the plans, arguing the project would use taxpayer funds to benefit private institutions like Tulane and "wealthy landgrabbers," while displacing hundreds of Black residents and business owners. OTAGNO president James Comiskey implored the city council to oppose the measures: "I hope you will stay with me and the people against the millionaires." In a direct echo of what Black leaders argued in the 1930s against the city's WPA-funded "slum clearance" of Central City and Tulane Gravier, John Dowling stated it was "unconceivable" that properties in the neighborhood were considered "slums," claiming HEAL assessment of the neighborhood as containing many "substandard" structures in need of clearance was false.[23]

Casting its support behind urban renewal, the city council approved HEAL's two initial grants. The first for $480,000 was to study the proposed area, examining blight, need for housing, capital fund requirements, and the needs for medical and supporting facilities. The second was a $3.8 million grant to redevelop the first four acres of the medical complex. HUD approved the grants in 1971. HEAL prepared to apply for a Neighborhood Development Program (NDP) urban renewal grant through HUD. NDP's primary goal was blight abatement, with grants to local governments for improvement and clearance projects. The new grant would fund clearance and redevelopment for an additional 114 acres, with plans to apply for future grants to fund the redevelopment of the remaining 172 acres in the area. At the time, residences containing 250 families—215 Black and thirty-five white—occupied 245 dwellings in the 114-acre area targeted by the NDP grant. The grant identified 233 of the units as having "deficiencies." Despite the earlier promises that it would not displace residents, HEAL would use its eminent domain power to remove those families and redevelop the properties. It also planned to remove seventy-nine Black-owned businesses. In addition to the general objective of "abatement of blight," the applicants also highlighted the second NDP objective "to expand and solidify an economic base for the total city which will encourage further development of those areas surrounding the NDP project." HEAL projected that the medical complex would create 900 full-time positions for low- and moderate-income New Orleanians, with preference going to the residents of Tulane Gravier. HEAL also noted in its application that it had formed a project area committee featuring property owners and some tenants of Tulane Gravier—with their inclusion only after protests from OTAGNO over not being included in the process—as well as representatives from the hospitals, medical schools, and other direct beneficiaries. While heavily tilted in composition toward proxies for the involved medical institutions, the application stated the committee was "representative." The HEAL application addressed the displacement of the 250 mostly Black families. HEAL argued that "any minority group concentrations will be dispersed through relocation activities to suitable, safe, and standard living conditions throughout the area," a dubious claim given the decades-long effort of excluding African Americans from the most desirable neighborhoods and the city-sanctioned placement of health hazards near Black-majority blocks. HEAL promised not to relocate the families into already-existing minority concentrations, but offered no specifics on where they would end up.[24] The application also stated that all the institutions involved in the process "do not discriminate," despite the fact that all three of the primary institutions—Charity, Tulane, and LSU—and secondary institutions like Hotel Dieu had pending lawsuits and investigations for their failures to comply with federally mandated desegregation and nondiscrimination. This cast serious doubt on HEAL's claim that the medical complex would provide "extensive opportunity" for employment for low-income residents.

The federal government never approved the application, due to a combination of factors. The lawsuits and investigations over discrimination may have led to the rejection, although there is no record of why the federal government denied the application. But grassroots activism certainly helped delay the application. OTAGNO protested the displacement of the residents and businesses. This opposition forced the city council to temporarily withhold its approval as the two sides negotiated, a necessary step before a citywide voter referendum on submitting the application to HUD. Although the city council ultimately voted to support the grant, over the objection of the residents, the delay meant the voter referendum did not occur until December 1971 and HEAL did not submit its grant until 1972.[25] By that period, the Nixon administration had largely gutted urban renewal and other Great Society projects. If Louisiana had lifted its ban on receiving federal grants earlier or never enacted it in the first place, or if residents had not organized to oppose the application, then HEAL probably would have led to the displacement of hundreds of African Americans and creation of significant medical complexes that the proponents described as already happening in places like Houston and Birmingham.

Regardless of the project's failure, HEAL's application is important to consider as it demonstrates the continual effort to expand the historically white Medical District and the pervasive attempts to displace Black residents. It also reveals the government mechanisms and funding sources that allowed the racialized health care system to perpetuate post-integration. HEAL's vision of a modern medical district would have to wait until post–Hurricane Katrina to be realized, but the effort continued unabated for decades, and HEAL did help fund the first major step in the 1970s, the creation of Tulane University Hospital.

Tulane University Hospital

Although the 1972 HUD grant failed, HEAL successfully passed a $37.5 million tax-exempt bond for Tulane in 1975 that covered most of the projected $43.4 million cost of its proposed hospital. Beyond HEAL, several other factors greatly aided the university in the construction of the hospital, advantages unavailable to Black medical institutions like Flint Goodridge. Tulane negotiated property exchanges with the city by trading property it controlled elsewhere in the city—Tulane was one of the city's largest property owners—for desired lots for the hospital and medical school. Tulane gave property to the city in March 1973 in exchange for the latter closing the road on South Liberty Street between Tulane Avenue and Cleveland Street, allowing Tulane to connect the lots it owned there. Thus, the school used its connections and wealth to gain favorable concessions from the city. These gestures stood in sharp contrast to the city's continual use of municipal powers to curtail Flint Goodridge's growth.[26]

The federal government had been helping to fund the medical school since the early twentieth century, with grants to promote medical and public health research through the U.S. Public Health Service, the National Institutes of Health, HEW, and other federal agencies. Tulane used these funds not only to pay for research, but also to build or renovate many of its buildings on the main campus and the downtown medical school campus. When Tulane sought to build a new medical science education building in 1971, it successfully applied for a HEW grant that covered two-thirds of the projected $25 million cost. Despite its $51 million in endowment, every year the school received special improvement grants from HEW available to medical schools in "financial distress." Tulane received $680,000 in 1972 and $865,000 in 1973 due to losses the school reported for raises, rising insurance costs, and reduction in income from clinic Medicare patients.[27] This ability to apply for federal grants extended to the new hospital, offering a valuable source of funds that were unavailable to nonuniversity hospitals like Flint Goodridge, which had lost its affiliated medical school with the forced closure of Flint Medical College decades earlier. Due to its prominence and connections, Tulane garnered financial support from its many wealthy supporters. Composed primarily of business leaders, the Tulane Board of Governors solicited millions in donations from their own and other companies and large funding sources. By March 1975, the board reported they had requested funding from thirty-six organizations and raised more than $17 million in its drive, which was directed by a nationally renowned fundraising consultant group. As a result, Tulane turned down low-interest commercial loans and even a tax-exempt financing offer from Goldman Sachs. While philanthropic groups like the Rosenwald Fund aided the construction of Flint Goodridge's new hospital in the 1930s, the hospital continually struggled financially and had no consistent large-scale financial backer after the Rosenwald Fund shuttered in 1943.[28]

Adding to Tulane's economic advantage was its development of the hospital in conjunction with a hospital company. In the 1970s, for-profit hospital companies grew, lured by the ever-increasing profits of health care. These companies offered financial management and stability for independent hospitals, emphasizing efficiency and cost control.[29] Tulane board members met with representatives from four hospital companies. Tulane negotiated with each to secure the best deal, ultimately signing a partnership with Hospital Affiliates International (HAI) in 1972. No such organization was willing to help the management of Flint Goodridge; in fact, the hospital corporation that eventually purchased Flint only did so to take its bed licenses.

Tulane purposefully avoided serving low-income patients from its inception. When local activists approached the hospital about including a badly needed community mental health center and offered $1.1 million from the National Institute of Mental Health, the board members voted in November 1971 to exclude the project, stating that "Community Health Centers are financial drains."[30] Tulane's hospital initially submitted a bid to take over the services offered by the Public Health Service hospital; however, it ultimately abandoned the idea because, according to the board, "HEW guidelines, recently received, indicate that Tulane could not receive sufficient revenue," and instead recommended Charity take on the services.[31] When board members met with representatives of HAI in July 1971, they told the company the proposed hospital was a good investment as they would keep "low-income patients at a minimum" by sending any such individuals to the nearby Charity, a practice known as "dumping" and later declared illegal by Congress.[32] Tulane's stated goal to exclude low-income patients succeeded despite violating the bed quota established under the Hill-Burton Act. Under this formula, New Orleans was already considered over-bedded for the non-indigent population with 3,374 beds in private hospitals in Orleans Parish. Ignoring these statistics and Tulane's explicit mission, the state granted Tulane Hospital's 154 bed licenses in the same period that it rejected Hill-Burton funding and additional bed licenses for Flint Goodridge. This mirrored the 1950s when the state rejected Flint Goodridge's Hill-Burton application, despite the need for beds for Black residents, and instead awarded funding to whites-only hospitals like Ochsner, despite New Orleans being over-bedded for whites; little had changed since the Jim Crow period.[33]

Hospital planners projected that initially only half of Tulane's patients would come from Orleans Parish, with another one-third from areas surrounding the city and 16 percent from elsewhere. They expected the numbers from Orleans Parish to decline and usage from the white flight suburbs to increase over time. Thus, the hospital they envisioned was not designed to meet the needs of the community, particularly Black residents, as seen in Tulane's low Black patient numbers. Again, this marked a sharp contrast with Flint Goodridge, an institution that treated mostly low-income patients, many from Central City and other predominantly Black neighborhoods, a majority using Medicare or Medicaid, and all Black. In addition to adding more beds to service an already over-bedded population, critics worried that the hospital would further hurt low-income and minority patients as Tulane, its students, and physicians focused their time and attention on the patients at their hospital and decreased attention on patients at Charity, therefore depleting the already declining quality of care.[34]

The focus on upper-income, insured, predominantly white patients partially reflected underrepresentation of African Americans in Tulane's leadership, a vestige of its policies into the mid-1960s. Civil rights leader and future mayor Ernest Morial joined the Tulane University Medical Center Board of Governors in 1971, as did Henry Braden—former chief of medicine at Flint Goodridge—in 1974 after Morial resigned. However, leadership remained predominantly white. In addition to the mostly white board, almost all high-level hospital administrators were white. After Morial's resignation, outside of Braden, the hospital and clinic had virtually no African Americans in leadership positions.[35] The university's overall governing body, the Board of Administrators, did not have a Black member until 1978, when Braden replaced a resigning member convicted of bribery. The medical school remained predominantly white as well. Despite a 1968 grant from the Macy Foundation to initiate a program to recruit minority medical students, with later funding from the Sloan Foundation, the National Institutes of Health, and the J. Aron Charitable Foundation Inc., by 1971 the medical school only had seven Black students and was more than 98 percent white; the school made gradual improvements but was still more than 95 percent white in 1974.[36]

The state approved the hospital's bed licenses, and the hospital opened in summer 1976. By 1977, revenue already exceeded costs. In addition to "dumping" low-income and Medicaid and Medicare patients at Charity, physicians would also "skim" patients from Charity, taking patients that needed expensive procedures that would result in large reimbursements and transferring them to Tulane. Over the next three decades, Tulane University Hospital proved its planners correct, as it brought in valuable revenue to the university. In fact, only one other hospital, Ochsner Foundation Hospital, consistently made an annual profit in the thirty years leading up to Katrina.[37]

Charity Hospital, the De Facto Black Hospital

While Tulane University Hospital thrived, the other hospital Tulane affiliated with, Charity, experienced a decline similar to Flint Goodridge. Ironically, in the same period in which Black patients and employees fought the hospital over discrimination, Charity became a Black-majority hospital for the first time as white patients left when the hospital integrated. By the end of the 1960s, a hospital that had been 60 percent white patients in the early 1960s had more than 75 percent Black patients. As this occurred, the state cut funding dramatically, leading to a 43 percent drop in hospital interns from 1967 to 1971, hospital moratoriums on buying needed equipment and repairs, closing of beds, and staff reductions, which all forced the hospital to turn away many patients and led to a general decrease in quality of care.[38]

After integration, the state passed legislation that allowed it to use Charity as a cash cow. One bill permitted the state Department of Hospitals to siphon money collected from surgeries done for injuries incurred during accidents—Charity had one of the leading surgical centers in the state and would accept money from paying patients for some procedures not available elsewhere—to use for its research and training fund. Similarly, the state took half of the money that the federal government allocated in reimbursement for Charity's Medicare and Medicaid patients and distributed it elsewhere. In 1970, additional funding cuts led to an acute crisis. That May, the hospital closed

454 beds and administrators and state leaders discussed shutting down the hospital altogether. The Human Relations Council, the NAACP, and other community organizations formed a coalition to secure hospital funding. Private hospitals wrote resolutions of support as they feared the closing of Charity would force them to care for indigent patients. The coalition mobilized media attention, pressured state politicians, organized mass rallies, and wrote their own legislative bills, which they sent to members of the state legislature. Their efforts led state legislators to introduce five new bills: to give Charity immunity to lawsuits; to allow Charity to keep all the money allocated by the federal government for Medicare and Medicaid treatment; to allow Charity to keep money from other sources like student nurse tuition, fees for legal reports, and soft drink machines; to allow the hospital to keep the money from operations for accidents; and a $3 million bond to improve the intensive care areas. The legislature approved all five bills, but funding shortfalls continued in the following decades for the hospital.[39]

Court Cases and Federal Investigations

By the end of the 1960s, little had seemingly changed in Black access to health care. Most Black residents still used Charity and Flint Goodridge, and the historically white private hospitals stayed mostly white. Tired of waiting for federal enforcement of integration and nondiscrimination, residents turned again to grassroots action and litigation. In 1969, the Human Relations Council found that Charity and other area hospitals, including the just-opened Methodist Hospital, still labeled their blood by race. This practice was legal under a 1958 Louisiana state law but was outlawed by the 1964 Civil Rights Act. The group filed complaints with HEW, but no change occurred. Finally, in 1972, following repeated warnings that the federal government would end all funding to every hospital in the state, the state removed the blood labeling legislation.[40]

In 1970, a group of Black women, aided by the NAACP, the National Tenants Organization, the People's Action Center, and the National Legal Program on Health Problems of the Poor, initiated a groundbreaking case with national implications. The group, with Rosezella Cook as lead plaintiff, sued ten New Orleans hospitals and the Louisiana state Department of Hospitals for violation of Title VI of the Civil Rights Act, the Hill-Burton Act, and the Medicare and Medicaid Acts. They also sued HEW for failure to enforce the laws. The hospitals had refused admittance to the women for acute health problems because they could not pay the admission fee. All were covered by

Medicaid, which would have paid the fee and other charges for services. However, in violation of the law, all ten hospitals refused to accept Medicaid patients. Additionally, by refusing to provide free care for at least some patients, the hospitals violated the public service provision of the Hill-Burton Act. The women also alleged racial discrimination.[41] The resulting case, *Cook v. Ochsner*, lingered in the court for the next two decades. In 1972, the Eastern District of Louisiana found that the secretary of HEW had failed to enforce the public service provision of the Hill-Burton Act by allowing the hospitals to refuse to admit Medicaid patients. That same year, the plaintiffs and the hospitals reached a consent decree in which the hospitals agreed to begin treating Medicaid patients. However, in 1973, plaintiffs presented evidence that the hospitals had ignored the consent decree, and the district court found them to be in violation in 1975, although appeals continued from some hospitals until the late 1980s.[42]

In 1974, after years of pressure from the NAACP as well as increasing attention due to the *Cook* case, HEW conducted a three-year study of New Orleans that documented the system was virtually the same in 1978 as prior to 1966. They found that 75 percent of all Black patients used either Flint Goodridge or Charity. Despite African Americans comprising more than 55 percent of the city's population, the other hospitals admitted few Black patients and Medicare and Medicaid patients. Many of the Black patients who used the historically white hospitals were individuals of higher income. Discrimination in employment continued as well, with few or no Black doctors in the private hospitals and only one white doctor still on staff at Flint Goodridge by 1978; additionally, most of the white doctors who had left Flint Goodridge had dropped their Black patients altogether. Discrimination extended to other hospital positions as well, with racial sorting of African Americans into lower-paying positions and repeated complaints to the NAACP over mistreatment.

HEW's investigation found nearly every private hospital to be out of compliance with federal law. HEW charged seven hospitals in 1977 and 1978 with violating Title VI of the 1964 Civil Rights Act. One hospital settled, but the others remained defiant. HEW began procedures against three: Hotel Dieu, Mercy, and Southern Baptist. African Americans were 8.1, 6.5, and 2.8 percent of patients at each hospital, respectively, and 3, 0.8, and 0.4 percent of medical staff; none of the hospitals ever had a Black member of their boards of trustees. After the hospitals refused to follow through on a list of actions that HEW mandated, the agency began formal termination proceedings of federal funding in 1978. However, the statute stipulated that an administrative law judge review HEW's findings and then listen to the hospitals' appeals. In

1979, the judge struck down many of the requirements as onerous, including formal recruitment measures. The judge argued the dearth of Black physicians in the city made it too difficult to comply with the order. He also characterized the requirement that doctors take Medicaid patients as a condition of staff privileges as "inappropriate" and the mandated opening of outpatient facilities as too costly. The judge ordered the hospitals to remind staff that they could not discriminate, urged them to undertake informal recruitment of Black physicians, and consider adding Black board members. With these meek stipulations, he dismissed the termination of federal funds. The NAACP appealed the ruling and filed contempt charges against HEW for its failure to enforce Title VI. In response, the government set a timetable for the hospitals to comply with the original demands by HEW, although no real substantive changes or follow-up occurred.[43]

The *Cook* case led to some formal policy changes and restitution. HEW quantified the amount of free care—previously not specified—that hospitals that received Hill-Burton funding had to perform at a 3 percent minimum for twenty years after receiving the money. In 1979, most of the hospitals involved in the initial *Cook* case settled with the families of those denied hospital admission. The settlement also provided additional Medicaid and Medicare funding for Charity to open additional beds and hire more nurses. However, some hospitals continued their appeals. It was not until 1989 that West Jefferson General Hospital and East Jefferson General Hospital signed consent decrees to recruit Black physicians and give Medicaid patients full access to the hospitals.[44]

Despite these settlements, HEW's failure to require substantive changes or dole out real punishment perpetuated racialized health care. HEW also failed to enforce the 3 percent free care requirement. As a result, white doctors at historically white hospitals continued to send most poor, Black, Medicaid, and Medicare patients to Charity or Flint Goodridge. Ultimately, much like the period a century earlier during the federal occupation of New Orleans, the late 1960s and 1970s proved to be a period in which the possible dismantling of the racialized health care system did not occur. Lawsuits initiated by Black residents with the support of the NAACP, backed by legislation including the Civil Rights Act, forced hospitals to adopt nondiscrimination policies. However, the inability or unwillingness of the federal government to enforce compliance allowed the historically white hospitals to remain predominantly white in patient makeup and the physician staff.

It should also be highlighted that like the earlier period, doctors and administrators at the hospitals were significant actors in maintaining racialized health care. These individuals purposefully denied entrance to Medicare and Medicare patients, turned away most Black patients (especially low-income ones), discriminated against the Black patients they did admit, and discriminated in the hiring and treatment of Black employees. This outcome—the perpetuation of racialized health care—was not inevitable. In fact, the fight by civil rights organizations and the court victories and federal legislation should have led to the end of racialized health care. The purposeful and illegal decisions of administrators and doctors in New Orleans to maintain racialized health care, partially driven by the monetizing of health care that incentivized health care providers to exclude low-income or indigent patients, and coupled with the federal government's failure to enforce compliance with the law allowed the system to perpetuate. As a result, in the decades after the official desegregation of health care, two health care systems continued to exist: private hospitals for white patients, and the underfunded and understaffed Charity and Flint Goodridge for African Americans.

Grassroots Activism and Federal Programs

With the racialized system's continuation and the decline in funding, staffing, and services at Charity and Flint Goodridge, the racial health gap widened again in the post–Civil Rights period. Black residents continued to face negative social determinants of health. Poor-quality education made it difficult for Black residents to get jobs. Racial discrimination in employment hurt their ability to get employer-provided health care and the ability to pay for health care costs. Black New Orleanians faced continued problems of white violence, police harassment and brutality, and everyday racism, which all took mental and physical tolls on health. Exposure to air, soil, and water pollutants from factories, dumping grounds, the municipal incinerator, and other sources affected many Black residents due to their placement in or near Black-majority neighborhoods, the vestige of environmental racism that became codified with the zoning and housing policies in the 1920s and 1930s. Substandard housing conditions, including the public housing units—which were poorly constructed to begin with, and suffered from declining funding and maintenance by HANO post-integration as the units became mostly Black occupied—caused a myriad of health issues.

One significant issue in the public housing units, and in many rental units, was lead poisoning. In 1970, the New Orleans Health Department (NOHD) began testing for lead poisoning. The NOHD presented initial findings of high instances of lead paint in residences, mostly in low-income housing.

This led the city council to pass an ordinance banning lead-based substances.[45] In its 1973 annual report, the NOHD documented that 44.4 percent of 21,000 children tested had blood-lead levels of 40 μg/dL (micrograms per deciliter) or higher, considered unsafe by World Health Organization standards at the time.[46] Today, scientists consider a level of 10 μg/dL high and argue that any level including below 5 μg/dL can result in the associated negative health effects of lead poisoning including cognitive development problems, stunted growth, brittle bones, rotting teeth, anemia, renal impairment and kidney failure, hypertension, immunotoxicity, attention deficit hyperactivity disorder (ADHD), antisocial behavior, hearing loss, lack of impulse control, seizures, and death.[47] Because of the standards in the 1970s, the NOHD report did not document how many children had levels higher than 0 but lower than 40 μg/dL. However, thousands of children and adults likely suffered from lead poisoning throughout the twentieth century. Additionally, while the data did not reveal race, African Americans were most at risk for lead poisoning due to the effects of racism—including wealth inequality and employment discrimination—that made them more likely to work in jobs that exposed them to lead and live in low-quality rental units or public housing units, both of which had a high prevalence of lead paint.

All these factors, the nexus of negative social determinants of health, caused significant health problems for Black New Orleanians, as indicated by a 1973 NOHD report. Black residents suffered from significantly higher rates of maternal death (5.0 per 1,000 compared to a rate of nearly 0 per 1,000 for whites), stillborn babies (19.0 per 1,000 compared to a rate of 8.6 per 1,000 for whites), neonatal morality cases (21 per 1,000 compared to 11.3 per 1,000 for whites), and infant mortality cases (10.9 per 1,000 compared to 4.7 per 1,000 white residents). Problems were greatest for Black residents of Central City. That neighborhood had the highest rates of stillborn children and infant and child mortality. Over 20 percent of children in the area were born premature, and the neighborhood accounted for 24 percent of the city's stillbirths. Many children suffered from malnourishment, anemia, parasites, lead poisoning, diphtheria, and whooping cough. For adults, the rate of tuberculosis was double that of the rest of New Orleans, and the neighborhood accounted for half of the cases of sexually transmitted infections.[48]

Facing these obstacles, and with the continued resistance of the historically white health care system to integration, Black residents turned again to health activism and formed new organizations to push for health care outside of the hospitals, primarily in the form of clinics. This effort was part of a larger, national health activism movement in the 1960s and 1970s. While more renowned for their more radical efforts, organizations including the Black Panthers, the Young Lords, and the United Farm Workers all created their own health clinics nationwide to meet the unfulfilled health needs of their communities.[49] These groups critiqued the historically white health care system and challenged it by offering free care to individuals traditionally excluded from and exploited by that system. They all pressed for attention to health issues that especially impacted people of color—issues like sickle cell anemia, lead poisoning, and tuberculosis—and often employed attention-grabbing tactics—for example, the Young Lords' 1970 occupation of Lincoln Hospital in the Bronx to highlight the disparity in health care funding. As noted by historian Alondra Nelson in her work on the Black Panthers, these efforts, including the clinics, represented the emphasis on "community control and self-determinist ethics of 1970s nationalism."[50] Yet, as argued by Nelson and demonstrated in this work, these activities were a continuity with past activism, not a break with the past. The creation of clinics and the health care activism in Chicago, New York, California, and New Orleans drew inspiration from previous generations of health care activists who created Black clinics, hospitals, and medical schools and initiated public health campaigns.

In the late 1960s and 1970s, Black New Orleanians in the public housing complexes, Central City, Desire, and the Ninth Ward—the areas with the highest rates of poverty and health problems and the least access to health care—embraced the self-determination and community-centered health activism modeled, much like their forbearers who created Flint Goodridge in the 1890s, the Civic Ward League in the 1920s, and public housing tenant councils in the 1940s. Formed to represent the interests of the residents, the tenant councils featured health committees that carried out projects in the 1940s and 1950s including working with the NOHD to offer tuberculosis testing and public health education activities. In the 1960s, the tenant councils demanded permanent health clinics in the public housing units, particularly as most tenants had no access to a vehicle to drive to a doctor or hospital. Pressure from the councils finally led the NOHD to plan to build clinics in Calliope, Desire, Lafitte, Magnolia, St. Bernard, and St. Thomas housing projects in 1966. These clinics offered basic medical services, primarily provided by nurses, for several hours during the weekdays. However, the city council's repeated budget cuts to the Housing Authority—which it had done every year since the first move toward integration and the beginnings of the white exodus from HANO buildings—led to most clinics closing in 1970.[51]

The tenant councils found allies with Total Community Action Incorporated (TCA), a nonprofit community agency founded in 1964 to coordinate the federal war on poverty programs in New Orleans. TCA identified seven neighborhoods as target areas for distribution of federally funded services: Algiers-Fischer, Central City, Desire, Florida, the Irish Channel, the Lower Ninth Ward, and St. Bernard, with neighborhood development centers in each.[52] In addition to coordinating services like employment training, TCA committees—composed of neighborhood residents—pressed the NOHD to establish neighborhood clinics. In 1969, Central City's Economic Opportunity Committee wrote directly to the director of the NOHD, Rodney Jung, to ask for more services at Edna Pilsbury Health Center. The long list illustrated the need for care and community-centered activism. The committee wanted the incorporation of the ideas of neighborhood residents into health planning and the training of residents for work in the health care field. They wanted the placement of a Black physician, who could "relate with or represent the aspirations and needs of the poor," to serve as a representative on the Board of Health. They also needed weekend immunizations and evening testing programs for workers. They wanted the city to conduct health surveys of parasites, anemia, dental defects, and malnutrition in their neighborhoods. They found that a daily emergency clinic was essential, and they believed that residents trained and hired as sanitation inspectors and health educators could also provide much-needed employment. "The time has come," the committee wrote, "when our city and state must provide a better health service if we are to have a healthful community." They demanded a meeting within ten weeks and threatened protests if the department did not comply. That same year, the Desire Area Community Council also pressed the NOHD for health services, including a clinic with physicians.[53]

The tenant councils, the TCA-sponsored neighborhood committees, and allied activists pressed the city to apply for funding for clinics from the federal Model Cities program. Signed into law in November 1966, the legislation gave federal funding to select cities to create new antipoverty programs. While many whites opposed New Orleans joining the program, the lobbying by Black residents and politicians led the Schiro administration to apply for and receive Model City grants in late 1968.[54] Under Mayor Landrieu, from 1970 to 1973, Model Cities aid funded the building of community recreation centers, helped develop Black businesses, and improved Black participation in the construction industries, almost all under the auspices of newly formed predominantly Black organizations and nonprofits.[55] The largest component of the Model Cities program funded small clinics in the Desire-Florida and Central City neighborhoods and a full-service health clinic in Central City, subcontracted to and run by the Economic Opportunity Corporation (EOC).

As described by an organizational pamphlet, the EOC was organized in 1965 "to ensure that the Anti-Poverty Program provides the maximum possible participation of residents of Central City and that they best types of services are provided." The EOC formed "Action Committees" comprised of neighborhood residents and designed to "provide an opportunity for them to help themselves through self-help programs" in several areas: employment, business improvement, legal aid, welfare, education, housing, recreation, youth organization, and health services. These committees helped register residents to vote and find jobs, and referred them to social service agencies, among other activities. The health and medical service action committee's self-described mission was "to determine what needed medical services could be brought into the area by existing community resources and what new services need to be created to meet the needs of area residents." Initially, it focused primarily on connecting neighborhood residents to various health programs—including Medicaid and Medicare—and institutions, including doctor referrals. Under the Model Cities program, the EOC took a more direct role in administering the health clinic in Central City.[56] In 1972, Family Health Inc.—a nonprofit organization started in 1966 by Tulane University's Dr. Joseph Beasley and featuring clinics and family planning centers in Louisiana and Latin America—assumed direct administration of the Model Cities clinics.

During their four-year tenure, the Model Cities clinics provided health services desperately needed by the residents of the housing units and surrounding neighborhoods, particularly for acute health conditions and for maternal and infant care. By 1973, the clinics had served 130,000 people, with 49,000 residents receiving outpatient care. Physicians treated 88,000 residents, filled over 125,000 prescriptions, and ran 36,000 lab tests.[57] Perhaps most significantly, the clinics refocused after their first year from targeting acute problems to addressing chronic health conditions including hypertension, glaucoma, anemia, and malnutrition. With this focus, the sites became badly needed primary care clinics, as most low-income residents could not afford primary care. The clinics hired internists, pediatricians, dentists, ophthalmologists, counselors, and caseworkers, and provided free transportation for referral services at other health care institutions.[58] The clinics' prenatal, infant, and maternal care provided services previously unoffered by other clinics and only available for patients at Charity. Similarly, the clinics offered the only nonacute pediatric services, and the only dental care outside of Charity.[59] Encouraged by these successes, Black residents continued to press for further expansion of the clinics. In 1973, the Neighborhood Health

Council Concerning Health Services—representing residents of Algiers-Fischer, Carrollton, Mid-City, and Tremé, all neighborhoods outside of the Model Cities target areas—asked the municipal and state governments for support in adding Model Cities clinics to their neighborhoods as well.[60] However, within months of their request, the clinics began scaling back services and reducing staff, not adding new locations; within a year, the Model Cities program ended.

The Model Cities program faced numerous problems during its brief tenure, particularly redundancy, lack of cooperation, and fighting for control among the various agencies involved in the clinics and other health programs. A 1973 study conducted by the Public Development Assistance Foundation found a "complex web" of health services in New Orleans. The state government operated welfare, hospital, mental health, aging, and vocational rehabilitation districts that covered New Orleans, with its own leadership for each various district. At the municipal level, the NOHD, the Department of Welfare, the Council on Aging, the Community Action Agency, the City Demonstration Agency, the school board, the Housing Authority, and the City Planning Commission all carried out health activities. At the nongovernmental level, organizations like the TCA, the neighborhood councils, and the New Orleans Health Corporation all participated in health services. All the various groups administered mostly federally funded health activities and programs, but coordination and cooperation never occurred, leading to redundancy and inefficiency.[61] Additionally, many hospitals and physicians refused to take referrals for patients from the Model Cities clinics. Although the clinics established official contracts with some hospitals to deliver babies, they could only offer a small fee for services (a flat fee of $210), so most physicians refused to participate.[62] Family Health Inc. added financial scandal to its problems, with local, state, and federal investigations of the organization for misappropriations and bribery starting in 1973. As a result, the government stripped control of the health clinics from Family Health Inc.[63]

The death knell for the Model Cities clinics came from the federal government itself. In April 1973, the Nixon administration announced funding cuts for Model Cities as part of the gutting of the Great Society programs. In October 1973, the administration announced it would not renew funding for New Orleans clinics, and in 1974 it ended the Model Cities program altogether. The nonprofit New Orleans Health Corporation took over the significantly scaled-down clinics.[64] The clinics run by the NOHD at the public housing units met a similar fate. While tenant councils successfully pressed the NOHD to reopen clinics in several public housing units in the early 1970s, new HUD rules—ending the rent-free agreement for the clinics and banning further expansion of clinic space in the housing units—and continued budget cuts to the NOHD and Charity—which partially staffed the clinics—resulted in the discontinuance of most services and closure of most clinics again in 1972.[65]

The shortest-lived and most dramatically ended of the community clinics occurred with the New Orleans chapter of the Black Panther Party's People's Free Clinic. The chapter created its health clinic based on the model established by the national BPP in Oakland, initiated in 1970 and recommended for all its chapters. At these clinics, BPP members and volunteer medical professionals offered basic medical services, with a special emphasis on sickle cell anemia testing, an issue the organization argued that the government and the health care system largely ignored as it predominantly affected African Americans. Chapters also carried out health education workshops at churches, homes, and community centers. Members used their own vehicles to drive residents without transportation to their clinics, and they protested medical exclusion and exploitation. The New Orleans BPP established its free clinic first at a building near the St. Thomas housing units in May 1970; and then, when the landlord—a white district court judge—ordered its eviction after only weeks of occupancy, at the Desire housing site starting in July. The clinic offered basic medical treatment, booster shots for children, and sickle cell anemia screening, in addition to a free breakfast program that provided free meals for children that year. They also offered classes on self-determination and organized neighborhood cleanups.[66]

Many whites viewed the BPP as militant, subversive, and threatening. The police chief told Mayor Landrieu that the free breakfast program was a front to "reach young children with their hate philosophy" against the police and the "white race."[67] The police carried out surveillance of the BPP's headquarters and attempted to infiltrate the organization. Three weeks after the BPP moved into Desire, the police successfully pressured the landlord to evict the group. A week prior to the eviction date, members of the BPP discovered that two attendees at their meeting that day were undercover police officers; after a physical scuffle, the two officers escaped. Sanctioned by Mayor Landrieu, the police announced the following morning they intended to raid the house. BPP members barricaded themselves in the building and refused the order of the assembled force—over 100 local and state officers, plus armored cars—to surrender. The police lobbed tear gas and opened fire, shooting over 30,000 rounds of ammunition in thirty minutes. Somehow, no one inside was injured and the police arrested thirteen members of the BPP. Other members opened a new headquarters in a nearby apartment. Three weeks later, police and tanks arrived to evict the members, which led to a violent confrontation between the police and hundreds of Desire residents who supported the BPP. Police officers shot five residents and burned the BPP headquarters to the ground. Thus, after only several months of operation, the local government ended the BPP's health clinic.[68]

The Model Cities, public housing units, and BPP clinics provided much-needed health services during their brief existences for many of the city's most disadvantaged residents. The clinics provided not only treatment for acute health problems, but also desperately needed preventative health care. These clinics could have combined with the legally required integration of hospitals to help end the racialized health care system and close the racial health gap in New Orleans. However, like the period in the 1860s and 1870s when the Freedmen's Hospital and Charity's adoption of a nondiscrimination policy opened health care for the first time to many African Americans, the promises of better health services and improved health for Black residents never came to fruition. In fact, in the following decades Black health declined. While the mortality gap had nearly closed by the end of the 1960s, by the end of the century Black New Orleanians again suffered from a mortality rate double that of whites. Chapter 8 explores Black health and health care in the last decades of the twentieth century.

CHAPTER EIGHT

Black Health Care in the Age of Abandonment, 1975–2005

Like James Newman a generation earlier, William Adams was a leader of the city's Black medical field, as the chief of staff at Flint Goodridge, and the larger Black community, through his work with the NAACP and the New Orleans Improvement Association. In May 1958, Adams testified before the House Committee on Interstate Commerce's hearings on amendments to the Hospital Construction Act. Adams spoke of the many barriers Black doctors faced and his determination to practice in New Orleans and also help lead the fight for equality:

> The many restrictions which have been placed upon the Negroes of the state are under attack and your humble servant is now one of the plaintiffs in the bus desegregation case. Although you know that the physician has his hands full, we are trying to put ourselves in line with the community, to see what we can do toward helping to lead our people out of the morass in which they find themselves. We are not compelled to stay in the South. Many of us can practice elsewhere and some are able to financially able to leave, but we feel that you cannot solve a problem by running away from it, so we tried to stay.[1]

For over five decades, Adams stayed in New Orleans and worked at Flint Goodridge. He remained with the hospital for its move to Central City, through its early uncertainty, its successes and expansion, and its losses and reductions since the late 1960s, all while maintaining his role as a civil rights activist.

By 1983, though, the eighty-two-year-old Adams warned that he might have reached a breaking point. That year, Dillard University sold Flint Goodridge to National Medical Enterprises, Inc. (NME), a hospital corporation. Dillard made this sale even though it had twice agreed to sell the hospital to a group of fifty Black physicians, including Adams, who had promised to keep the hospital open. After NME offered more money up front—although less money overall—Dillard instead pulled out of the deal and sold the hospital to NME. Adams and members of the staff feared the worst, that NME would shut the hospital down. Adams also feared he might have to move out of New

Orleans to find a new hospital that would grant him admitting privileges, necessary to have clients as a surgeon. Beyond these personal concerns, Adams lamented the economic impact of the loss of hundreds of Black jobs and the adverse effect on the Black community. "It will have a bad effect on the Black morale because everybody likes to feel like they own something," he told PBS reporters in February 1983. He believed the hospital's closure would be especially difficult for Black youth who aspired to one day be a doctor at Flint Goodridge. In his opinion, the closing of the hospital would result in "nothing for the Black children to look up to, to look forward to, to say one of these days I can be part of this thing." As a boy growing up in New Orleans, Adams had that dream, had that place to look up, and had been part of "this thing" for nearly 20,000 days. Like Adams predicted, though, those days were numbered. In May 1985, NME closed the hospital and distributed its bed licenses to the other hospitals it controlled in the region.[2]

This chapter examines Black health care in New Orleans in the age of crisis, from the late 1970s until Hurricane Katrina. It explores the factors that led to the decline, sale, and closure of Flint Goodridge, primarily the hospital's declining finances due to low levels of reimbursement from Medicare and Medicaid, inability to attract donors or investors, and lack of government funding. This chapter also explores the growing corporatization of health care. While Flint Goodridge became a victim of this process, hospitals like Tulane and Ochsner thrived because they served a wealthier, whiter clientele and received support from hospital companies and continued aid from HEAL. Finally, this chapter details the further decline of Charity, principally caused by the state's continued reduction in funding. By the 2000s, Charity provided care for 75 percent of the city's Black hospital patients as both quality of care at the hospital and the racial health disparity worsened.

Flint Goodridge's Decline

By 1977, 56 percent of patients at Flint Goodridge used Medicare or Medicaid.[3] Over the next four years, that figure climbed to 70 percent.[4] The high percentage of patients on Medicare and Medicaid caused revenue to plummet. Every year of the 1970s until its final closure in 1985, the Board of Management reported that actual cost of care for Medicaid and Medicare patients far exceeded government compensation. In response, administrators attempted nearly annually to negotiate with the government to increase the compensation amount. Although often successful in gaining modest increases, the increased amounts still did not meet the costs to the hospital. Additionally, because every patient's case required an individual claim, approved payment to the hospital occurred months after the actual expense, if at all. Often, claims became bogged down in bureaucratic wrangling or rejected by the government. While Medicare and Medicaid partially helped the hospital sustain as paying patients left, the delayed, underpaid, or denied compensation for procedures led to increasing annual losses. By 1981, the hospital reported that the government owed it an estimated $600,000 for unpaid or partially paid claims.[5]

The use of the hospital primarily by Medicaid and Medicare patients also further stigmatized the hospital. Ironically, the 1969 expansion report noted the worry that many Lower Ninth Ward residents—primarily working class—would not use the hospital because they had an "image of our institution as being concerned only with middle-class needs."[6] Few in the city made this claim by the mid-1970s. Indeed, the 1977 report by HEW's Office of Civil Rights noted that most New Orleanians thought of Flint Goodridge—and Charity—as the "hospitals for the poor."[7] Other factors hurt the hospital as well, such as the declining reputation of care as the institution's dire financial situation prevented the acquisition of needed equipment and kept staff numbers low. The declining reputation of the surrounding neighborhood, as the Magnolia Projects became infamous for high crime and drug use, kept away patients. Patients also faced difficulty in reaching the hospital due to lack of public transportation to Flint Goodridge, desperately needed in a city where many residents did not own a car. Additionally, fees that were annually raised to offset losses and competition for paying patients—and nurses—kept patient numbers low.[8] These problems drove away many of the higher-income, paying patients. As noted by physician George Thomas Jr. in a 1986 interview, even though most Black residents wanted to sustain the hospital, "nobody wants to make the sacrifice . . . they don't want to put themselves at risk to support Black institutions."[9]

The hospital carried out several measures to cut costs and increase revenue. It rented out properties and subcontracted food and laundry services. In 1971, the hospital closed the outpatient clinic and reduced spending and staff for the emergency room. In 1972, it closed the third floor and seventeen total beds, followed by the closure of the childcare center in 1973. The hospital began replacing full-time workers with part-timers and further reduced each department to "absolutely necessary personnel." Still short on funding, the hospital began borrowing hundreds of thousands from local banks at high interest rates and unsuccessfully applying for more federal grants. None of these measures made a significant impact.[10]

The hospital still tried to meet its three main goals. To address its first goal of training Black medical professionals, Flint Goodridge served as a medical training center for students of Meharry Medical College and Dillard's registered nursing program. The hospital also started new partnerships with several local programs. It offered experience for a licensed practical nursing program with the Orleans Parish School Board, Delgado Community College's radiology program, the Tulane School of Public Health and Social Work, and Xavier University's College of Pharmacy in the 1970s and 1980s. Through these programs, Flint Goodridge provided invaluable opportunities for Black medical professionals, still severely underrepresented in the health care field.

To address its second goal of addressing public health issues, Flint Goodridge tackled problems that particularly afflicted the Black community. In 1971, the hospital began offering weight loss clinics to address issues like diabetes and hypertension. In 1972, it partnered with the federal government to offer screening and education on sickle cell anemia. In many ways, Black New Orleanians needed the hospital more than they had in decades, as white flight drained municipal resources and deindustrialization and the oil bust of the 1980s drove up rates of unemployment and poverty, with an accompanying rise in health problems.[11] With 58 percent of families living below the poverty line, Central City proved to be perhaps the hardest hit neighborhood, and Flint Goodridge's leaders argued that the hospital "must re-establish itself as a needed community center" in an area "characterized by unemployment, underemployment, lack of quality education and training; inadequate housing, social services, health facilities, and plagued by drugs and crime." Ultimately though, the community outreach and public health initiatives of the period paled in comparison to the hospital's earlier efforts in the 1930s, 1940s, and 1950s due to the hospital's financial woes.[12]

The hospital's ability to reach its third goal, traditional hospital care for as many Black patients as possible, gradually withered. From a high of 164 patient beds in the early 1960s, budget shortages led the hospital to cut the number of beds to eighty-one by 1980. Flint Goodridge was operating on fumes. The hospital owed over $500,000 to vendors, over $600,000 to Dillard, nearly $400,000 to the Internal Revenue Service (IRS), and hundreds of thousands to local banks.[13] Financially burdened by the hospital's mounting debt, Dillard's leaders decided to end its affiliation with Flint Goodridge in 1981 and sell the hospital. Initially, Dillard struck a deal for $1.5 million with Doctor Hospitals Group, Inc. (DHGI), a group of fifty local Black doctors that planned to keep the hospital open. Dillard reneged on the deal after Humana offered $2 million but renewed its agreement with DHGI in April 1982 when DHGI increased its bid to $3.2 million, with $2 million up front and $500,000 due within six months. Representatives of DHGI told the *Times Picayune* that although they planned to convert the hospital to a "for-profit" model, they would continue operating Flint Goodridge as a "patient-care oriented" facility and keep the hospital as the "base for Black medicine in New Orleans."[14] Dillard president Samuel Cook told the *Louisiana Weekly* that ten other groups had submitted higher bids, but the school chose DHGI because its "main concern was to keep the hospital in the community." The other groups, Cook detailed, were primarily interested in acquiring the hospital for its coveted 128 bed licenses and transferring them to another hospital.[15] Despite this pledge to keep the hospital in the community, Dillard again voided the contract when the university demanded DHGI immediately pay the $500,000 originally agreed due in six months. Only able to raise $300,000— from the physicians themselves—Dillard cancelled the contract in June 1982. The two sides began negotiating again in October, but instead Dillard sold the hospital in January 1983 to NME, a medical conglomerate with five hospitals in New Orleans and more than forty nationwide, for $1.8 million. NME senior vice president Gerald Stevens stated that among "different avenues" the company was considering leasing the hospital to Black doctors "so they can continue the heritage." For three years, the hospital hung in limbo, with minimal staff and a small operating budget.[16] Flint Goodridge's staff fought to keep the hospital open. They contacted physicians and emergency rooms to ask them to send their patients to the hospital and serviced the community with health fairs where they provided free vision, hearing, sickle cell, and diabetes testing.[17]

In April 1985, DHGI made a final offer for the hospital, reaching an agreement with NME to buy, renovate, and operate the hospital for $4.2 million; as happened earlier, though, NME backed out and in May 1985 shut the hospital down. NME's leadership argued that declining admission numbers made running the hospital financially unfeasible; critics claimed NME never invested enough money into the hospital. NME transferred the bed licenses to other hospitals it controlled. Ninety years after first starting as the one-room Phyllis Wheatley Sanitarium, Flint Goodridge Hospital permanently closed its doors.[18] Unsurprisingly, the sale caused controversy in the Black community. President Cook defended the deal. Cook cited the reason as primarily financial, although he admitted the hospital had actually made a profit the last couple of months before the sale. Cook argued the financial losses resulted from several factors. Desegregation of the city's formerly all-white hospitals drew away upper-income Black patients. The high number of individuals covered by Medicaid and Medicare—90 percent by the 1980s—diminished patient fees. Cook also argued that "tragic mismanagement" and "financial irregularities" by the hospital's administrators further drained the coffers. Cook claimed that Dillard held onto the hospital "for sentimental reasons" despite losses and that although Dillard had made "concessions" during twenty months of negotiations with DHGI, their offers had not been "serious." Cook also attributed the hospital's demise to "the loss of broad of community support," blaming Black residents for not further using or contributing to the hospital: "If the Black community is not willing to pay the price to support it, and if the Black doctors aren't going to put patients in, what can we do?" Although "painful" to let it go, Cook argued that the effect on the Black community would be "more philosophical and psychological than practical."[19] Others vehemently disagreed. Keith Butler, a local investment banker who attempted to aid the doctors' group in raising money, told the New York Times that the sale was "part of a continuing pattern, a demolition of minority businesses that once thrived in the deep segregated South." Group member Dr. Dwight McKenna argued the failed bid "spelled the death knell for Black medicine in this community."[20] In many ways, Butler proved correct. Flint Goodridge's closure proved to be part of the "death knell for Black medicine," not just in New Orleans, but throughout the country as many Black hospitals shut down. Between 1961 and 1988, forty-nine Black hospitals closed nationwide, most the victims of the same problems that plagued Flint Goodridge, which was one of seven Black hospitals closed in 1985 alone.[21]

Corporate Health Care

What befell Flint Goodridge Hospital reflected the larger racialized health care system. While Black hospitals like Flint Goodridge and public hospitals like Charity struggled to remain solvent, private corporate hospitals prospered. A 1984 study found that investors earned a return of 25 percent on hospitals.[22] By 1980, corporations that owned multiple hospitals controlled 30 percent of hospital beds in America, and the numbers increased in the following years.[23] Many of the companies adopted a "polycorporate structure," with a parent company owning hospitals to maintain its tax-exempt status but owning other for-profit ventures.[24] Beyond hospitals, companies invested in other health care ventures like nursing homes, and the newly formed health maintenance organizations (HMOs) and preferred provider organizations (PPOs), which were backed by the Nixon administration. Hospitals attempted to create "integrated delivery systems" by buying suburban hospitals and private practices, with physicians at those facilities referring their patients to the main hospital, where they received specialized care.[25] Independent hospitals increasingly turned to hospital companies as federal funding decreased and costs increased—driven by rising prices for medical equipment and new technology. Others unable to secure hospital company support closed. As a result, the number of hospitals declined 17 percent nationwide from 1980 to 2000. In the 1990s and early 2000s, surviving independent hospitals turned to local hospital systems through mergers to compete with the larger medical companies.[26]

New Orleans experienced these shifts, including the growing presence of hospital companies. This could be seen not only in HAI's investment in Tulane's hospital in the early 1970s, but also in hospitals throughout the city, which became increasingly owned by large hospital corporations.[27] By the 2000s, national hospital companies Universal Health Services and Tenet and regional companies like Tulane/HCA and Ochsner owned most of the hospitals in the area. These companies benefited greatly from public–private partnerships and arrangements, primarily in the form of tax-exempt bonds to build new hospitals. Other hospitals created their own hospital systems in New Orleans. In 1990, the Board of Trustees approved the establishment of the Touro Infirmary Foundation. In 1994, Touro formed its own HMO. Touro continued to operate as its own entity, occupying increasingly large swaths of what had become known as the Touro neighborhood in Uptown.[28]

Funding from HEAL also allowed both Tulane and Ochsner to grow significantly. Through HEAL, taxpayers funded not just the hospitals themselves, but the infrastructure that supported the hospitals, and indirectly the resulting gentrification of the surrounding areas. HEAL passed tax-exempt bonds of $3.3 million in 1973 for Tulane's hospital to build a parking deck, $31.3 million for hospital expansion in 1985, and $9.8 million in 1998 for expansion of the parking deck. In 1995, HEAL issued a $56.2 million bond to expand the Ochsner Medical Foundation Hospital. Not only outside of the Medical District, the hospital existed just outside of city bounds in Jefferson, and had no connection to the proposed New Orleans Medical Center Complex. Nevertheless, HEAL justified the tax-exempt support of the private hospital as an economic boost for the region, as Ochsner projected to add

880 new jobs, as well as bring in an estimated 144,000 new patients from outside of the area. By the early 2000s, Ochsner had become the region's largest medical system and the area's biggest employer, with more than 7,000 employees. However, while both hospitals created large numbers of jobs, as acknowledged by HEAL, most of the higher-wage, high-skilled positions went to individuals from outside of New Orleans. While this brought in some higher-income residents, many chose to live in the suburbs, bringing tax benefits primarily to white areas. In contrast, as noted by HEAL, the "less skilled tend to come from the local community." These low-paying jobs offered salaries comparable to domestic or service sector work. Additionally, to accommodate the hospitals' growth, local governments paid for expanded municipal services but received no direct tax benefits from the hospitals due to their tax-exempt status.[29] Finally, patients at both Tulane and Ochsner remained predominantly white, upper-income individuals, many from outside of the New Orleans area.

The Widening Gap in the Two-Tiered System

While these two institutions thrived and New Orleans's health care economy grew, the gap in the two-tiered health care system widened. In the 1980s, the Reagan administration began gutting New Deal and Great Society programs aimed at helping those in need, exacerbating the differences in the two-tiered health care system. As problems worsened for low-income residents, hospitals that served Black patients shuttered. Two served limited clientele: the Illinois Central Railroad Company closed its employee hospital in 1970, and the federal government closed the Marine Hospital in 1981. A significant loss occurred with the shuttering of Bywater Hospital. Started as a small, private, whites-only hospital in the Bywater neighborhood in the 1940s, the owners sold it to Lifemark Company in 1972 as the neighborhood become predominantly Black with white flight. In the 1970s, the hospital was the closest hospital for the mostly Black residents of St. Claude, the Upper Ninth Ward, the Lower Ninth Ward, and the increasingly Black-majority Bywater. In 1982, Lifemark closed the hospital and converted it to a private drug rehabilitation center to make a larger profit.[30]

As these hospitals closed, Charity and the NOHD's remaining clinics treated even more low-income Black residents, even as these clinics too declined. While residents and tenant councils pressed the city for more clinics, budget constraints—driven largely by the city's shrinking tax base due to white flight—forced the NOHD to operate the existing clinics as "multi-service centers" that covered multiple neighborhoods. This presented problems as many low-income residents had no access to a car and New Orleans had an underdeveloped, underfunded public transportation system. The NOHD noted that "geographical distance and inadequate transportation" to clinics and Charity worsened health problems as they "resulted in neglect of simple health problems with attention being given only to severe and acute health needs as they present themselves to the hospital."[31] In 1975, the NOHD estimated that 92,000 people lived in service areas of their "multi-service centers." The 95 percent Black clientele had an average median family income of $3,140. Only 15 percent could even partially pay for medical care. The NOHD envisioned these service centers as the main entry point into the medical system. They would provide basic primary care, with consultation and further care provided by Charity, as well as 100 private physicians that would receive reimbursement from the NOHD.[32]

Budget constraints and other problems limited implementation of this program. When Dutch Morial became mayor in 1978, his transition team conducted a study of the NOHD and found a deeply troubled agency that was "not a modern department." Structurally, the NOHD suffered from deep fragmentation and a poorly designed administrative base. The agency had little to no liaison with other health-related agencies or the private health sector. The NOHD faced understaffing due to low salaries impacting the ability to fill vacancies. Budget constraints severely limited the agency's capabilities. The NOHD relied on federal funding for 90 percent of its budget and increasing cuts under Nixon—and later Reagan—devastated the agency. In client services, the NOHD offered no health education or preventative services, and the services it did offer duplicated many of those provided by Charity and the remnants of the New Orleans Health Corporation clinics. Jurisdictional and financial limits prevented the department carrying out rodent control in the infested public housing units. Morial's team rated the NOHD programs overall as "low quality." Unfortunately, the NOHD had little data gathering and evaluation to improve services or reduce redundancy. Morial's team made several recommendations to improve the NOHD. Among multiple ideas, they suggested modernizing and restructuring the department and improving coordination with other health-related groups. They also advocated for improving the city's health care for the prison population, better coordination and quality of care of mental health activities, and restarting the immunization program through the school system.[33]

Little changed in the ensuing years. In fact, the NOHD's services declined substantially over the next three decades. The budget problem proved to be perhaps the most significant issue. As tax revenue declined in the 1970s and 1980s with white flight and economic recessions, city funding decreased, increasing reliance on state and federal funding. However, the state also reduced funding, and federal funding varied under presidential administrations, with deep cuts under Reagan. The 1984 NOHD Budget Report Summary noted that funding cuts led to reduction in lead poisoning analysis and increased waiting times at clinics due to layoffs.[34] The 1985 NOHD budget statement to the city council predicted a "bleak financial future." The department noted decreased city, state, and federal funding even as the NOHD had taken on more programs. "It appears that the point of diminishing returns is near," it stated. "Further cuts will greatly influence marginal productivity due to burnout and stress." At the same time, it noted that residents placed greater demands on the department due to the region's economic downturn.[35]

In 1986, the state cut funding for Medicaid, Aid to Families with Dependent Children (AFDC), and food stamps, placing an even greater demand on the NOHD. Due to budget cuts, the NOHD announced it was closing the Mid-City and Guste Apartment clinics, as well as reducing sickle cells clinics and the nascent HIV/AIDS program.[36] Cuts in services continued in 1987 for programs for the elderly, tuberculosis patients, sexually transmitted infection patients, and pest control. Previously under the auspices of the police department, the city transferred the emergency medical services (EMS) program to NOHD, even as funding decreased; by 1986, New Orleans had the lowest per-capita EMS expenditure of any Southern city, with a budget of less than half that of other comparably sized urban centers, and still faced further cuts in 1987. As a result, New Orleans had the slowest emergency response time for any Southern city.[37]

That same year, federal funding for the NOHD reached a low of $899,000. In subsequent years, federal funding grew, but primarily in the form of grants for new programs. Overall funding declined again in the early 1990s due to state cuts. In 1991, the NOHD had a budget of $13.72 million for services for 496,938 people. In comparison, Atlanta's health department budget was $41 million for its 630,000 residents and Baltimore's health department's budget was $103 million for its 750,000 residents. With this funding, in addition to running clinics like the Delgado Clinic, which averaged 25,604 visits per year in the 1980s, the NOHD carried out communicable disease control, HIV/AIDS programs, Medicaid's Early and Periodic Screening, Diagnostic, and Treatment Program, lead poisoning testing, services for those affected by homelessness, the Drug-Free Program, rat control, hypertension programs, sickle cell programs, and many other services. The NOHD continued to apply and receive federal grants for new programs, but the funding was temporary and further spread its efforts thinner. The declining city budget offset many of these gains, thus even as the department gained federal and state grants in the mid- to late 1990s, it cut clinic staff and services.[38]

While the NOHD clinics slowly atrophied, Charity closed its system of satellite clinics altogether in the mid-1980s due to state budget cuts. Coupled with the closing of Flint Goodridge's and the Model Cities clinics in the 1970s, New Orleans had virtually no primary care options for low-income residents. "Decisions, personalities, circumstances, failed commitments, dwindling resources and the absence of critical community input and participation all combined to bring the resourceful primary health care era in New Orleans to an end," stated the NOHD. Even when the clinics did operate, they usually referred patients to Charity for further care. Patients had to then go through the afore-described byzantine process of the hospital determining their eligibility, and then go again for a referral, before finally being given an appointment. The time length from the initial referral to actual care was about two months in the 1970s; by the 2000s, it was six months. The 1991 NOHD report's conclusion decried health options for the city's poorest and minority residents: "the current state of health affairs in New Orleans is bleak at best."[39]

As in earlier periods, community organizations attempted to fill the void. In 1972, civil rights leader Oretha Castle Haley founded the New Orleans Sickle Cell Anemia Foundation. The group initiated sickle cell public awareness campaigns and fundraising drives, which it used to create a mobile unit that offered detection and genetic counseling services throughout Louisiana. It also held a research symposium in conjunction with Tulane, LSU, and Charity, and created a sickle cell library.[40] In 1987, the St. Thomas Housing Redevelopment Council—a public housing tenant council—worked with Sisters of Charity nuns to create the St. Thomas Health Services Clinic with some physicians from Ochsner volunteering their services. In 1998, a coalition of local musicians led by the Union of New Orleans Musicians American Federation of Musicians (AFM) Local 174-96 and faculty from LSU—with support from Tulane, Loyola University's School of Nursing, radio station WWOZ, the Daughters of Charity, the Performing Arts Medicine Association, and several Mardi Gras krewes—established the New Orleans Musicians' Clinic in the LSU Health Sciences Center. The clinic provided services for local musicians.[41] However, community organizations and the NOHD clinics could not adequately meet the health care needs of low-income residents. Charity served as the main health care option for these New Orleanians. When Flint shut its doors in 1986, most patients transferred to Charity, which was struggling due to the state's repeated budget cuts and the renewal of the practice of siphoning federal funding intended for reimbursing care provided for the hospital's Medicaid and Medicare patients. The building and equipment deteriorated, leading the hospital to lose accreditation repeatedly throughout the 1980s, and the quality of care decreased significantly.

Charity's experience in the period reflected the larger struggle of urban public hospitals in the United States, which also treated most cities' minoritized, low-income, uninsured, and Medicaid/Medicare patients. Many private hospitals "dumped" Medicaid and Medicare patients and patients whose insurance ran out on public hospitals like Charity as private hospitals focused on making a profit. With budget lines for advertising, larger rooms, advanced equipment, and better overall conditions, owner-invested hospitals drained public hospitals of paying patients, thus further undermining their precarious financial situation and widening the already existing health care gap. As a result, those who needed care the most received treatment in distressed hospitals. Many low-income patients, especially the uninsured, used emergency rooms for primary medical care, further draining public hospital resources.[42]

Federal legislation attempted to address some of these problems. Congress passed the Emergency Medical Treatment and Active Labor Act in 1986, which made it illegal for hospitals to "dump" Medicaid/Medicare patients in public hospitals and expanded Medicaid eligibility in 1988. However, the practice of "dumping" continued, and even with Medicaid expansion, only 19 percent of New Orleans residents were eligible in a city with a poverty rate of 28 percent. This mostly resulted from state policy, which kept the maximum income threshold for Medicaid at the second lowest level for any state.[43] Moreover, the NOHD assessed that most residents did not know about their eligibility under the expansion due to a lack of a public information campaign on that or any of the Medicaid services. Additionally, while 1,254 physicians citywide were licensed to offer services for Medicaid patients in 1991, only fifty-eight doctors treated Medicaid patients, a reflection of inaccessibility and unwillingness of many physicians to become involved in Medicaid services.[44] Furthermore, many New Orleanians had no health insurance through their employer. Nearly 21 percent of residents, predominantly African Americans, had no health insurance at all. Twice as many Black residents were uninsured compared with whites.[45]

With these conditions, two-tiered health care persisted. Insured, middle- and upper-income, mostly white residents received primary care from private physicians and through HMOs. For hospital care, they used predominantly white, investor-owned, high-quality hospitals like Ochsner and Tulane. In contrast, the NOHD clinics, community clinics, and Charity provided care to the uninsured, Medicaid and Medicare recipients, the low-income, and mostly Black residents. New Orleans leaders recognized the existence of this health care divide. In its 1991 annual assessment, the NOHD wrote: "the network of health care services available to citizens of New Orleans is stratified much as the demographics and income indicators suggest. The poor and near poor use free or subsidized services for mostly episodic, rather than continuous care. As a result, much of their health care needs are met in emergency rooms." The NOHD reported that low-income patients primarily used Charity's emergency room for health care. Many low-income residents also used the emergency room as their primary pediatrics care; over half of outpatient patients were thirteen or younger. The heavy reliance on the emergency room for all medical conditions, coupled with reduced staffing due to budget cuts, resulted in an average emergency room wait time of twelve hours at Charity.[46]

Low-income Black patients also increasingly used the emergency room at the Methodist Hospital in New Orleans East. As previously detailed, hospital founders and city leaders envisioned the hospital playing a significant role in promoting the white suburb within city bounds. However, the demographics of New Orleans East shifted in the 1980s as middle-class African Americans seeking a suburban lifestyle moved to the area and large-scale apartment complexes began accepting housing vouchers for low-income residents. This transition, as well as the loss of higher-paying petroleum, port-related, and manufacturing jobs, led to a second wave of white flight, as whites moved to suburbs outside of New Orleans East in the late 1980s and 1990s, making the area majority Black by 2000. With this shift, low-income residents began increasingly using the emergency room at the Methodist Hospital, the only hospital in the area. By the time of Katrina, the former white flight hospital had become the second most used hospital by Black residents.[47]

Charity remained the primary source of health care for Black residents. The NOHD reported that Charity admitted 169,397 patients in 1990. Of these patients, 75 percent were people of color, with 67 percent African American and 6 percent Latino. The hospital and its clinics had 375,000 outpatient visits. Of this group, over 87 percent were people of color, with 80 percent Black and 5 percent Latino.[48] With this increased usage, overcrowding, and long waits, a change needed to happen. Either Charity had to expand, or private hospitals needed to accept more low-income patients. Not surprisingly, the leaders of the private hospitals and the OPMS favored the former. In a 1983 report, the OPMS Charity Hospital Study Committee examined whether the city still "needed" Charity. In a survey of eleven private hospitals, only seven stated they provided "some care" for low-income residents, and only two hospitals indicated they would be willing to accept more low-income patients if Charity closed. Rather than push these hospitals to take more low-income patients to relieve the burden of the already overcrowded Charity—which had 1,642 beds despite having a "utilizable capacity" of 900 and still continually turned away patients, including for needed surgeries—the OPMS recommended that Charity add an additional 1,200 beds. The OPMS called for upgrades and renovations of every basic structure, equipment, the emergency room, plumbing, electrical, and sterilization equipment, all described as in "dire need." It recommended the administrative system be completed "overhauled" as it had "little accountability, low morale, lack of productivity, and no long-range planning."[49]

The 1983 report also cited the joint administration by LSU and Tulane, which "frequently had competing interests," as one of the main issues. Under their 1974 agreement with the state to run the hospital, LSU and Tulane could prevent any programs or activities at Charity Hospital that they viewed as counter to their interests. For example, when Tulane established its own hospital, the university directed the revenue-producing research projects it had previously carried out at Charity to its own hospital and fought to prevent similar research projects from being awarded to Charity, preventing badly needed income for the hospital.[50]

To counter this problem of administration, the state legislature created the Louisiana Health Care Authority (LHCA), which assumed control of all nine hospitals in the statewide Charity system in 1991. In the "strategic report" it issued to the state legislature, the LHCA identified New Orleans's Charity Hospital's biggest problems, many the same identified by the OPMS eight years earlier. The continuing underfunding had led to reductions in the number of medical residents. Low salaries drove away many employees. Due to understaffing, patients faced long waits for procedures. Much of the equipment was outdated or damaged and needed upgrades and repairs. In fact, the LHCA argued that the entire building should have been replaced thirty years earlier. All these issues negatively impacted quality of care.

As if to underscore its point, in 1991 Charity lost its hospital accreditation due to its problems, nearly forcing its closure. In 1992, the LHCA purchased Hotel Dieu from the Daughters of Charity, intending to include it in the New Orleans Medical Center Complex. The LHCA changed the name from Hotel Dieu to the University Hospital, with the intention of using that and not

Charity as the main teaching hospital and announced plans to close Charity within the following five years. In the interim, the LHCA asked the accreditation commission to allow Charity to continue operating without making improvements the commission mandated to restore accreditation as they estimated the costs to exceed $20 million. However public backlash over the willingness of the LHCA to allow patient care in a facility deemed unsafe forced the LHCA to carry out the improvements and the commission restored the hospital's accreditation in 1994. The spending on the improvements also halted the construction of a critical care tower next to the University Hospital, intended to placate physicians at LSU who wanted their own space to treat private patients, mostly "skimmed" from Charity. Ultimately, the state legislature rejected the idea of closing Charity.[51]

In 1997, citing poor leadership, excessive spending, the purchase of the Hotel Dieu, and the creation of high-paying "unnecessary" positions for cronies, the state legislature voted to abolish the LHCA and turned administration of the Charity system over to LSU. LSU again reached a partnership arrangement with Tulane to coadminister Charity. However, both schools focused primarily on their own hospitals: Tulane on the Tulane University Hospital, and LSU on the University Hospital, which they used for their paying patients. Both schools also continued to "dump" low-income patients on Charity and "skim" the high-reimbursement patients from Charity for their own hospitals. In addition, Charity continued to suffer from state siphoning of its Medicaid and Medicare reimbursement. Congress awarded Disproportionate Share Hospital (DSH) funding for the statewide Charity system to help offset the costs of providing care for so many Medicaid and Medicare patients, reaching $4.2 billion annually by 1994. However, the funding did not go directly to Charity, but rather to the state Department of Health and Hospitals (DHH). The DHH reallocated funding to other projects, including for private psychiatric facilities. The state also used part of the funding to pay for budget shortfalls in other areas. Congress passed legislation to attempt to prevent this practice by the states and threatened to cut all DSH funding to Louisiana due to its misuse. Under Governor Mike Foster, Secretary of Health and Hospitals Bobby Jindal negotiated a deal with the federal government to only reduce the funding by $400 million—still a devastating loss that hurt Charity's patients—and pledged to end the practice of reallocating the funding. However, the practice continued in the following years.[52]

By the 1990s, Charity had become the embodiment of the abandonment of the public health care system. Rather than address the hospital's needs, which resulted in near-perpetual crisis, state leaders and hospital administrators carried out superficial measures that fixed none of the problems. In 1999, the state stripped administrative co-control of Charity from Tulane, blaming the school for the hospital's failures. That same year, a state budget deficit almost resulted in the closure of 15 percent of beds, averted only by the influx of money from a settlement with tobacco companies. The legislature prevented a mandated closing of the hospital due to the missed deadline that year to install fire sprinklers by writing new legislation that gave the hospital until 2005, with funding for the improvements finally occurring in 2002. Budget cuts from the legislature continued nearly every year, even as the federal government increased DSH funding, with money continuing to be diverted to other projects or budget shortfalls in other areas. These cuts occurred even after the legislature ordered Charity and the other hospitals in the Charity system to assume control of—and payments for—hospital care for prisoners. In 2003, when the DHH diverted $334 million of DSH funding intended for the Charity system, the legislature cut Charity's funding by $27 million, leading to the elimination of fifty-nine jobs, the diabetic clinic, nine operating rooms, and the W-16 walk-in clinic, which annually provided free care for over 40,000 patients.[53]

Some emergency room patients from Charity ended up at the reopened Bywater Hospital. In 2003, a group of local physicians purchased the former Bywater Hospital from Lifemark—still being used a drug rehabilitation facility—and reopened the hospital. From 2003 to 2005, the emergency room at the Bywater Hospital admitted 10,000 primarily low-income, uninsured Black patients. However, due to low finances as an independent hospital, the Bywater Hospital closed in March 2005.[54]

As state cuts further eroded patient care at Charity, the state and LSU sought to decrease services and patient numbers, rather than restore funding. In 2003, pushed by LSU, the state legislature passed Act 206, which established a new means test for use of Charity. Patients now had to be below 200 percent of the federal poverty threshold to receive treatment. This legislation led to a slight reduction in patient usage at Charity at the expense of care for residents who fell slightly above the cutoff point. Additionally, the bill authorized LSU to cut spending at Charity by up to 35 percent without permission from the legislature.[55] By 2004, the average wait time for emergency room services was twelve hours and for an appointment at a clinic it was six months.[56] Despite this, in a survey on potentially closing the Charity system and pooling the money to provide care for the indigent in other hospitals, over 91 percent of New Orleanians favored keeping Charity open.[57]

Increased oil revenues buoyed Charity's budget for 2004 and 2005. Additionally, the new administration of Governor Kathleen Blanco finally ended the practice of diverting DSH funding, further shoring up the hospital's finances. Nevertheless, LSU continued to push for closing Charity, arguing the conditions at the hospital would again lead to the loss of accreditation. The legislature threatened to decrease funding for LSU if hospital administrators did not address the long waiting period and the closure of beds—by 2005, the hospital was down to 700 beds—a situation the legislature partially created through years of diverting the federal DSH funding. Critics lambasted LSU's administration of Charity, arguing the school was more focused on providing training for its medical students than for patient care.[58] Unperturbed, in May 2005, LSU released a report that proposed closing both Charity and the University Hospital and building a new academic university hospital, despite the lack of political support for the plan.[59] By 2005, African Americans comprised 75 percent of Charity's patients. Eighty-five percent of patients earned less than $20,000 annually, and over half had no medical insurance—other hospitals in the city averaged only 4 percent of patients without insurance, and combined served 17 percent of uncompensated cases, compared with the 83 percent provided for by Charity.[60]

As the gap in the two-tiered health care system widened, the racial health gap increased, exacerbated by increasingly negative social determinants of health for the Black population including low-quality education and high dropout rates in the underfunded public school system; high Black unemployment—triple the rate of whites—and underemployment as the loss of higher-paying port-related manufacturing and transportation jobs were replaced with low-paying jobs in the service sectors; Black median income half that of whites; a Black poverty rate more than triple that of white residents; residential segregation and racial concentration of poverty; increasing crime, drug, homicide, and incarceration rates; and the HIV/AIDS epidemic.[61]

Health hazards, which the 1929 Comprehensive Plan and other policies codified, continued to severely impact Black health. Several environmental racism issues witnessed increasing attention in the 1980s and 1990s. Starting in the 1980s, grassroots activists began using the term "Cancer Alley" to refer to the eighty-five-mile stretch from Baton Rouge to New Orleans that contained over 130 petrochemical plants and refineries. Annually, these sites produced millions of tons of hazardous waste and contained hazardous waste incinerators and chemical landfills. Studies began linking working for and living near these sites and the state's high rate of cancer, the second highest in the nation.⁶² In 1994, residents filed class action lawsuits against the municipal government for building the HANO subdivisions Gordon Plaza and Press Park in the 1960s and 1970s atop the ninety-five-acre Agriculture Street Dump in the Desire neighborhood. That same year, the U.S. Environmental Protection Agency declared the toxic area a Superfund site.⁶³ Also in 1994, residents of the public housing units filed a class action lawsuit against the city for decades of lead poisoning. Since the 1970s, tenants reported hundreds of cases of lead poisoning directly to HANO, but the agency refused to act, leading to a series of lawsuits and federal investigations and culminating in the class action suit in 1994.⁶⁴ Both the lawsuits for Gordon Plaza and the housing units lingered in the courts for decades.

All these negative social determinants of health led to high Black rates of diabetes, heart disease, stroke, cancer, infant mortality, maternal mortality, asthma, lead poisoning, and HIV/AIDS; a rate of mortality double that of whites; and low life expectancy.⁶⁵ With Black health and health care at a new nadir by the new millennium, New Orleans desperately needed a radical change. In 2005, Hurricane Katrina fundamentally altered health care, explored in the concluding chapter.

Conclusion
Black Health and Health Care after Katrina

Malik Rahim had been an activist for nearly four decades by August 2005. Born in 1947 in the Algiers neighborhood of New Orleans, Rahim descended from a lineage of activists, including his grandparents who were members of the Universal Negro Improvement Association and African Communities League and contemporaries of Queen Mother Moore, the Louisiana-born civil rights leader and Black nationalist. Rahim dropped out of high school to join the Navy in 1965. During training in Los Angeles, Rahim became involved with Maulana Karenga's pan-Africanist US Organization. After a tour of combat in Vietnam, Rahim returned to New Orleans in 1967 and helped lead the local chapter of the Black Panthers. With the BPP, he helped run the free breakfast program, neighborhood cleanups, community patrols, and the health clinic in the Desire housing projects. Wounded by police during the "Showdown at Desire," a jury acquitted Rahim of attempted murder charges. As a community organizer in California in the 1980s, Rahim fought for affordable housing and tenants' rights. In the 1990s he returned to New Orleans where he established a housing and job training program for ex-offenders and fought against the death penalty and to release the Angola Three.[1]

Rahim's experiences as an activist and community organizer served him well in the aftermath of Hurricane Katrina. A week after the hurricane made landfall, Rahim, Scott Crow, Sharon Johnson, and Ferris Bowles started the Common Ground health clinic in Algiers. As told by Rahim in a 2006 interview, the group started the clinic to provide care for Black residents abandoned by the federal government and threatened by armed vigilante groups of whites that refused to let them cross over the bridge into Gretna:

> Right after the hurricane, we came to the realization that the city wasn't going to provide any services. The first couple of days we was doing rescues, then we moved into doing relief work, cooking food for the people that was coming across, trying to feed them, giving them water, I'm talking about those that was escaping the flooding. Once they walked across the bridge, Gretna, and the Jefferson Police, and the Jefferson Parish police, would turn Blacks around. If you was white, you was able to find refuge in Gretna, but if you was Black, you wasn't able [to] even enter,

you couldn't pass through it. They were literally quarantining, and they would literally tell you, "Take your Black ass back to the Ninth Ward." We knew that we had to develop some type of lasting mechanism to assure that everyone that is in need of aid would receive that aid and that we could learn and develop a mechanism to make sure that this never happened again. So under that environment of blatant racism and total abandonment by the federal government, we founded Common Ground.[2]

Volunteers rode bikes around the area to see if residents needed care. They found not just acute issues from the storm, but also widespread chronic health issues afflicting low-income residents. Activists set up the clinic first in a mosque and later in a former corner store, with Rahim using personal contacts to get physicians to volunteer at the clinic. In the first two months of operation, 4,000 people visited the clinic. In November 2005, Common Ground became a registered 501(c) nonprofit. The clinic also started providing vaccinations and health services for immigrant laborers involved in the rebuilding efforts. In 2006, they started the Latino Outreach Project, which provided a weekly health clinic in Central City.[3] By the end of 2008, over 1,000 health care providers had volunteered their services at the clinic.[4]

As iterated by the founding members, the Common Ground clinic built on decades of Black health activism and self-care in light of official neglect. Rahim traced his experience with the BPP clinic as foundational for starting Common Ground's clinic:

Well, to start a health clinic or a first aid station wasn't nothing, because this is things that we did in the Panther Party. So I knew that after seeing that this city was without health care, that it was something that had to be developed . . . I knew that it could be done cause we had health program[s], so it wasn't nothing for me to make a call for health care professionals because I knew that they was out here. I knew the doctor that had been in the Party, working with us in Oakland. I made a call out to her, she called other health care professionals, told me she couldn't come right then but she was gonna make sure that others came. So it wasn't nothing to start the health care program and health clinic that eventually became a health clinic, the first aid station . . . Everything that we did was based upon self-sufficiency, so it wasn't nothing to start or to reestablish, because I knew that it was workable. I could've been in the Ninth Ward doing all kind of things because of the fact that most of the residents, the young adults in the Ninth Ward today, I fed their parents.

You know, they came to our breakfast program. They had their first taste of political education through us. Even though they might not remember me by name, "Oh, he was one of them Panthers? Oh yeah, man."[5]

For Rahim, his experience with the BPP showed that activists could start a health clinic. Rahim was also able to utilize some of his contacts with the BPP to find doctors to staff the clinic and establish trust with clientele of the clinic due to the BPP's previous work.

The establishment of the Common Ground health clinic represented many of the changes and continuities in health care in post-Katrina New Orleans. As detailed in this chapter, Katrina, or rather the opportunities presented by the disaster, led to one of the most significant changes in the city's history of health care: the shuttering of Charity. Although ready to reopen just weeks after the storm, LSU administrators chose purposefully to keep the hospital closed in what became a successful bid to finally replace the institution with a modern university hospital. This chapter explores that decision, the process that led to the federal government's funding of the project, and the impact of this transformation, including the loss of access to health care for many low-income, Black residents, and the displacement of hundreds of Black families and businesses to build the University Medical Center as part of the BioDistrict. Akin to previous periods like post–Civil War and Civil Rights years, an opportunity to erase racialized health care existed and evaporated. Instead, clinics like Common Ground and others provided care for low-income, Black residents, building on hundreds of years of Black health activism. This chapter also explores the roles of federal programs like the federally qualified health centers (FQHCs) and the expansion of Medicaid in increasing access to health care, and the factors that contributed to the perpetuation of racial health disparities. This dynamic—of positive improvements by health activists countered by steps to continue racialized health care, with the state and federal government often helping fund both elements—proved to be the mark of the decade and a half after Katrina and the legacy of hundreds of years of racialized health care in New Orleans.

Impact of Katrina and the Failure of the Levees

The inundation of New Orleans from Hurricane Katrina and the failure of the federal levee system led to a severe crisis for the health care system and set in motion a radical transformation. Flooding displaced nearly 4,500 physicians from the Greater New Orleans area and caused the closure of every hospital in the city, with only three hospitals in the suburbs—Ochsner, East Jefferson, and West Jefferson—staying open.[6] Although Charity suffered the least amount of flooding of any city hospital, water in the basement led to the loss of primary power and forced the hospital to rely on diesel generators and hand-pumped devices. For five days, 360 patients and 1,200 staff members waited for rescue, while helicopters hired by the companies that owned the city's private hospitals evacuated those institutions. Physicians brought the most critically ill patients to the rooftop of the Tulane University Hospital parking garage, where helicopters hired by Tenet rescued that hospital's patients and staff. Despite the higher need, Tenet refused to take the Charity patients. As stated by Ben deBoisblanc, chief of Charity's medical intensive care unit: "I saw 100 helicopters land and take off and people walking onto those helicopters . . . and fly off while I'm there on the rooftop bagging critically ill patients." At least one Charity patient died on the rooftop during the twelve hours they waited. Finally, after a total of five days, army helicopters landed to rescue the critical patients, and a mix of airboats—operated by volunteers and the Department of Wildlife and Fisheries—and trucks evacuated the remaining patients and staff. DeBoisblanc iterated the anger and frustration that many at Charity felt about the delayed evacuation: "It's a travesty how this hospital for indigents was being treated."[7]

That anger only intensified in the coming months as LSU officials fought to prevent Charity's reopening. Following the evacuation, military units pumped out the water and cleaned the hospital. An inspection by the Army Corps of Engineers revealed the building to still be structurally sound and ready to reopen in late September. Staff reported to open, but administrators ordered them to leave and keep the hospital closed. LSU's leaders claimed the hospital was unfit to reopen, defying the assessment of the military and hospital staff. Signaling its intentions, in late September 2005, the Louisiana Department of Health and Hospitals refused to accept $340 million in Federal Emergency Management Agency (FEMA) public assistance funding from the Department of Defense to carry out repairs at Charity. The reasons soon became clear: LSU's leaders and political allies viewed this as their best opportunity to finally replace Charity with a new university hospital.[8]

The closure of Charity severely limited the availability of hospital beds and disproportionately impacted low-income residents and those with chronic health problems. With the main hospital closed, staff opened the Spirit of Charity clinic, which operated out of a tent first in the convention center, then in a mall, and later in a building next to the Superdome. The clinic provided only limited care, with no services for patients with chronic health problems. Other hospitals took on some of Charity's former patients. Overall, six months after the storm, Greater New Orleans had 1,984 beds in use, down from 4,083 before Katrina. Staffing shortages prevented the use of all beds at the still open or recently reopened hospitals. With LSU keeping Charity closed, Touro, which reopened 28 days after Katrina, East Jefferson and West Jefferson hospitals witnessed significant jumps in use of their emergency rooms as patients that previously used Charity turned to emergency rooms as their only source of health care. Touro, for example, had a 50 percent increase in emergency room visits in 2006. After Tulane Hospital reopened in February 2006, uninsured patients made up about 12 percent of patients for the year.[9]

The increased number of uncompensated cases led to operating losses for all these hospitals. In response, the state legislature reallocated $120 million previously designated for the Charity system and raised Medicaid rates by 4 percent. West Jefferson, East Jefferson, Ochsner, Tulane, and Touro collectively reported more than $212 million in operating losses for 2005. Special payments from the state and federal government offset much of the expenses for 2006, resulting in a net loss of nearly $29 million. The following year was worse, as costs increases led to over $145 million in losses for 2007. With Charity still closed, the two-tiered health care system had suddenly changed, forcing suburban and private hospitals to provide significantly more care for low-income and indigent patients and incur the associated losses. However, unlike the state's decades-long pilfering of federal funding intended to reimburse Charity for its uncompensated or undercompensated care, federal and state funding to offset the losses at the suburban and private hospitals passed and spared them financial pitfalls. Additionally, many former Charity patients lacked transportation to Touro—located uptown—or the hospitals in the suburbs. As low-income individuals, many of Charity's patients were the least likely to return from their displacement as many lacked the needed financial resources. These two factors limited the number of low-income and indigent patients at the private and suburban hospitals assuming some of Charity's patient load.[10]

In November 2006, LSU finally reopened part of the New Orleans Medical Complex; instead of reopening Charity, they chose to use federal aid to open part of University Hospital, the institution they had used for their paying patients prior to Katrina. Additionally, instead of the 575 beds in use prior to the storm, the hospital initially only used eighty-five beds. In February 2007, still operating at partial capacity, the University Hospital assumed the designation as the city's primary trauma center, which was previously provided by Charity. From nearly 1,300 beds combined between Charity and university hospitals prior to Katrina, the public hospital system operating inside of the city bounds now totaled just eighty-five beds.[11]

LSU's refusal to open Charity led to protests and grassroots response. Residents and local activists, including Charity employees, organized and formed the group Save Charity Hospital. Creating a coalition with other community organizations, the groups tried to pressure LSU to reopen the hospital. Despite protests, LSU and its allies began pushing for a new university hospital that would replace Charity and serve as the centerpiece of a medical and bioscience district in New Orleans. Weeks after Katrina, the state legislature passed a bill that authorized the creation of the Greater New Orleans Biosciences Economic Development District, a direct descendant of HEAL. Beyond the funding of Tulane University Hospital, Ochsner's expansion, and several smaller projects, HEAL largely lingered in the years before Katrina. In 1993, a group of architects and planners created the master plan for the New Orleans Regional Medical Center. The plan created a governing commission, identified partner institutions, formulated funding schemes, and projected job growth and economic impact of an expanded medical and bioscience district. This led to no changes, however. In 1999, Governor Foster's administration crafted the Louisiana master plan for economic development titled *Louisiana Vision 2020*. This plan identified the medical field as one of the state's "technology clusters" that would grow and diversify the state's economy, with New Orleans as a focal point. In 2002, New Orleans updated its 1993 plan for the Medical Center, now titled the *Comprehensive Plan for the New Orleans Biomedical Research and Development Park*. In 2004, the mayor's Office of Economic Development contracted with Greater New Orleans, Inc.—a private, regional economic development organization—to help plan the biomedical district with representatives from the Downtown Development District, LSU, Tulane, the University of New Orleans, and Xavier University. This contract with Greater New Orleans, Inc. and the name change of the planned area—from the Medical Center to the Biomedical Research and Development Park—reflected the larger shift in vision on health care. In the 1960s and 1970s, the state agency HEAL had focused primarily on growing the Medical District through the expansion of local health institutions—the state-funded Charity and LSU medical school and the private Tulane University School of Medicine and Hospital, Hotel Dieu Hospital, Ear, Eye, Nose, and Throat Hospital, and Ochsner. In the 2000s, the city and state handed over leadership from the state agency to a private economic development organization and placed greater emphasis on attracting outside biomedical companies. This transition represented an even greater revelation of the neoliberal approach to the health care economy and urban governance in general. After Katrina, the state legislature passed a bill authorizing the formal creation of the Greater New Orleans Bioscience Economic Development District. Similar to HEAL, a board of commissioners directed the district, with twelve representatives from Greater New Orleans Inc., LSU, Tulane, Ochsner, Delgado, the Community Council, the Business Council of New Orleans, the New Orleans Chamber of Commerce, and the Louisiana Department of Economic Development. This body also possessed many of the previous powers of HEAL: they could sell bonds, ask voters for increases in property taxes, purchase land without paying property tax, and take land through eminent domain.

With the passage of the legislation for the medical and bioscience district, proponents turned to creating the new university hospital and discussions over redesigning the larger statewide Charity system. In 2005, the Louisiana Department of Health and Hospitals organized a meeting of 100 public and private health care stakeholders that led to the formation of the Greater New Orleans Health Planning Group. Members included representatives from Louisiana Blue Cross Blue Shield, the Louisiana Department of Health and Hospitals, the Louisiana Public Health Institute, LSU, Tulane, the NOHD, and the U.S. Public Health Service.[12] Thus, many of the organizations like LSU and Tulane that had advocated for replacing Charity for decades now would decide the fate of that hospital and the other hospitals in the Charity system. With input from the Rand Corporation, they produced the *Framework for a Healthier Greater New Orleans*. The framework made several recommendations. First, the plan advocated addressing many of the negative social determinants of health that accounted for persisting racial health disparities. The framework called for a "health neighborhood design" that included rebuilding neighborhoods with sidewalks, recreation spaces, access to healthy foods, and "conditions that promote safety." Second, to directly address environmental health problems, the framework advocated reduction of exposure to hazardous sources, safe drinking water, reduced pollution, and improved sewage and waste management. Third, the framework recommended improving access to primary health care to lessen the reliance on hospital care. To achieve this goal, the plan called for several changes to the health care structure that had plagued New Orleans in the pre-Katrina period, including improved services offered by the NOHD, expanded health education, neighborhood-based and comprehensive primary clinics affordable to all residents, and integrated health care with better collaboration and coordination between various health care institutions and professionals. Finally, the framework addressed the hospital system. The group called for "access to quality hospital and specialty care regardless of their income or health insurance." They noted that Charity had "responsibilities for care of low-income and uninsured persons" but that "it may not have to remain the domain of a public/state facility."[13] Although not explicitly stating their endorsement for LSU's long-hoped university hospital, the framework tacitly endorsed the end of the public Charity Hospital and the transition to a private hospital. This was not surprising, considering representatives of LSU and their allies served on the planning group. However, if all the elements had been addressed—including reducing negative social determinants of health, providing preventative and primary care for all residents, and ensuring that all residents could use the private hospitals—then the post-Katrina period could have witnessed the end of the two-tiered health care system and a significant decrease in racial health disparities.

Ultimately, though, the policy makers focused almost exclusively on replacing Charity with LSU's university hospital as the main solution, eschewing the work to address social determinants of health or improve low-income health care access. Many of the same representatives from the Greater New Orleans Health Planning Group—including those like LSU and Tulane with direct interests in replacing Charity—joined Governor Blanco's task force on health care, which more explicitly endorsed the opening of a new university hospital. This group worked with PricewaterhouseCoopers to create a report on redesigning low-income health care service in the state. Leaked in spring 2006, the report stated that New Orleans had too many acute care beds prior to Katrina, and it questioned the need to reopen Charity. After public blowback, the final report supported the building of an academic medical center under LSU's administration to replace Charity, with the university giving up control of the other hospitals in the statewide Charity hospital system. The Louisiana Recovery Authority endorsed this plan in June 2006.[14]

After the publication of this report, U.S. Health and Human Services Secretary Mike Leavitt asked the state to form a task force to redesign the state's charity hospital system in hopes of eliminating two-tiered health care. In response, Governor Blanco formed the Louisiana Health Care Redesign Collaborative, which started meeting in July 2006. In addition to many of the same members as the earlier groups, the task force included state legislators, health care industry representatives, and representatives from Ochsner. Blanco instructed the group to include a new LSU university hospital and Veterans Affairs (VA) hospital as part of its final plan. The group proposed creating a state-subsidized program called the Health Insurance Connector. Enrollees could have income up to 300 percent of the federal poverty level and could use the subsidy to participate in an employer-sponsored plan, buy their own insurance as an individual, or buy into the state's Medicaid program. Patients would have a "home" hospital or clinic that would provide their primary care. This "home" institution would also coordinate referrals with each participating hospital using the same record-keeping system to maximize efficiency and reduce duplication of services. As such, the plan represented an attempt at "integrated health care" for the uninsured, similar to the setup of hospital systems like Ochsner. Secretary Leavitt told members of the Louisiana Health Care Redesign Collaborative repeatedly that he wanted to eliminate the two-tiered health care system that existed prior to Katrina. The federal government countered the state's plan in January 2007 with a proposed statewide insurance program for half of uninsured Louisianans, with funding from the DSH and Medicaid covering other residents through managed care programs.

While officials debated the various proposals, LSU moved forward with its own plan to create a new university hospital, finding a partner with the VA hospital. Prior to the storm, the VA hospital existed adjacent to Charity on Perdido Street. Like Charity, the VA hospital received flood damage, and the federal government decided not to reopen the hospital, originally built in 1951. Ochsner lobbied the government to move the hospital adjacent to its main campus in Jefferson, and other politicians pushed for moving the hospital to other locations in Louisiana or outside of the state. In 2006, the municipal government released the Unified New Orleans Plan, mandated by FEMA and HUD for the city to receive federal funding. That plan, approved by those agencies, detailed neighborhood recovery proposals, including building the VA and University hospitals on a shared thirty-seven-acre area half a mile from Charity's location on Tulane Avenue currently occupied by residences and businesses. LSU quickly signed a memorandum of agreement with the VA to create a shared building that would contain housekeeping, the cafeteria, and an energy plant, believing this would help strengthen its position in pushing for its own hospital. However, Mayor Nagin threatened to deny $75 million in HUD funding for the VA hospital unless it agreed to move to another thirty-acre site, separate from Charity Hospital and further into the residential area of the Tulane Gravier neighborhood. LSU would keep the original thirty-seven-acre site solely for its hospital, and thus the proposed thirty-seven acres became sixty acres. In 2008, the Department of Veterans Affairs signed a memorandum with the city for the hospital. To build the VA hospital—originally projected to cost $625 million but ultimately totaling $1.2 billion—the city planned to use its municipal eminent domain power to seize property and raze homes and businesses. As in the case of HEAL's plan to displace Black residents and businesses in 1971, residents organized against this effort and sued the city in 2009 for signing the memorandum of agreement with the VA hospital without required public hearings or approval by the city council and in violation of the city charter.[15] In response, in 2010 the city planning commission and the city council exempted the relocation of the VA hospital from the city's master plan. This allowed the municipal government to approve the proposal without going through public meetings or receiving any form of public input—including the opportunity for residents to voice opposition or suggest alternate sites—which was mandated under the master plan.[16]

With the full backing of the city and state leaders, LSU turned toward securing its own new hospital. The administrators of LSU remained determined to use DSH funding—which covered 67 percent of Charity Hospital's costs prior to Katrina—to support their new hospital even as the federal government proposed ending that allocation and instead using that funding for the statewide insurance program for the uninsured. State leaders ultimately rejected the federal government's plan; as noted by political scientist Mary Clark, those who benefited from maintaining the current system—state leaders who wished to continue to control and redistribute federal DSH funding—resisted the federal efforts, as did LSU and its allies who wanted to use DSH funding at its new hospital. In April 2007, LSU announced a proposed $1.2 billion, 484-bed hospital (up from the $650 million, 350-bed proposal in 2004). To afford the hospital, LSU needed disaster funding from FEMA, $300 million that HUD had already designated for the Louisiana Recovery Authority, as well as state allocations and bonds. LSU, Tulane, and their political allies successfully pressured the state legislature and HUD to approve the reallocation of the agency's funding.[17] Next, they had to secure FEMA's funding. In late 2005, FEMA estimated that Katrina caused $23.9 million in damage to Charity, less than one-tenth of LSU's estimate of $257.7 million in damage. LSU's administrators pushed for the higher amount to support their claim that Charity should not be repaired but rather had to replaced, as federal regulations stipulated that costs had to exceed 51 percent of the building's value for replacement. Charity staff and military officers later accused LSU of hiring individuals who purposely trashed the hospital to convince federal officials that Charity was unfit for reopening.[18] Governor Blanco backed LSU's call for a new hospital over the objections of the city council and local activists. In 2008, after a joint study between FEMA and the state, the former raised its estimates to $150 million, while LSU upped its estimate to $492 million. FEMA concluded that the damage did not exceed the 51 percent threshold and that LSU and the state were attempting to use federal funding to pay for long-deferred repairs and upgrades. LSU appealed FEMA's estimate in March 2009. With lobbying from Senator Mary Landrieu and Congressman Anh Cao, the state successfully won an arbitration appeal in 2010, securing its 2008 call for $475 million from FEMA. Forty years after LSU helped push through HEAL legislation with a desired end of building a new university hospital as part of an expanded medical district, it finally secured funding to accomplish its goal.[19]

In 2011, contractors broke ground on the University Medical Center hospitals. In 2012, LSU transferred management of the still under-construction University Medical Center and the old University Hospital to LCMC Health, the hospital company that also managed Touro. With LCMC's takeover, the University Hospital became a privately administered hospital. While the construction of LSU's new University Medical Center continued, the old University Hospital maintained its role as the city's public hospital and only level 1 trauma center, despite only having 235 beds in operation by 2014. On August 1, 2015, nearly a decade since LSU closed Charity Hospital, the new University Medical Center opened. With the hospital's opening, LCMC closed the University Hospital. In November 2016, the VA hospital—formally the Southeast Louisiana Veterans Health Care System Veterans Medical Center—opened its 1.7 million square foot institution. The opening of the University Medical Center and the new VA hospital marked the formal advent of BioDistrict New Orleans. The 1,500-acre district included the two hospitals, and extended to Carrollton Avenue, Earhart Boulevard, Iberville Street, and Loyola Avenue, occupying a large swath of Mid-City, the Medical District, and Gert Town. In addition to hospitals, the medical schools, and bioscience companies, planners stated the district would also have a projected 29,000 square feet of retail space and amenities like green space and bike lanes to attract workers. Leaders estimated the BioDistrict would produce $9.6 billion in earnings in its first twenty years and create more than 17,000 jobs. By the 2010s, New Orleans increasingly relied on the growing health care sector as a key driver of the local economy.[20]

Yet, as developers, politicians, and hospital leaders celebrated their success in finally replacing Charity and fulfilling HEAL's fifty-year quest to establish a biomedical district, others decried the process and the negative impact on low-income residents. In a repeat of the WPA-sponsored "slum clearance" of

Black residences and businesses in the Tulane Gravier neighborhood in the 1930s to build the last Charity Hospital, the city and state used their eminent domain power—again, supported by federal funding—to raze 265 homes and dozens of businesses in the predominantly Black upper Mid-City neighborhood for the University Medical Center New Orleans (UMCNO) complex. They did so even after a 2009 state legislature–sponsored study by the Foundation for Historical Louisiana and the RMJM Hiller architectural firm found that the Charity Hospital structure was still sound and could be renovated and reopened within three years for $550 million—less than half the $1.2 billion for the UMCNO—without displacing any residents.[21]

Additionally, local officials and residents never voted on LSU's plan for the Medical Center, and the planners incorporated no feedback from residents at the handful of public meetings. As stated by Sister Vera Butler of St. Joseph's Church on Tulane Avenue: "a few neighborhood meetings were held in 2008 and 2009, and conversations were going on but it was difficult to get any concrete information. There was never a point person you could go to. You couldn't find out who to ask, who to call." Instead, the designers used the plans developed prior to Katrina, and then expanded in 2007. The displacement of the 265 families and dozens of businesses drastically altered the makeup of the neighborhood, which was predominantly Black and low income. Some of the displaced residents had only recently moved back into their homes after rebuilding, including using Road Home funding, a short-lived federal program that aimed to help Louisianans repair or rebuild homes damaged or destroyed during Katrina.[22]

Many of the families had resided in the neighborhood for generations. As told by Sister Butler: "You had people living here whose grandparents had grown up here. . . . But they've now gone to Gentilly, Jefferson Parish and out of state. It's a scattered, broken community now."[23] Many displaced residents faced difficulty in finding new homes. The area had some of the lowest property values and rents in the city. When forced out through eminent domain, the city and state gave homeowners the market value of the property prior to the start of development. In the wake of the storm, housing prices had increased and affordable housing had decreased, and many residents could not find new homes. In addition to directly displacing those individuals, the building of the two hospitals and the creation of the BioDistrict started a significant process of gentrification in the neighborhood and the surrounding areas. The planners of the hospitals and the districts not only created spaces for the hospitals and other biomedical sites, but they also closed streets, created green spaces, and developed new housing units to attract doctors, medical students, and biomedical workers. The resulting increase in property taxes and rents forced many other residents to leave the increasingly unaffordable area. Scholars Eric Joseph van Holm and Christopher Wyczalkowski identified the neighborhood as one of areas that had the highest level of gentrification in the decade after Katrina.[24]

Beyond the displaced residents, the shift from Charity to the UMCNO affected tens of thousands of other low-income, predominantly Black residents through the change in the hospital's mission. As stated by LSU Health Sciences Center Chancellor Dr. Larry Hollier in 2006, administrators were "absolutely committed to keeping us away from the charity model" and instead were interested in following the "academic center model." In fact, LSU focused on rebranding the hospital by dropping the "Charity" name in an attempt to remove the "stigma" and become known as a "destination" hospital where patients from throughout the region, the country, and internationally would come for specialized care. The mission and vision statements of the UMCNO reflected this shift, with the former stipulating that "UMCNO will provide exceptional patient-centered care and a world-class academic experience through advanced research, leading technology and innovation" and the latter holding that the hospital would be the "destination choice for exceptional health care."[25] As required by its state contract, the UMCNO patient mix had to include at least 20 percent uninsured individuals. However, this marked a drastic change from its pre-Katrina mission to only provide care for uninsured or individuals under 138 percent of the federal poverty level. LSU had been pushing to allow paying customers to use Charity Hospital prior to the storm without success. In the wake of the disaster, it finally succeeded in changing the allowable patient mix. This change occurred on top of the sharp reduction in beds, from over 1,300 between Charity and the University Hospital to 446 by 2018 at the UMCNO. With a 60 percent reduction in inpatient beds and a turn toward attracting paying patients and serving as a "destination hospital," the UMCNO now serves only a fraction of its traditional patient population, predominantly low-income, Black New Orleanians.

Methodist Hospital underwent a similar transformation. The 181-bed hospital, which had become the city's second largest Black patient–serving hospital in the two decades leading up the storm, closed during Katrina and did not reopen, leaving the predominantly Black New Orleans East without a hospital for nearly a decade after the storm. In 2014, LCMC Health—which operated the UMCNO—opened the New Orleans East Hospital on the site of the former Pendleton Memorial Hospital. The eighty-bed hospital—a reduction in beds of 56 percent from the pre-Katrina hospital—served an area with 80,000 residents.[26]

Primary Clinics and Federal Funding

One positive change for low-income residents post-Katrina was the expansion of primary care clinics. After the storm, the St. Thomas Community Health Center expanded its services with a $500,000 disaster grant. By the end of 2005, the clinic saw 120 patients a day and provided services on a sliding scale, with free care for indigent residents. The clinic moved to a new location on Magazine Street, renovated in 2012 with an $850,000 Community Development grant from the city. By 2015, 45,000 patients a year visited St. Thomas's clinics. In 2017, St. Thomas opened the Heart and Vascular Center on Magazine Street and another clinic on St. Bernard Avenue.[27] Other community-based clinics grew or started in post-Katrina New Orleans. In addition to the previously detailed Common Ground clinic, the New Orleans Musicians' Clinic expanded, supported by the New Orleans Musicians' Assistance Foundation, a 501(c) nonprofit started in 2005. It later moved to the LSU Health Faculty Practice Clinical building on St. Charles Ave.[28]

Federal funding helped fuel the growth of primary care clinics. In 2007, Congress appropriated $100 million in the form of a "primary care stabilization grant" to help low-income residents who surpassed the state's income threshold for Medicaid—the second lowest in the nation—get primary care. Local proponents created the Greater New Orleans Community Health Connection (GNOCHC) in 2010 to coordinate efforts to lobby the federal government for additional funding and create a shared pool for grant money. Through a mix of local, state, and federal funding—primarily Medicaid funding—the GNOCHC distributed money to low-income residents to cover primary care, but not hospitalization or medications. By 2014, over 53,000 residents had enrolled in the GNOCHC program, which covered 97,000 clinic visits that year.[29]

The funding not only helped residents, but also supported clinics like St. Thomas and Common Ground. Both became FQHCs. The FQHC program provided funding to eligible community-based health care organizations that provided primary care services in underserved areas in the form of grant money and Medicaid reimbursement. By 2016, New Orleans had twelve organizations with the FQHC status with forty clinic locations.[30] Additionally, the Affordable Care Act provided more funding for community-based health centers. In 2017, including the forty FQHC clinics, over seventy community health centers provided services for over 59,000 residents.[31]

State funding continued to undermine efforts to further help low-income residents. The state used federal Community Development Block Grant funding to cover its share of the costs of the GNOCHC program. However, as enrollment grew and required additional state funding, Governor Jindal's administration refused to support more state spending, leading to the near ending of the GNOCHC in 2014. The passage of the Affordable Care Act offered health insurance for many previously uninsured residents, leading to significant reductions in the uninsured rate, although Black residents still had an uninsured rate of 16 percent in 2014, down from 32.3 percent in 2009–2011, compared to the white rate of 11 percent in 2014, down from 16.6 percent in 2009–2011.[32]

Under the Affordable Care Act, in 2014 the federal government offered additional funding to expand Medicaid to individuals that made up to 138 percent of the federal poverty level, but the Jindal administration refused to accept the money.[33] As a result, thousands of low-income residents that slightly exceeded the federal poverty level—ranging from an individual making $11,670 to a household of four with an income of $23,850—were not eligible for federally subsidized health care and thus largely unable to access health care. Under the administration of the new governor John Bel Edwards, Louisiana finally accepted the federal Medicaid expansion. Going into effect in July 2016, this change automatically enrolled the GNOCHC participants— over 63,000 by that point—in Medicaid. This expansion shrank the uninsured rate in New Orleans to 11.5 percent in 2017. Overall, in New Orleans in 2017 Medicare provided health insurance for 6.5 percent of residents and Medicaid for 23.3 percent of residents, with 51.2 percent of residents covered by employers.[34] The rise of the FQHC clinics led to a significant change for the health department. Starting in 2010, the NOHD shifted from its previous role as the primary provider of clinics for low-income residents to a more policy-focused mission. Since then, the NOHD has focused on implementing federal programs like the Healthy Start Initiative that targeted areas with high percentages of low-weight newborns.[35]

Mental health services remained severely lacking, which was especially problematic as many survivors of Hurricane Katrina suffered from posttraumatic stress disorder and other mental health issues due to the disaster. Even prior to the storm, New Orleans lagged behind other cities in providing mental health care and hospitalization. Scholars posited that prior to Katrina, New Orleans lacked adequate mental health services and psychiatric beds in hospitals, with an estimated need of an additional 226 beds.[36] Katrina exacerbated these problems, as the city had 39 percent fewer adult and 25 percent fewer child psychiatric beds a decade after the storm, with most beds lost at Charity Hospital.[37] Even as the city faced these severe shortages, the Jindal administration closed the New Orleans Adolescent Hospital and made additional cuts to psychiatric beds at DePaul Hospital and a reduction in mental health services for prisoners.[38] In addition to fewer hospital beds, many psychiatrists did not return to the city. In 2005, 196 psychiatrists practiced in the city; in 2010, only sixty-five practiced, and only three of these accepted Medicaid patients.[39] As happened in most areas of health care, the decline in mental health beds and services disproportionately impacted low-income, Black residents.

In addition to the radical changes to the post-Katrina health care system, many of the social determinants of health worsened for Black residents. As white, upper-income residents moved to the city and began buying houses in formerly predominantly Black, low-income neighborhoods, New Orleans underwent increasing gentrification and residential racial concentration. In the decade after Katrina, sixty-two census tracts significantly gentrified.[40] Gentrification paired with increased racial concentration as neighborhoods like the Bywater, Carrollton, the Irish Channel, the Marigny, St. Roch, Uptown, Mid-City, Algiers Point, and Milan became more white, while New Orleans East and Gentilly became more Black.[41] The racial makeup of the city as a whole changed; by 2015 more than 100,000 African Americans had not yet returned to the city, while the white population returned to near pre-Katrina levels, shrinking the Black percentage from 67 to 59 percent, and increasing the white percentage from 27 to 31 percent.[42] Many of the economic indicators for Black residents became worse in the years after Katrina. The economic gap widened between Black and white residents, as Black income and unemployment worsened while both numbers improved for whites.[43] Black New Orleanians became increasingly concentrated in low-paying employment sectors, primarily hospitality and service jobs, as rent and housing prices increased with gentrification and the city's demolition of public housing units.[44] African Americans had poverty rates six times higher than whites, with poverty concentrated in predominantly Black neighborhoods like Central City, Desire, and the Seventh Ward.[45] Beyond poverty, Black residents disproportionately faced many other problems that negatively affected health including poor-quality housing, low levels of education, lack of access to grocery stores, high rates of crime victimhood and incarceration, and continued exposure to environmental hazards.[46]

The continuance of these negative social determinants of health led to the persistence in the racial health gap in the post-Katrina period. In 2013, Black New Orleanians suffered from hypertension or high blood pressure at a rate 65 percent higher, asthma at a rate of 70 percent higher, and diabetes at a rate 40 percent higher than whites.[47] By 2016, Black residents were six times more likely than whites to contract HIV/AIDS and twice as likely to die from the virus.[48] This mortality gap existed for other diseases as well: African Americans were 1.33 times as likely to die from heart disease; 1.55 times as likely to die from cancer; 2.32 times as likely to die from kidney disease; three times as likely die as an infant; and three times as likely to die from diabetes. Overall, Black residents were 1.37 times more likely to die at any age than whites.[49] The NOHD calculated for the period from 2008 to 2010 that African Americans had an overall avertable death rate of 30 percent, meaning that if they had the same death rate as whites, 30 percent of Black deaths would not have occurred.[50]

The culmination of these health factors led to significantly lower life expectancies for Black New Orleanians, particularly those in the neighborhoods with the highest concentrations of Black residents and poverty rates. Using numbers from 2010–2015, the U.S. Small-area Life Expectancy Project found that the residents of the Hoffman Triangle neighborhood (adjacent to Central City), a predominantly Black low-income neighborhood, had the lowest life expectancy of 62.3 years of age and Lakeview had the highest at 88.1 years of age. All the neighborhoods with high life expectancy were predominantly white and had low levels of poverty; neighborhoods with the lowest life expectancy were predominantly Black and low income.[51]

Summary

The continuation of the racial health and mortality gap attests to the perpetuation of a racialized health care system, one with deep historical roots tied to the larger system of white supremacy. From the founding of New Orleans, two health care systems have existed: one for whites, and another for African Americans. In the earliest system, African Americans suffered from exclusion and exploitation. Enslavers based their decisions to seek medical care for enslaved people on a cost–benefit analysis: the potential loss of investment—money spent to purchase the enslaved person as well as the loss of value of future labor—versus the cost of medical treatment and the likelihood of success. Doctors too viewed enslaved individuals through a similar financial lens: income from treating enslaved people at "slave hospitals"; professional advancement from creating medical procedures or gaining proficiency in a medical procedure they did not already possess by experimenting on enslaved patients; and standing from running a medical school that utilized Black bodies in hospitals as teaching cases and Black corpses for anatomical lessons. For enslavers and physicians alike, slavery proved profitable, and physicians and hospitals played a key role in upholding the slave system, with arguments of racial inferiority used to justify slavery and doctors treating enslaved people to prevent the spread of disease, increase the prices of slave traders, back redhibition policies, and return enslaved people to labor. In return, money from treating enslaved people—paid by slave traders and enslavers—sustained the burgeoning health care system in New Orleans, allowing it to prosper by the Civil War.

The Civil War disrupted these two systems, slavery and the health care sector. The conflict and federal occupation presented a potential turning point for Black health care. The creation of the Freedmen's Hospital and the end of racial discrimination at Charity opened access to health care for African Americans. However, the promise of this crucial turning point quickly vanished. The end of Reconstruction—which included the closing of the Freedmen's Hospital, the return to power of the Democrats, and the decisions by white leaders to maintain racialized health care—ended this brief point of more equal access and led to the institutionalization of Jim Crow, including in health care. The newly formed OPMS instituted a whites-only member clause, all private hospitals refused to admit Black patients, and Charity resegregated. In the post–Civil War period, the racial health gap widened dramatically. Black life expectancy fell below white life expectancy as the Black mortality rate doubled that of whites.

In the early twentieth century, New Orleans initiated public health campaigns and municipal improvements to support newly emerging economic systems: trade with Latin America and tourism. However, these efforts primarily benefited white residents and excluded African Americans. Akin to earlier periods, racist ideas helped support the larger system of Jim Crow, as whites used supposed public health concerns to justify segregation. Thus, in the late nineteenth and twentieth centuries, public health and Jim Crow became part of a self-reinforcing cycle. Segregation and other elements of Jim Crow and white supremacy created negative social determinants of health: lack of access to health care; unemployment and economic inequality; overcrowded and low-quality housing; neighborhoods without services; exposure to health hazards; underfunded and dilapidated schools; violence at the hands of police officers and white residents; everyday stress from discrimination; and other factors, all products of white supremacy, that led to higher rates of disease and mortality. Instead of addressing the underlying issues, white officials used the racial health disparities to support their notions of Black inferiority and the need to segregate and spatially contain Black residents.

Excluded from the historically white health care system and facing these negative social determinants of health, Black New Orleanians fought for improved health. Building on the earlier efforts of enslaved and free individuals to provide care for themselves, African Americans in the late nineteenth and twentieth centuries became doctors and lay healers; started medical colleges—the attempts at Straight University and New Orleans University doomed by the illegal denial of state funds, and later Flint Medical College—built Flint Goodridge Hospital; created an alternate Black medical district in Central City; and carried out public health campaigns. In response, white leaders forced the closure of Flint Medical College, removed Black medical institutions from the growing medical district in Tulane Gravier, used municipal powers to restrict the expansion of Flint Goodridge, and refused to desegregate the health care system.

With pressure from federal court rulings and legislation like the Civil Rights Act of 1964, African Americans finally succeeded in ending legally sanctioned segregation in health care, marking another potential turning point for Black health and health care. By the late 1960s, Black health care and health activism reduced the Black mortality gap from more than double that of whites as late as 1930 to only 10 percent higher. Court-ordered integration and growth of NOHD, community-based, and Model Cities clinics should have led to the further closure of the racial health gap and equal access to health care.

Yet, racialized health care and racial health disparities not only persisted, but intensified in the following decades as historically white hospitals continued to deny admission to Black patients or hire Black doctors, private hospitals dumped Medicare and Medicaid patients on Charity and Flint Goodridge, and funding for Charity, the NOHD, and the Model Cities clinics evaporated. Like other cities, New Orleans experienced a boom in the health care economy in the latter decades of the century and the health care sector became an increasingly important component of the economy. Buoyed by taxpayer bonds and government funding, white-flight hospitals helped support white suburban growth. While hospitals like Ochsner—which received federal Hill-Burton and state HEAL funding—and Tulane—also a recipient of HEAL aid—prospered, Flint Goodridge—denied additional Hill-Burton funding and HEAL aid—and Charity struggled financially, with the former closing in 1985 and the latter serving as the de facto Black and low-income hospital. Negative social determinants of health also worsened in the decades after integration with growing economic inequality.

The post-Katrina health care system changed drastically. In a controversial move, LSU refused to reopen Charity, and instead used political lobbying to secure funding to build its long-desired University Medical Center, opened in 2015 with a new mission that purposely abandoned the charity model. Primary care clinics grew, helped by federal funding, and the eventual expansion of Medicare too increased health care for low-income residents. Yet the racial health gap and racialized health care remain. As this work has demonstrated, the persistence of this inequality was not inevitable. Crucial turning periods after the Civil War, the Civil Rights period, and post-Katrina could have led to the end of racialized health care. Instead, purposeful decisions by health care and municipal leaders, with support from state and federal officials and funding, prevented the abolishment of this system and led to the institutionalization of racism in health care, despite efforts by Black activists.

Recommendations

Although racialized health care and racial health disparities are deeply entrenched, studying the history of these inequalities allows us to see steps that can and must be taken to make improvements. As the BioDistrict becomes one of the centerpieces of the health care system and as the city increasingly focuses on the health care economy as a financial boon, several matters should be considered. First, the health care field has deep historical ties to supporting a racist hierarchy. Health care professionals need to incorporate this history into their training—for example, classes on the subject in medical schools—as well as instruction on health equity. Fortunately, the People's Institute for Survival and Beyond, based out of New Orleans, offers training on equity, which it has provided for the staff of the NOHD and other clinics. Other health care institutions should utilize these workshops.

Second, efforts to educate individual health care workers, to have them modify their behaviors and attitudes, is not enough. Institutions, including the hospitals and medical schools detailed in this work, need to address and eradicate the racism embedded in their policies, practices, and cultures. The allegations against Ochsner detailed in the introduction to this work—the involuntarily discharging of twenty-five Black COVID patients from the hospital to die at home in summer 2020—attest to the perpetuation of institutional bias in hospitals. Contemporary studies have found inequity in the quality of health care—for example, less time in clinical evaluations, disbelief and dismissal of health complaints, and continued belief in notions of scientific racism including higher Black tolerance of pain, all resulting in less treatment and procedures for patients of color versus whites.[52] This has exacerbated the existing health inequity and led to lower levels of satisfaction in and trust of health care among people of color. As argued by scholars Paris Adkins-Jackson, Rupinder Legha, and Kyle Jones, institutions need to assess the bias in their systems, institute reporting mechanisms, hold offenders accountable, and institute anti-racist policies to change existing racist practices and health care cultures.[53]

Medical schools must address institutional bias too. For example, in October 2020, Dr. Princess Dennar, Tulane University School of Medicine's first and only Black woman program director, filed a lawsuit against the school for discrimination against her and Black residents she supervised. In February 2021, the school removed Dennar from her position as the director of the pediatrics residency program, an action Dennar alleged occurred in retaliation for the lawsuit. After Dennar's suit and removal, dozens of students and alumni went public with their own complaints of discrimination. In July 2021, the Accreditation Council for Graduate Medical Education placed the school on probation while they investigated the allegations. While some complaints alleged actions by specific individuals at the school, the whole of the complaints reveal the larger issue of institutional racism. In February 2021, sixty residents signed a letter that argued the allegations—including underrepresentation of students of color due to the use of a ranking tool for potential students that devalued education at HBCUs and bias in the interviews and other stages of the application process, failure to recruit or promote people of color to associate or full professor positions and program director roles, giving Black residents more difficult clinical workloads than whites, the failure to discipline professors and administrators over abuse and discrimination claims, and daily microaggressions against students of color—demonstrated the "deeply entrenched structural racism and bias within Tulane University and within the halls of our hospitals."[54] The health care system in New Orleans is no longer led by explicit racists like Emmett Lee Irwin and others detailed in this work. However, institutional racism still plagues health care institutions and must be addressed. Pledges of commitment to diversity and inclusion are not enough. Like hospitals, medical schools must confront their institutional racism and adopt anti-racist policies.

Third, the health care field needs to address the underrepresentation of African Americans in positions like physicians and surgeons. This needs to start with medical schools, which need to improve the dismal number of Black students. African Americans make up over 32 percent of Louisiana's population but only 4 percent of medical students.[55] Preliminary research has found that increasing the number of Black doctors can have significant positive impacts on improving use of preventative services and a corresponding decrease in mortality.[56] Thus, increasing the number of Black doctors will benefit both practitioners and patients.

Fourth, city leaders must recognize that reliance on a health care economy is often problematic. A 2017 study found that the Greater New Orleans area had the largest growth in hospital jobs in any metropolitan area in the United States in the previous decade, and projected the health care sector in New Orleans would see the largest growth of any sector in the following decade.[57] Proponents of the health care sector's expansion argue the field's growth will create not just more jobs, but jobs with higher wages. This is partially true as the mean hourly wage for individuals with occupations identified as health care practitioners and technical occupations and health care support occupations—a total of 58,900 people employed in both fields combined, representing 11.4 percent of all jobs in the area—is $28.65 in the New Orleans area, compared to $24.05 for all occupations. However, wide disparity in pay exists in the field. Individuals in the first health care occupation cluster—practitioner and technical occupations—make $35.59 an hour on average in comparison to $12.98 for those in support. Within the two broad fields are wide disparities as well. Physicians make significantly more than other positions. For example, the forty family medicine physicians make $123.62 and the 110 general internal medicine physicians make $90.30 an hour. The 1,890 pharmacists make $57.37 an hour. The 860 nurse practitioners make $54.31 an hour. Registered nurses, the largest group with 14,290 people, earn $34.10 an hour. The 3,970 licensed practical and vocational nurses make $21.90. Those in the health care technical positions make even less: the 710 surgical technologists make $20.38; the 1,100 emergency medical technicians (EMTs) and paramedics make $19.17; the 1,700 pharmacy technicians make $17.64; and the 320 psychiatric techs make $13.63 an hour. Those in the second broad health field, support, earn the least, averaging $12.98 an hour. This includes 2,620 medical assistants earning $15.58; 4,790 nursing assistants earning $12.28; and 5,610 home health and personal care aides making only $9.90 an hour. These groupings also do not include individuals in other health care support roles, including maintenance, office, cooking, and cleaning staff at the hospitals, medical schools, and other medical institutions; most of these individuals make minimum wage of $7.25 an hour.[58]

While promoters of the health care economy trumpet the employment potential of the sector, most individuals working in health care earn below what is considered a living wage for New Orleans: $14.84 for a single adult with no children; $30.94 for an adult with one child; $37.57 for an adult with two children; and $47.61 for an adult with three children.[59] Additionally, the health care field is rife with racial sorting. As noted, African Americans are underrepresented in higher-wage physician positions and overrepresented in low-wage technician and support positions. Promoting the health care sector as job creation therefore is not enough. Health care institutions must increase pay to a living wage and provide more training and opportunities for advancement for underrepresented groups for this job growth to be equitable.

Fifth, as detailed in this book and other works, the expansion of health care institutions has caused displacement of people of color and low-income residents and gentrification. The threats of these impacts will only worsen as New Orleans increasingly focuses on promoting the health care economy, primarily through the form of the BioDistrict. In August 2021, the chairman of the BioDistrict lobbied the city council for support in designating the BioDistrict as a "tax increment financing district," which would give the BioDistrict agency annual city and state tax revenue projected to exceed $2 million annually. The BioDistrict Board, comprised of representatives appointed by the city mayor, governor, leaders of Tulane and LSU's medical schools, and economic development agencies, would guide how the money is spent, with planned goals of grants for bioscience companies, infrastructure projects, construction of new buildings for the medical schools, and "blight removal" on Claiborne Avenue.[60] This proposal epitomizes the Medical District's deeply troubled history of structural racism. White leaders used the concept of "blight removal" to displace Black medical institutions; Black doctors, dentists, and pharmacists; and Black residences, schools, churches, and businesses in the early twentieth century to expand Charity Hospital and LSU, with financial backing from the federal government. They attempted the same tactics in the late 1960s with HEAL and displaced hundreds more Black residents after Katrina to create the new University Medical Center, VA hospital, and the BioDistrict, again with federal funding. Now, they seek again to carry out these efforts, targeting an area—Claiborne Avenue—impacted by the building of the I-10 overpass in the 1960s. Proponents use color-blind terms like "economic development" and "blight removal" to mask the racism embedded in these efforts and within the institutions guiding and benefiting from these decisions. But the history of the Medical District, of the historically white medically institutions, and racialized health care in

New Orleans is clear and poignant and must not be repeated. The promotion of the health care economy must not come at the expense of those displaced by expansion. Health care and city leaders must address displacement and gentrification caused by health care institutions and must incorporate citizen input in decision-making and on leadership boards like the one guiding the BioDistrict.

Sixth, displacement and gentrification are just two of many of the negative social determinants of health that leaders must address. Inequality in access to education, lack of safe and affordable housing and neighborhoods, economic instability and wealth inequality, lack of access to recreation spaces, exposure to health hazards, racism, and other factors have exacerbated the inequality in access to health care and perpetuated the racial health gap as seen in the significantly higher rates of disease and mortality for Black residents versus whites.

While fixing systemic and institutional racism is a monumental task, leaders must recognize that failing to do so is literally killing Black New Orleanians and lowering their life expectancy. This work has identified the crucial turning points in the history of the racialized health care system, moments where leaders could have dismantled that system. It is my hope that by studying this history and analyzing these lost points of potential change, the leaders of New Orleans today—both inside and outside of the health care system—can make the changes necessary to finally end the city's racialized health care system and push for health equity.

Appendix

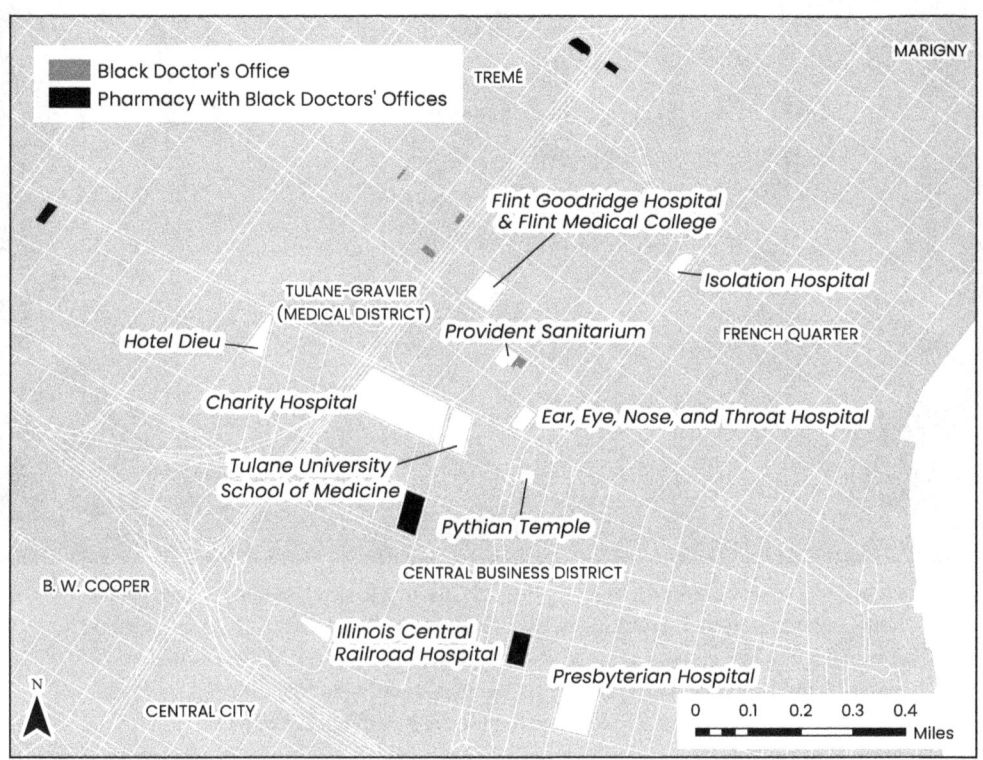

MAP A.1 The Medical District in 1913.

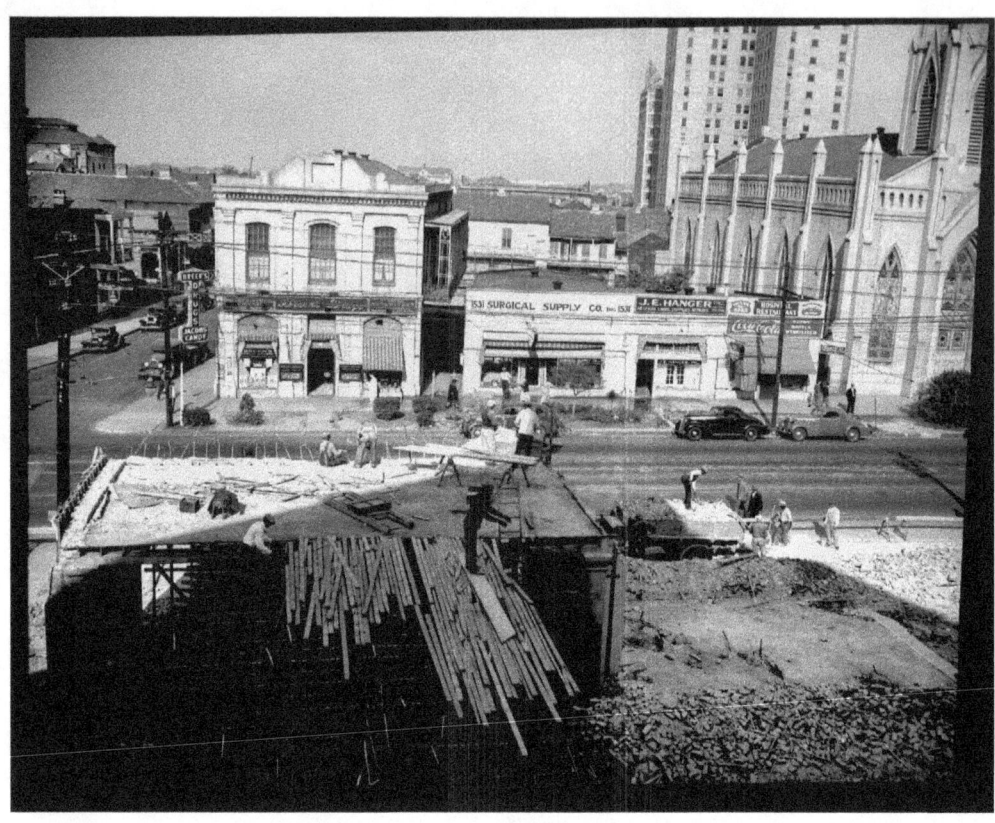

FIGURE A.1 WPA workers deconstruct the old Charity Hospital building in 1936 (WPA Photograph Collection, City Archives, New Orleans Public Library). The neighborhood surrounding the hospital was a mix of Black residences, stores, and St. Mark's Baptist Church. Administrators used WPA "slum clearance" funding to raze the neighborhood, displacing the Black residents and businesses for the new medical complex.

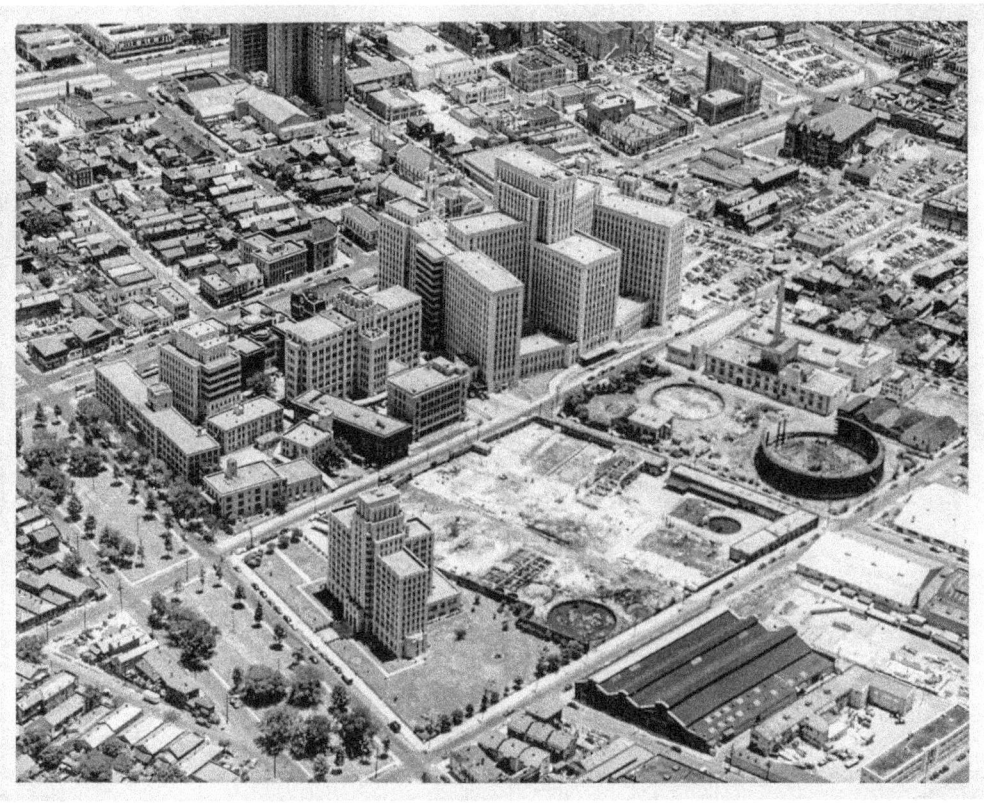

FIGURE A.2 Aerial view of the Charity Hospital complex in 1948 (General Photographs Collection, City Archives, New Orleans Public Library). Buildings for the Charity Hospital complex, Tulane University School of Medicine, and Louisiana State University Medical School replaced the razed Black residences and businesses.

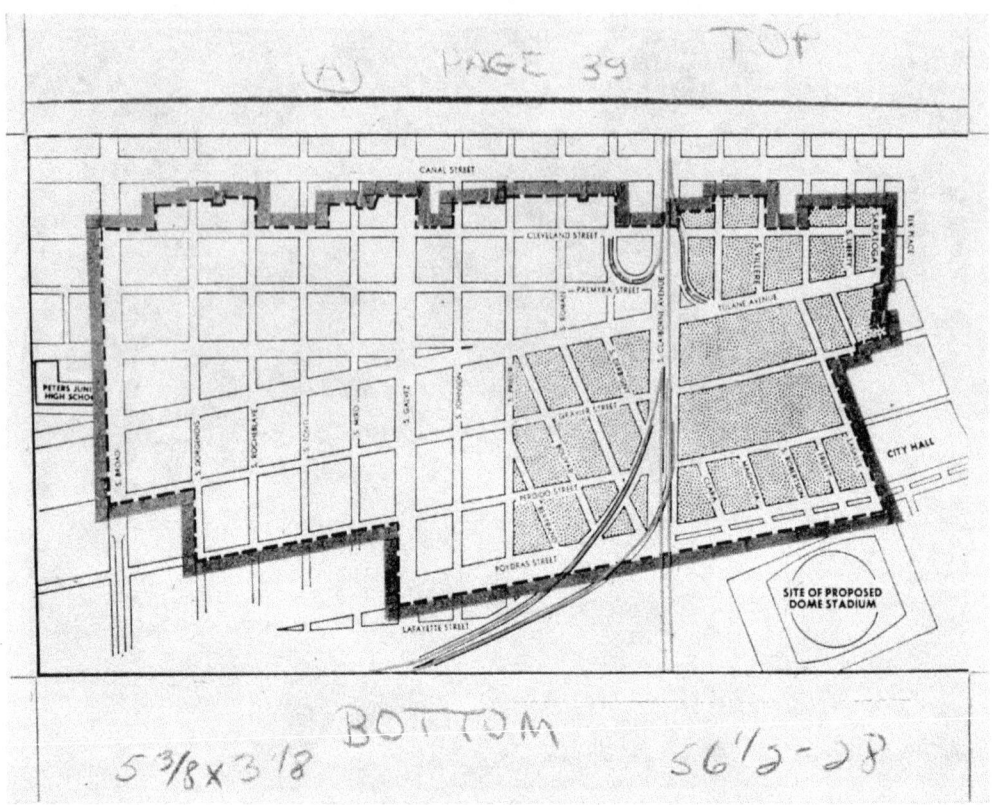

FIGURE A.3 Map showing the area encompassed by the Health Education Authority of Louisiana (HEAL), 1973 (City Archives, New Orleans Public Library).

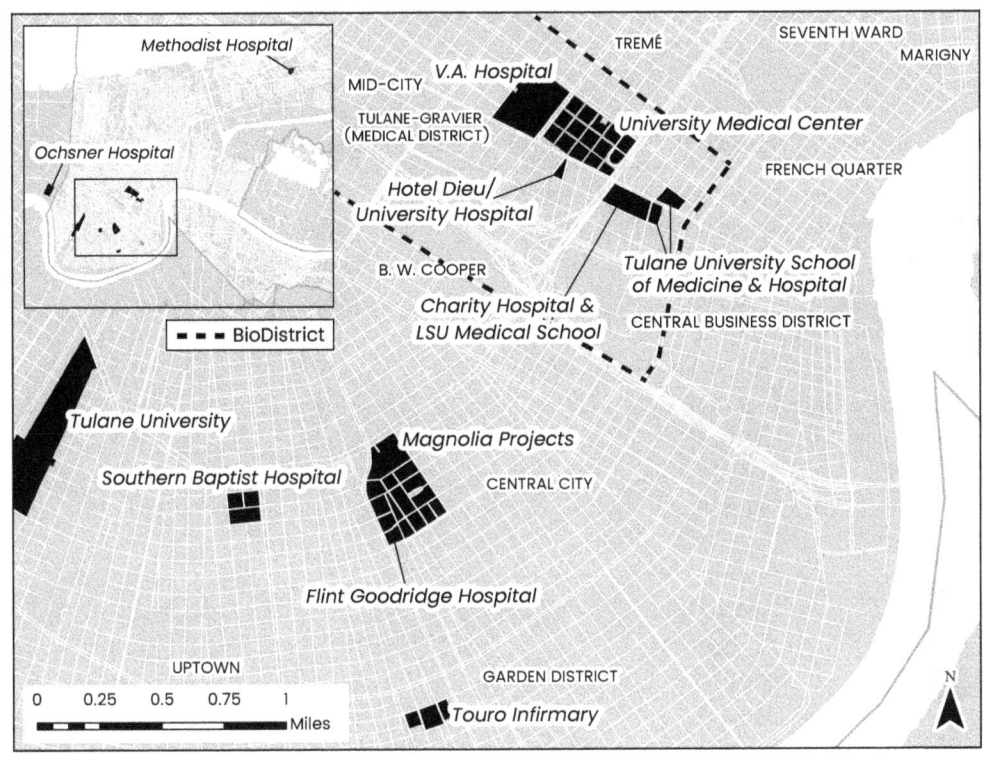

MAP A.2 Select New Orleans medical institutions.

TABLE A.1 Population of New Orleans, 1769–2019

Year	Total Black Population	Enslaved Population	Free People of Color Population	Total White Population
1769	1,326	1,227	99	1,803
1791	2,651	1,789	862	2,386
1805	4,671	3,105	1,566	3,551
1810	10,911	5,961	4,950	6,331
1820	22,134	14,946	7,188	19,244
1830	28,545	16,639	11,906	21,281
1840	42,614	23,348	19,226	59,519
1850	28,029	18,068	9,961	91,431
1860	25,523	14,484	10,939	149,063
1870	50,456			140,923
1880	57,617			158,473
1890	64,491			177,376
1900	77,714			209,390
1910	89,262			249,813
1920	100,930			285,884
1930	129,632			329,130
1940	149,034			345,503
1950	181,775			388,670
1960	233,514			394,011
1970	257,478			335,993
1980	308,149			249,366
1990	307,728			189,210
2000	325,942			135,956
2010	206,871			113,428
2019	230,418			128,871

Sources: Population figures 1791–1860 from Sumpter, "Segregation of the Free People of Color," 23. Population figures 1870–2000 from Campanella, *Geographies of New Orleans*. Data for 2019 from U.S. Census "Bureau Population Estimates 2019."

TABLE A.2 Number of Black and white medical doctors and ratio of doctors to population, 1791–1940

Year	*Number of Black medical doctors	Ratio of Black doctors to Black residents	Number of white medical doctors	Ratio of white doctors to white residents
1791	1	1 per 2,651	8	1 per 298
1805	0		12	1 per 296
1810	0		39	1 per 162
1820	0		45	1 per 423
1830	0		62	1 per 456
1840	0		113	1 per 527
1850	4	1 per 7,007	224	1 per 408
1860	6	1 per 4,254	301	1 per 495
1870	14	1 per 3,604	239	1 per 590
1880	16	1 per 3,601	256	1 per 619
1890	18	1 per 3,583	281	1 per 631
1900	21	1 per 3,701	382	1 per 548
1910	42	1 per 2,125	488	1 per 512
1920	29	1 per 3,480	555	1 per 515
1930	47	1 per 2,758	708	1 per 465
1940	39	1 per 3,821	855	1 per 404

*Excludes dentists and other nonmedical doctors.

Sources: Compiled from census records and city directories. Numbers for 1890 from Savitt, "Entering a White Profession," 511.

TABLE A.3 New Orleans mortality rates by race, 1810–2020*

Year	Black mortality rate per 1,000	White mortality rate per 1,000
1810	40.88	58.6
1845	22	25.1
1850	52.10	62.08
1856	35.66	32.98
1860	52.79	41.99
1861	37.16	31.58
1863	59.5	37.3
1864	81.75	42.14
1865	60.88	33.31
1866	65.66	36.77
1870	50.74	30.62
1880	34.3	22.96
1890	37.88	24.96
1900	34.44+	20.56
1910	32.86	17.25
1920	23.1	12.59
1930	23.53	11.32
1940	20.53	14.59
1950	12.13	10.04
1960	11.4	9.8
1970	10.06	9.15
1980	—	—
1990	—	—
2000	—	—
2010	9.4	6.86
2015–2020	8.88	6.81

*Numbers prior to 1910 may include nonresident deaths.

+ In 1900, a significant difference existed between the Black mortality rate listed in the records of the City Board of Health and data from the U.S. Census Report. The latter listed the Black mortality rate at 41.11, compared with the City Board of Health's statistic of 34.44 per 1,000. In other years listed, the mortality rates are much closer aligned between the two sources.

—Until the mid 1970s, the New Orleans Health Department produced annual reports that listed mortality by race. The department did not respond to requests for data from the period 1980–2000.

Sources: Compiled from U.S. Census Bureau reports and City Board of Health reports. Data for 1861–1866, Blassingame, *Black New Orleans*, 242. Numbers for 2010 from New Orleans Health Department, *Health Disparities in New Orleans*, 3. Numbers for 2015–2020 from National Institute on Minority Health and Health Disparities, "Death Rates Table 5 Year Average."

Notes

Abbreviations for Archives

ARC   Amistad Research Center, Tulane University, New Orleans
CANOPL City Archives, New Orleans Public Library
CHC   Charity Hospital Collection, Rudolph Matas Library of the Health Sciences, Tulane University
FGHC   Flint Goodridge Hospital Collection, Dillard University, New Orleans
LCUNO   Louisiana Collection, University of New Orleans
LRCTU   Louisiana Research Collection, Tulane University
NARA   Records of the Bureau of Refugees, Freedmen, and Abandoned Lands, National Archives and Records Administration, Washington, D.C.
NOHD   New Orleans Health Department Collection, City Archives, New Orleans Public Library
OPMS   Orleans Parish Medical Society Collection, Louisiana Research Center, Tulane University, New Orleans
TUHC   Tulane University Hospital Collection, Louisiana Research Collection, Tulane University

Introduction

1. May 9, 1974, Report of M. A. Galathe to the NAACP, Louisiana Chapter of the NAACP Collection, ARC.
2. Waldman and Kaplan, "Sent Home to Die."
3. Louisiana Department of Health, "Louisiana Coronavirus Information."
4. Lahut, "Fauci Says the Coronavirus Is 'Shining a Bright Light' on 'Unacceptable' Health Disparities for African Americans."
5. Evans et al., *Social Determinants of Health and Crime in Post-Katrina Orleans Parish*, 16.
6. Centers for Disease Control and Prevention, "CDC Research on SDOH."
7. Artiga and Ortega, "Key Facts on Health and Health Care by Race and Ethnicity."
8. Rudowitz et al., "Health Care in New Orleans Before and After Katrina."
9. Stephens, *Governor's Health Care Reform*.
10. Horowitz, *Katrina: A History, 1915–2015*, 147.
11. Bonilla-Silva, "More than Prejudice," 76, 77, 82.
12. Hirsch, *Making the Second Ghetto*, 5–6.
13. Hine, *Black Women in White*; Gamble, *Making a Place for Ourselves*; McBride, *Integrating the City of Medicine*; Savitt, "Entering a White Profession"; Smith, *Sick and Tired of Being Sick and Tired*; Long, *Doctoring Freedom*; Ward, *Black Physicians in the Jim Crow South*.
14. Wailoo, *Dying in the City of the Blues*; Roberts, *Infectious Fear*.

15. See Hogarth, *Medicalizing Blackness*; Owens, *Medical Bondage*; Schwartz, *Birthing a Slave*; Washington, *Medical Apartheid*.

16. Connor, "The University That Ate Birmingham"; McKee, "The Hospital City in an Ethnic Enclave"; Simpson, *The Medical Metropolis*; Winant, *The Next Shift*.

17. Roberts, *Infectious Fear*; Shah, *Contagious Divides*.

18. See Vidal, ed., *Louisiana: Crossroads of the Atlantic World*; Adams and Sakakeeny, eds., *Remaking New Orleans*.

19. See, for example, Florida, "Where Eds and Meds Industries Could Become a Liability."

Chapter One

1. Northup, *Twelve Years a Slave*, 75.
2. Northup, *Twelve Years a Slave*, 85.
3. Northup, *Twelve Years a Slave*, 177–178.
4. Starr, *The Social Transformation of American Medicine*, 72. For more on the origins of American hospitals, see Rosenberg, *The Care of Strangers*.
5. "Treaty of the Company of the Indies and the Ursulines," September 17, 1726; "The State of New Orleans État de la Louisiane," June 1720, Archives du Ministère de la Guerre, Library of Congress; Strange, *Vital Negotiations*, 173.
6. Stange, *Vital Negotiations*, 175.
7. "Last Will and Testament of Jean Louis," November 16, 1735, Records of the French Superior Council in New Orleans, Louisiana State Museum Historical Center.
8. Salvaggio, *New Orleans' Charity Hospital*, 14.
9. Orders by Governor Antonio de Ulloa, March 20, 1766, Rosemonde E. & Emile Kuntz Collection, LRCTU.
10. Fossier, "The Charity Hospital of New Orleans."
11. Hall, *Africans in Colonial Louisiana*, 60.
12. Byrd and Clayton, *An American Heath Dilemma*.
13. Hall, *Africans in Colonial Louisiana*, 77.
14. Klein et al., "Transoceanic Mortality," 113.
15. Salvaggio, *New Orleans's Charity Hospital*, 7.
16. Stange, *Vital Negotiations*, 147.
17. Hall, *Africans in Colonial Louisiana*, 77–80.
18. Hall, *Africans in Colonial Louisiana*, 89.
19. "Louisiana's Code Noir 1724." From B. F. French, *Collections of Louisiana* (New York: D. Appleton, 1851).
20. Salvaggio, *New Orleans' Charity Hospital*, 6–7; Cruzat, "The Ursulines of Louisiana."
21. "Document Freeing Marie Arain," March 10, 1744, Master Calendar Collection, Louisiana State Museum Historical Center.
22. "March 29, 1770 Sale of Slave," Index to Spanish Judicial Records, *Louisiana Historic Quarterly* (1924): 323–324.
23. "The Constitution for the New Hospital of Charity," 1793, Medical Documents Collection, LRCTU.
24. "1791 New Orleans Census," CANOPL.

25. "Action to Take Possession of the Administration of the Charity Hospital of Saint Charles," 1794, Medical Documents Collection, LRCTU.

26. Rothman, "Before the Civil War, New Orleans Was the Center of the U.S. Slave Trade."

27. For more on yellow fever, see Willoughby, *Yellow Fever, Race, and Ecology in Nineteenth-Century New Orleans*. See also Olivarius, *Necropolis*.

28. Hogarth, *Medicalizing Blackness*, 20.

29. Willoughby, *Yellow Fever, Race, and Ecology in Nineteenth-Century New Orleans*, 90.

30. Anthony Peniston, "Memoir on the Races of Mankind," *New Orleans Medical News and Hospital Gazette* 5, no. 2 (July 1859).

31. Hogarth, *Medicalizing Blackness*.

32. Haynes, *Noah's Curse*.

33. Samuel D. Cartwright, "How to Save the Republic, and the Position of the South in the Union," *DeBow's Journal* 11, no. 2 (1851): 184–197

34. D. Warren Brickell, "Epidemic Typhoid Pneumonia Among Negroes," *New Orleans Medical News and Hospital Gazette* 3, no. 1 (February 1856).

35. *A Digest of the Ordinances and Resolutions of the General Council of the City of New Orleans* (New Orleans, 1845), 28, Records of the City Councils, CANOPL.

36. Tansey, "Bernard Kendig and the New Orleans Slave Trade."

37. Fett, *Working Cures*, 20; Covey, *African American Slave Medicine*, 31.

38. "Health," *New Orleans Medical News and Hospital Gazette* 1, no. 1 (March 1854): 20.

39. Johnson, *Soul by Soul*, 120, 210.

40. Johnson, *Soul by Soul*, 142, 181.

41. "178 Sugar and Cotton Plantation Slaves," 1855 Pamphlet, Antebellum Period Collections, Louisiana State Museum Historical Center.

42. Johnson, *Soul by Soul*, 131

43. Johnson, *Soul by Soul*, 146.

44. "1791 New Orleans Census," CANOPL.

45. 1830 Federal Census.

46. Johnson, *Soul by Soul*, 103.

47. Johnson, *Soul by Soul*, 102.

48. Klein et al., "Transoceanic Mortality," 113.

49. Mintz, "Childhood and Transatlantic Slavery."

50. See Schwartz, *Birthing a Slave*.

51. Tadman, "The Demographic Cost of Sugar."

52. Covey, *African American Slave Medicine*.

53. For more on the health of enslaved people in Louisiana, see Bankole-Medina, *Slavery and Medicine*.

54. Fogel, *Without Consent or Contract*, 137.

55. Rao, "On Long-term Mortality Trends in the United States, 1850–1968," 409.

56. Sumpter, "Segregation of the Free People of Color," 33.

57. Marcus Christian and the Members of the Dillard Unit of the Louisiana Writer's Project, "Slave Health, Remedies, and Hospitalization" in *The Negro in Louisiana* (1942), 13. Marcus Christian Collection, LCUNO.

58. Covey, *African American Slave Medicine*, 36; Fett, *Working Cures*.

59. Kenny, "A Dictate of Both Interest and Mercy?," 7.

60. Russell, *My Diary North and South*, 258.

Chapter Two

1. Erasmus D. Fenner, "Specimens for the Museum of the New Orleans School of Medicine," *New Orleans Medical News and Hospital Gazette* 7, no. 2 (April 1860): 131.

2. Kenny, "A Dictate of Both Interest and Mercy."

3. Matas, *History of Medicine in Louisiana*, 201.

4. Pritchett and Yun, *The In-Hospital Mortality Rates of Slaves and Freemen*, 6.

5. Matas, *History of Medicine in Louisiana*, 229.

6. T. G. Richardson, "Report of Stone's Infirmary, for the year ending August 31st, 1860," *New Orleans Medical and Surgical Journal* 7, no. 18 (1861), 201–224.

7. Matas, *History of Medicine in Louisiana*, 230.

8. Matas, *History of Medicine in Louisiana*, 230.

9. Kenny, "A Dictate of Both Interest and Mercy," 26.

10. Kenny, "A Dictate of Both Interest and Mercy," 37.

11. Matas, *History of Medicine in Louisiana*, 231.

12. Pritchett and Yun, *The In-Hospital Mortality Rates of Slaves and Freemen*, 5.

13. Pritchett and Yun, *The In-Hospital Mortality Rates of Slaves and Freemen*; Admission Book of the Touro Infirmary 1855–1860, CANOPL.

14. Kenny, "A Dictate of Both Interest and Mercy," 33.

15. Kenny, "A Dictate of Both Interest and Mercy," 46.

16. Salvaggio, *New Orleans' Charity Hospital*, 12.

17. Johnson, *Slavery's Metropolis*.

18. Charity Hospital Papers, Louisiana State Museum Historical Center.

19. "Board of Administrators Report 1832 and 1857–1861," CHC.

20. "Charity Hospital Board of Administrators Annual Report 1849," CHC.

21. Brian H. Oviedo, *National Register of Historic Places Inventory/Nomination Form: The Houmas* (Washington, D.C.: National Park Service, 1979).

22. "Charity Hospital 1912 Annual Report," CHC.

23. de Grummon, *Renato Beluche*, 162–167; *The Josefa Segunda*, 18 U.S. 5 Wheat. 338 338 (1820).

24. "Charity Hospital Board of Administrators Annual Report 1843," CHC.

25. Starr, *The Social Transformation of American Medicine*, 44.

26. "Annual Circular of the Medical College of Louisiana for the Session of 1838 & 1839," Stanford E. Chaille Papers, LRCTU.

27. Stanford E. Chaille, "Historical Sketch, of the Medical Department of the University of Louisiana," 1861, Stanford Chaille Papers, LRCTU.

28. "Erasmus Darwin Fenner," *Transactions of the American Medical Association* XXIX (Philadelphia: Collins, 1878): 646.

29. "Medical School Statistics for 1858–59," *New Orleans Medical News and Hospital Gazette* 6 (May 1859): 230–231.

30. "4th Annual Circular and Catalogue of the New Orleans School of Medicine," June 1860, Stanford Chaille Paper, LRCTU.

31. Despite a ban on Black students, both schools regularly had Latin American students.

32. D. Warren Brickell, "Introductory Lecture" November 8, 1857, Stanford Chaille Papers, LRCTU.

33. Kenny, "Specimens Calculated to Shock the Soundest Sleeper." For more on these practices and other ways that early medical schools contributed to white supremacist racial science, see Willoughby, *Masters of Health*.

34. E. D. Fenner, "Elephantiasis," *New Orleans Medical News and Hospital Gazette* 4 (August 1857), 322.

35. D. Warren Brickell, "Introductory Lecture" November 8, 1857, Stanford E. Chaille Papers, LRCTU.

36. D. Warren Brickell, "Epidemic Typhoid Pneumonia Among Negroes," *New Orleans Medical News and Hospital Gazette* 3, no. 1 (February 1856), 540.

37. Samuel Choppin, "Charity Hospital," *New Orleans Medical News and Hospital Gazette* 1, no. 1 (March 1854), 19–20.

38. Cornelius Beard, "Resume of Practice, Hospital and Private," *New Orleans Medical News and Hospital Gazette* 5, mo. 2 (July 1859).

39. "H. P. Richard, "Atchafalaya," *New Orleans Medical News and Hospital* Gazette 3, no. 2 (July 1856): 356.

40. Owens, *Medical Bondage*.

41. Brickell, "Epidemic Typhoid Among Negroes," 540.

42. Many scholars have criticized Sims for his operations on enslaved women without their consent and his refusal to administer anesthesia. See, for example, Owens, *Medical Bondage*.

43. D. Warren Brickell, "Two Cases of Vesico Vaginal Fistula Cured," *New Orleans Medical News and Hospital Gazette* 5 (November 1858): 579.

44. D. Warren Brickell, "Veso Vaginal Fistula," *New Orleans Medical News and Hospital Gazette* 6, no. 1 (January 1859): 159.

45. Schwartz, *Birthing a Slave*, 278.

46. Brickell, "Typhoid Epidemic," 540.

47. D. Warren Brickell and E. D. Fenner, "Editorial," *New Orleans Medical News and Hospital Gazette* 2 (1855): 40.

48. Fett, *Working Cures*, 58; Covey, *African American Slave Medicine*, 43.

49. Wynes, "Dr. James Durham."

50. A. P. Tureaud and C. C. Haydel, "The Negro in Medicine in Louisiana" (1935), 3, A. P. Tureaud Collection, ARC.

51. Roudanez, "Grappling with the Memory of New Orleans."

52. Sumpter, "Segregation of the Free People of Color," 23.

53. City directories included Dr. Joseph Joly, a "mulatto" physician. His listed title of "Dr." indicates a medical degree, although where he attended school is unknown.

54. 1850 Census, 1861 New Orleans City Directory, CANOPL.

55. 1860, 1870, and 1880 Census.

56. 1851 New Orleans City Directory, CANOPL.

57. Hall, *Africans in Colonial Louisiana*, 58.

58. Long, *A New Orleans Voudou Priestess*.

59. Cornelius Beard, "Quackery Rampant," *New Orleans Medical News and Hospital Gazette* 7, no. 1 (January 1860): 394

60. D. Warren Brickell, "Two Cases of Vesico Vaginal Fistula Cured," *New Orleans Medical News and Hospital Gazette* 5 (November 1858): 579.

61. Sumpter, "Segregation of the Free People of Color," 33.

62. *Annual Report of the Board of Health to the General Assembly of the State of Louisiana, 1883–1884.*

63. Olivarius, *Necropolis*.

64. Campanella, "An Ethnic Geography of New Orleans."

Chapter Three

1. "Hotel Dieu Hospital Patient Registers 1858–1900," Hospital Records Collection, CANOPL.

2. "Hotel Dieu Hospital Patient Registers 1858–1900," Hospital Records Collection, CANOPL.

3. The War Department, *Reports of the Extent and Nature of the Materials Available for the Preparation of a Medical and Surgical History of the Rebellion* (Philadelphia: J.B. Lippincott & Co., 1865).

4. *Report on the Condition of the Freedmen of the Department of the Gulf, to Major General N.P. Banks, Commanding, by Chaplain T.W. Conway, U.S.A. Superintendent Bureau of Free Labor* (New Orleans: H.P. Lathrop, 1864), 9, African American Pamphlet Collection, Library of Congress.

5. Blassingame, *Black New Orleans*, 51.

6. For more on conditions in refugee camps, see Downs, *Sick from Freedom*. See also Long, *Doctoring Freedom*, ch. 2.

7. Blassingame, *Black New Orleans*, 61.

8. Blassingame, *Black New Orleans*, 122.

9. Samuel Thomas, "Miscellaneous Reports and Lists Relating to Murders and Outrages," March 9, 1867, NARA.

10. Blassingame, *Black New Orleans*, 242.

11. "Register of Contrabands in Corps d'Afrique, New Orleans, 1863," NARA.

12. Duffy, *The Samaritans*, 161.

13. "October 31, 1866 Report of the Operation of the Medical Department Bureau State of Louisiana for the Year 1866," NARA.

14. "Abstracts of Interments at Freedmen's Cemetery, New Orleans, Louisiana May 1867–July 1867," NARA.

15. "October 31, 1866 Report of the Operation of the Medical Department Bureau State of Louisiana for the Year 1866," NARA.

16. For more on problems with Freedmen's Hospitals and the Medical Division, see Downs, *Sick from Freedom*.

17. "October 31, 1866 Report of the Operation of the Medical Department Bureau State of Louisiana for the Year 1866," NARA.

18. "October 31, 1866 Report of the Operation of the Medical Department Bureau State of Louisiana for the Year 1866," NARA.

19. "New Orleans Riots," 39th *Congress Report* No. 216 February 11, 1867.

20. "Report of the Operation of the Medical Department Bureau State of Louisiana for the Year 1867," NARA.

21. "May 31, 1868 Report of Lucius H. Warren," NARA.

22. "August 31, 1868 Report of Lucius H. Warren," NARA.

23. "December 31, 1868 Report of Lucius H. Warren," NARA.

24. "December 31, 1868 Report of Lucius H. Warren," NARA.

25. "November 6, 1868 Report of Lucius H. Warren," NARA.

26. "History," Records of the New Orleans Field Offices, Bureau of Refugees, Freedmen, and Abandoned Lands, 1865–1869 (Washington: National Archives Trust Fund Board National Archives and Records Administration, 1987), 2.

27. "Charity Hospital Annual Report 1861," CHC.

28. "Charity Hospital Annual Report 1864," CHC.

29. For more on Reconstruction politics in New Orleans, see Nystrom, *New Orleans After the Civil War.*

30. "Charity Hospital Annual Report 1869," Charity Hospital Records, RMTU.

31. "Charity Hospital Annual Report 1877," Charity Hospital Records, RMTU.

32. "Reports of James T. Newman," American Missionary Association Collection, ARC.

33. "History," 2.

34. Marler, *The Merchants' Capital.*

35. "Important Meeting," *Times Picayune* July 30, 1875.

36. "Record of Patients in the Touro Infirmary of New Orleans, 1869–1891," Hospital Records Collection, CANOPL.

37. Matas, *History of Medicine in Louisiana,* 520

38. Kenny, "Specimens Calculated to Shock the Soundest Sleeper," 171.

39. "Erasmus Darwin Fenner," *Transactions of the American Medical Association* XXIX (Philadelphia: Collins, 1878): 646.

40. "Circular of the New Orleans School of Medicine, Course of Lectures for 1868–69," Stanford E. Chaille Papers, LRCTU.

41. "Medical School Catalogue," Stanford E. Chaille papers, LRCTU.

42. Savitt, "Straight University Medical Department," 177.

43. Savitt, "Straight University Medical Department," 185.

44. Savitt, "Straight University Medical Department," 185.

45. "The History of Flint Goodridge Hospital," 5 Marcus Christian Collection, LCUNO.

46. "The History of Flint Goodridge Hospital," 3, Marcus Christian Collection, LCUNO; Roudanez, "Grappling with the Memory of New Orleans."

47. Vincent, "Aspects of the Family and Public Life of Antione Dubuclet."

48. "Constitution and By-Laws of Les Jeunes Amis Organized Aug. 1, 1867, Incorporated March 2, 1875," Charles Rouseve Papers, LRCTU.

49. Blassingame, *Black New Orleans,* 168.

50. "Charity Hospital Annual Report 1877," CHC.

51. Citizens of New Orleans, Times Picayune September 13, 1874.

52. Alcee Fortier, ed., *Louisiana: Comprising Sketches of Parishes, Towns, Events, Institutions, and Persons, Arranged in Cyclopedic Form* Vol. 3 (New Orleans: Century Historical Association, 1914), 74–75.

53. "Address to the White League of New Orleans," *Times Picayune*, September 19, 1875.

54. Stanford Chaille, "Orleans Parish Medical Society History," 787, Stanford E. Chaille Papers, LRCTU.

55. African Americans made up a sizable portion of patients, comprising, for example, 45 percent of the hospital's 604 patients in 1890. Over 16 percent of patients came from Louisiana, and 84 percent of this group were Black. However, records do not specify residence; if all the Black Louisianans resided in New Orleans, the total in 1890 would have been eighty-one. It is unknown if the hospital treated Black patients in a separate space from white patients. "Marine Hospital Records, 1890," LRCTU.

56. "Charity Hospital Annual Report 1878, 1881," LRCTU.

57. Kenny, "Specimens Calculated to Shock the Soundest Sleeper," 173.

58. With the violence of 1874, the school system largely resegregated, a move retroactively permitted by the 1879 state constitution and mandated by the 1898 state constitution.

59. Finley, "Lynching"; Monroe Work Today, "Map of White Supremacy White Violence."

60. For more, see Prince, *The Ballad of Robert Charles*.

61. Blassingame, *Black New Orleans*, 242.

62. "The History of Flint Goodridge Hospital," 5, Marcus Christian Collection, LCUNO.

63. Hine, *Black Women in White*.

64. "The History of Flint Goodridge Hospital," 31, Marcus Christian Collection, LCUNO.

65. "The History of Flint Goodridge Hospital," 24, Marcus Christian Collection, LCUNO.

66. Hayes, "Emma Wakefield-Paillet, MD."

67. Rosenberg, "Martinet, Louis Andre."

68. Savitt, "Entering a White Profession," 510.

69. "The History of Flint Goodridge Hospital," 42, Marcus Christian Collection, LCUNO.

Chapter Four

1. "Dr. J. T. Newman, Dean of Negro Physicians," *Louisiana Weekly*, October 10, 1925; "Negro Hospitals, Medical Schools," *Times Picayune*, December 30, 1913.

2. "Council Kills Film Inspection," *Times Picayune*, November 30, 1912.

3. "Ordinance Creates Five New Precincts in City," *Times Picayune*, October 14, 1916.

4. "Sanitarium Bitterly Opposed Before Newman," *Times Picayune*, January 18, 1917.

5. "Would Widen Scope of Sunday Law," *Times Picayune*, February 28, 1917.

6. "Council Refuses to Delay Action in Station Matter," *Times Picayune*, March 14, 1917.

7. "Letter to the Editor," *Louisiana Weekly*, August 4, 1928.

8. Like many Black physicians of the period, Lord Beaconsfield Landry came from a prominent family. Formerly enslaved, Landry's father Pierre became the first Black elected mayor of a U.S. town, Donaldsonville, Louisiana, in 1868; he later was a state legislator and authored the bill to create New Orleans University, as well as serving on Flint Medical College's Board of Trustees. J. B. Landry's brother Eldridge graduated from Flint and ran his

own pharmacy in New Orleans. Another brother, Oliver, attended Flint until its closure, graduated from Meharry, and established a medical practice in Central City. L. B. graduated from Meharry; had a medical practice in Algiers; operated a free clinic for Black residents; taught at Flint; and authored a health column in the *Louisiana Weekly* titled "How to Keep Well" from 1926 to 1934. Frank Lincoln Mather, ed., *Who's Who of the Colored Race* (Chicago, 1915), 170.

9. "Letter Sent Editor on Hospital Stand," *Louisiana Weekly*, August 4, 1928.

10. In 1872, 178 hospitals operated nationwide. In 1910, over 4,000 hospitals existed. Starr, *The Social Transformation of American Medicine*, 178.

11. The New Orleans Sanitarium opened in 1886; Beard's Hospital in 1895; Dr. E. D. Fenner's Private Orthopedic Infirmary and Sanitarium for Sick Children in 1905; the New Orleans Dispensary for Women (later Sara Mayo Hospital) in 1905; and Brosnan's Hospital for the Injured in 1912.

12. "Petition of Mrs. Bella Levy Marouse and Dr. Percy L Querens," December 8, 1927, City Planning and Zoning Commission Records, CANOPL.

13. Carpenter, "Gateway to the Americas," 24.

14. Souther, *New Orleans on Parade*, 20.

15. Gotham, *Authentic New Orleans*, 77.

16. Bureau of the Census, "Mortality Statistics 1910" (Washington, D.C.: Government Printing Office, 1912), 12.

17. Williams, "Martin Behrman and New Orleans Civic Development"; "Disease Rates," New Orleans Sewerage and Water Board, Twenty-Sixth Semi-Annual Report (New Orleans 1912): 48–49.

18. Department of Commerce and Labor, Bureau of the Census, "Mortality Statistics 1905" (Washington, D.C.: Government Printing Office, 1907), 35.

19. Creighton Wellman, "The New Orleans School of Tropical Medicine and Hygiene," 1912, C. C. Bass Papers, LRCTU.

20. No. 609 C.C.S. 1922, Commission Council Series, CANOPL.

21. No. 11271 C.C.S. 1929, Commission Council Series, CANOPL.

22. Klein, *A History of LSU School of Medicine New Orleans*, 1–5.

23. Miller, "Urban Blacks in the South."

24. Colten, "Basin Street Blues."

25. Ordinance No. 8037, September 16, 1924, CANOPL.

26. City Zoning Commission, Major Street Improvements 1927, Chapter VII, "The Process of Planning," 2, CANOPL.

27. Savitt, "Entering a White Profession," 510.

28. Abraham Flexner, "Medical Education in the United States and Canada: A Report to the Carnegie Foundation for the Advancement of Teaching" (New York: Carnegie Foundation, 1910), 233. "History of Flint Goodridge Hospital," 19.

29. Robert Elijah, "Flint Goodridge Hospital Dedicated," *Southwestern Christian Advocate*, March 9, 1916, Robert Elijah Jones Papers, ARC.

30. "Charity Hospital and Segregation," *Louisiana Weekly*, April 24, 1926.

31. "Leading Negro Citizens Ask for Removal of Jim Crow Law," *Louisiana Weekly*, May 15, 1926.

32. Gaines, *Uplifting the Race*.

33. For more on this generation of New Orleans Civil Rights leaders, see Decuir, "Attacking Jim Crow." See also Devore, *Defying Jim Crow*.
34. Lincoln, "The History of Tulane University's School of Medicine's Involvement with Charity Hospital."
35. "The New Charity Hospital," *Louisiana Weekly*, September 19, 1936.
36. "Charity Hospital 'Remedies' Congestion," *Louisiana Weekly*, November 30, 1937.
37. Campanella, *Cityscapes of New Orleans*, 53.
38. See the map on University of Richmond, "Mapping Inequality."
39. Starr, *The Social Transformation of American Medicine*, 111
40. "New Orleans as a Medical Center," C. C. Bass Papers, LRCTU.
41. "Inaugural Address of Emmet Irwin," January 6, 1931, OPMS.
42. "The New Charity Hospital," *Louisiana Weekly*, April 4, 1935.
43. "Temple Leased for Hospital," *Louisiana Weekly*, October 3, 1936.
44. "Temple Still Belongs to Pythian Grand Lodge," *Louisiana Weekly*, June 9, 1937.
45. Claire Perry and George Sessions Perry, "Penny a Day Hospital," *The Saturday Evening Post*, September 2, 1939.
46. "An Evidence of Racial Solidarity," *Louisiana Weekly*, December 24, 1938.
47. John Rousseau, "Charity Patients 'Jim Crowed' in Own Section," *Louisiana Weekly*, June 15, 1936.
48. Carrier, *Charity*, 30.
49. Washington, *Medical Apartheid*, 237.
50. "Miss Kate Gordon Promoted to National Leadership," *Times Picayune*, July 7, 1921.
51. Larson, *Sex, Race, and Science*, 109.
52. Kemp, "Jean and Kate Gordon," 391.
53. L. L. Lumsden, "A Survey of Tuberculosis in Louisiana," *Public Health Bulletin* 219 (April 1935): 202.
54. Rudolph Matas, "The Surgical Peculiarities of the Negro," *Transactions of the American Surgical Association* XIV (1896).
55. Louisiana Board of Health, *1906–1907 Annual Report*.
56. "A Gilt-Edged Investment," *Times Picayune*, July 17, 1917.

Chapter Five

1. "Bishop Jones is Hailed as Super Citizen; 'Hospital Will Defy Death Rate'—Ward," *Louisiana Weekly*, October 31, 1931.
2. "The Origin, Development and Achievements of the N.O. Federation of Civic Leagues," *Louisiana Weekly*, June 30, 1934.
3. For more, see Gamble, *Making a Place for Ourselves*.
4. "Dr. T. Restin Heath, Flint-Goodridge Supt., to Quit," *Louisiana Weekly*, March 20, 1926.
5. "Hospital Situation is Acute," *Louisiana Weekly*, August 21, 1926.
6. "A Hospital Tangent," *Louisiana Weekly*, September 5, 1926.
7. "The Uncharitable Hospital," *Louisiana Weekly*, May 8, 1926.
8. "The New Hospital," *Louisiana Weekly*, September 25, 1926.
9. "Help Yourself," *Louisiana Weekly*, October 26, 1926.

10. "To Build a New Hospital," *Louisiana Weekly*, September 25, 1926.

11. "Citizens Back the Hospital," *Louisiana Weekly*, November 6, 1926.

12. "Hospital to be Erected Soon," *Louisiana Weekly*, May 28, 1927.

13. "CCS 9594," Synopsis of Ordinances, Commission Council Series, CANOPL.

14. "CCS 10014," Synopsis of Ordinances, Commission Council Series, CANOPL.

15. Cherrie, "A Black Physician in the Jim Crow South."

16. "Observe Negro Health Week in Schools," *Louisiana Weekly*, April 12, 1930.

17. H. W. Knight, "Flint-Goodridge Hospital," *Journal of the National Medical Association* 22, no. 3 (1930): 130–131, 131. R. B. Eleazer, "Flint Goodridge Hospital," *The Crisis* 40, no. 7 (July 1933): 151.

18. Flint Goodridge Hospital, "Health Hazards of New Orleans (1929)," Hospitals Subject Files, CANOPL; "Crowd Turns Out for Corner Laying Ceremony," *Times Picayune*, October 24, 1929.

19. "Dedication," *Times Picayune*, January 31, 1932.

20. "Asks Reason for Ban on Physicians," *Chicago Defender*, December 6, 1930; "Council Approves Site for Dillard University," *Louisiana Weekly*, December 20, 1930.

21. Flint Goodridge Hospital, "Health Hazards of New Orleans."

22. Eleazer, "Flint Goodridge Hospital," 151.

23. Knight, "Flint Goodridge Hospital," 130; "Hospital Campaign," *Louisiana Weekly*, May 10, 1930.

24. For more on these hospitals see Gamble, *Making a Place for Ourselves*.

25. Richardson, "Albert W. Dent."

26. "Will W. Alexander to W. W. Brierley," July 7, 1932, American Missionary Association Collection, ARC; 1933 Charity Hospital Annual Report, LRCTU.

27. Eleazer, "Flint Goodridge Hospital," 151; "Asks Reason for Ban on Physicians," *Chicago Defender*, December 6, 1930.

28. "Embree Replies to N.Y. Doctors on Hospital," *Louisiana Weekly*, January 10, 1931.

29. Flint Goodridge Hospital, "Health Hazards of New Orleans."

30. Gamble, *Making a Place for Ourselves*, 109.

31. Flint Goodridge Hospital, "Health Hazards of New Orleans."

32. "Superintendent's Report 1944," American Missionary Association Addendum Series A Subseries Dillard, ARC.

33. A. W. Dent, "The Role of a Negro Clinic in the Control of Tuberculosis in a Large Southern City," *Transactions of the Thirty-Seventh Annual Meeting of the National Tuberculosis Association* (1941); AMA Addendum Series A Subseries Dillard, ARC.

34. Claire Perry and George Sessions Perry, "Penny a Day Hospital," the *Saturday Evening Post*, September 2, 1939.

35. Perry and Perry, "Penny a Day Hospital."

36. Smith, "Black Communities Mobilize."

37. "The History of Flint Goodridge," 53, Marcus Christian Collection, LCUNO.

38. Perry and Perry, "Penny a Day Hospital."

39. "Flint Goodridge Hospital Advances," *Louisiana Weekly*, June 27, 1936.

40. "Superintendent's Report 1944," AMA Addendum Series A Subseries, ARC.

41. "1936: Report on City Subsidies to Private Agencies 1936 Budget Department of Public Welfare," Council of Social Agencies of New Orleans Records, LRCTU.

42. Dent, "The Role of a Negro Clinic."

43. Hine, *Black Women in White*, 70–71.
44. Radford, *Modern Housing for America*.
45. "Slum Clearance for New Orleans," *Louisiana Weekly*, April 10, 1937.
46. "Not the Proper Location," *Louisiana Weekly*, December 25, 1937.
47. "Opposed to Proposed Site," *Louisiana Weekly*, February 26, 1938.
48. Woodruff, "High Lead Levels."
49. "Superintendent's Report 1944," AMA Addendum Series A Subseries, ARC. For more on Dillard's nursing program, see Hine, *Black Women in White*, 77–83.
50. Hine, *Black Women in White*.
51. "Flint Goodridge Hospital: A Financial War Casualty," Press Release April 3, 1947, FGHC. "Cites Hospital's Endowment Need," *Times Picayune*, April 3, 1948; "Financial Support Sole Need of Flint Goodridge," *Pittsburgh Courier*, June 10, 1950.
52. "Superintendent's Report 1944," AMA Addendum Series A, Subseries Dillard, ARC.
53. "Flint Goodridge Plan Acclaimed," *Times Picayune*, April 15, 1947; "Superintendent's Report 1944," AMA Addendum Series A, Subseries Dillard, ARC.
54. "Flint Goodridge Ranks with Best Hospitals in Country," *Louisiana Weekly*, March 11, 1950; Edgar Stern, "Statement," March 1, 1952, FGHC.
55. "Study of Flint Goodridge Hospital by Dr. F. C McLean & Dr. P. M. Murray Feb 15–17, 1955," Peter Marshall Murray Papers, Howard University.
56. "Letter A. W. Dent to Edgar Stern," January 2, 1952, FGHC.
57. "Testimony of Dr. William Adams," House Committee on Interstate and Foreign Commerce Hearing on the Hospital Construction Act Amendments, May 5–8, 1958, Hearings Volume 4 (Washington: Government Printing Office, 1958), 73.
58. "Flint Goodridge Plan Acclaimed," *Times Picayune*, April 15, 1947.
59. "Superintendent's Report 1944," AMA Addendum Series A Subseries Dillard, ARC; "Flint Goodridge Hospital Report to Its Friends," 1952, Council of Social Agencies of New Orleans Records, LRCTU.
60. In 1947–1948, there were 495 Black medical students in the South, all at Howard and Meharry. In comparison, 8,608 white medical students were studying in the South, with 953 in Louisiana. In the North, Midwest, and West, there were 93 Black medical students and 18,318 white medical students. Cornley, "Segregation and Discrimination in Medical Care in the United States," 1077.

Chapter Six

1. "Statement of Jessie Frohm," August 6, 1953, NAACP Collection, LCUNO.
2. "Growth Pamphlet," Rosa F. Keller Papers, CANOPL.
3. Thomas, *Deluxe Jim Crow*, 177.
4. "A Summary Statement on Inter-Group Racial Problems in New Orleans (A Plan for Dealing with Them)," J. Harvey Kearns Executive Director Urban League of Greater New Orleans, 1961, NAACP Collection, LCUNO.
5. "Rosa Keller to DeLesseps S. Morrison," April 30, 1958, DeLesseps S. Morrison Collection, CANOPL; Haas, *DeLesseps S. Morrison*, 255; Keller, *Memoirs*, 11.
6. "Rosa Keller to Mayor DeLesseps Morrison," April 30, 1958, DeLesseps S. Morrison Records, CANOPL.

7. Haas, *DeLesseps S. Morrison*, 75–76.
8. "Expansion," Flint Goodridge Subject File, CANOPL.
9. "Memorandum Rosa Keller to All Workers in the Special Gifts Division," March 19, 1958, Mayor Chep Morrison Records, CANOPL.
10. "Minutes of the Board of Management," May 22, 1961, FGHC.
11. "Minutes of the Board of Management," January 26, 1970, FGHC.
12. "Orleans Parish Medical Society Minutes," February 1, 1954, OPMS.
13. "Untitled Document," Rosa F. Keller Papers, CANOPL.
14. "Interview of George Thomas Jr.," February 15, 1986, George Thomas Jr. Papers, ARC.
15. "OPMS Meeting Minutes," November 14th and 22nd, OPMS.
16. "Affidavits Hit at Integration," *Times Picayune*, December 11, 1955.
17. "Jury Trial of Bus Suit Asked," *Times Picayune*, February 9, 1957.
18. "Irwin Attacks Drive of NAACP," *Times Picayune*, February 15, 1958.
19. "Racial Fences Commended by Council Leader," *New Orleans States-Item*, May 26, 1958.
20. "Tribute," *New Orleans States-Item*, November 25, 1957.
21. More overtly, in 1981 Ochsner wrote a blurb for the revised edition of Wilmot Robertson's *The Dispossessed Minority* (self-published in 1972), a diatribe that promoted a racial hierarchy with the "superior" Nordic/Aryan race at the top and "inferior" African Americans at the bottom, as well as promoting the segregation of African Americans into communities kept physically separate from whites, akin to the apartheid state in South Africa. Ochsner hailed the book as "one of the greatest books I have ever read." Carpenter, "Social Origins of Anti-Communism," 126.
22. Fairclough, *Race & Democracy*, 168.
23. Fairclough, *Race & Democracy*, 169.
24. "Field Training Report," March 24–May 29, 1947; Small Collections, ARC.
25. "A Pattern of Gross Indifference," *Louisiana Weekly*, July 30, 1963.
26. "Statements by Katherine London, Marie Williams, and Marguirite Brown," April 9, 1951, NAACP Collection, LCUNO.
27. For more on the "Group," see Decuir, "Attacking Jim Crow."
28. Ward, *Black Physicians in the Jim Crow South*, 289.
29. "Back American Way is Appeal," *Times Picayune*, September 10, 1956.
30. Emanuel and Tureaud, *A More Noble Cause*, 127.
31. Emanuel and Tureaud, *A More Noble Cause*, 137; "LSU Medical School Admits First Negro," *Louisiana Weekly*, May 25, 1965; Mohr, *Tulane*, 240.
32. A 1959 survey found that only 6 percent of hospitals in the South were integrated; over 33 percent admitted no African Americans, and the rest treated Black patients in segregated sections. The survey also found only 25 percent of Southern hospitals granted staff privileges to Black doctors. "U.S. Hospitals and the Civil Rights Act of 1964."
33. "U.S. Hospitals and the Civil Rights Act of 1964."
34. "Board of Management Minutes," February 21, 1963, FGHC.
35. "Petition to the Greater New Orleans Community," (Undated), Ernest "Dutch" E. Morial Papers, ARC. For more on the efforts of Civil Rights activists in New Orleans, see Rogers, *Righteous Lives*.
36. "Hospitals Using U.S. Funds Must Desegregate Says Court," *Louisiana Weekly*, March 7, 1964.

37. "NMA Doctors Urged to Support Cause, Fight Hospital Bias," *Louisiana Weekly*, February 23, 1963.

38. "Silence," *Louisiana Weekly*, April 5, 1964.

39. "Action to Mix Charity Filed," *Louisiana Weekly*, July 23, 1964.

40. "Charity Board Desegregates TB Ward," *Louisiana Weekly*, October 28, 1964.

41. "Drop Barriers at Charity," *Louisiana Weekly*, January 9, 1965.

42. "Order Charity Hospitals' Desegregation," *Louisiana Weekly*, December 12, 1965.

43. A handwritten note on the back of the letter—either by Jung or Schiro—included the question "must we hire n——s?" next to a picture of a rifle. "Letter Rodney C. Jung to Mayor Victor Schiro," February 9, 1965, New Orleans Health Department Collection, CANOPL.

44. "First Complaints Filed Under Title 6 of Civil Rights Act," *Louisiana Weekly*, February 27, 1965; "Record Number of Complaints Made Against Southern Hospitals," *Louisiana Weekly*, April 24, 1965.

45. Cornley, "Segregation and Discrimination in Medical Care in the United States," 1077.

46. "OPMS Meeting Minutes," December 10, 1956, OPMS.

47. "Testimony of Dr. William Adams," House Committee on Interstate and Foreign Commerce Hearing on the Hospital Construction Act Amendments, May 5–8, 1958, Hearings Volume 4 (Washington: Government Printing Office, 1958), 73.

48. For more, see Washington, et al., "Segregation, Civil Rights, and Health Disparities."

49. "OPMS Meeting Minutes," June 8, 1965, Orleans Parish Medical Society Collection, LRCTU.

50. "Waiting Room Bias Outlawed by Civil Rights Act," *Times Picayune*, September 15, 1965.

51. "OPMS Meeting Minutes," August 26, 1965, Orleans Parish Medical Society Collection, LRCTU.

52. "Petition of a Group for Better Health Services," *Times Picayune*, June 15, 1966.

53. "Report of the Committee for Better Health Services," April 1966, NAACP Collection, LCUNO.

54. Jeff Gordon, "Are You Strong Enough to Be Sick," Human Relations Council April 1969 Newsletter, NAACP Collection, ARC; Dan Bloomenthal, "Poor People's Panacea," Human Relations Council June 1969 Newsletter, NAACP Collection, ARC.

55. "1963," Charity Hospital Folder, Mayor Victor Schiro Collection, CANOPL.

56. "Human Relations Council, July 1969 Report," NAACP Collection, ARC.

57. "Petition of a Group for Better Health Services," NAACP Collection, LCUNO.

58. Salvaggio, *New Orleans' Charity Hospital*, 192.

59. "Report," May 25, 1966, NAACP Collection, LCUNO.

60. "Complaint of Victoria Jones," October 11, 1966, NAACP Collection, LCUNO.

61. "Complaint of Eliza Reynolds," September 29, 1968, NAACP Collection, LCUNO. For more on the history of police brutality in New Orleans, see Moore, *Black Rage in New Orleans*, and Adler, *Murder in New Orleans*.

62. "Report," May 25, 1966, NAACP Collection, LCUNO.

63. "Complaint of James Sanders," April 30, 1968, NAACP Collection, LCUNO.

64. "Home for Incurables Reports," New Orleans Social Council Collection, LRCTU.

65. "Ellis Hull Jr. Report," April 24, 1966, NAACP Collection, LCUNO.
66. "Report," April 10, 1968, NAACP Collection, LCUNO.
67. "Concerned Negro Nurses at VA Hospital," June 1, 1968, NAACP Collection, LCUNO.
68. "OPMS Meeting Minutes," April 11, 1967, Orleans Parish Medical Society Collection, LRCTU.
69. Lincoln, "Tulane University School of Medicine and Charity Hospital."
70. Campanella, *Cityscapes of New Orleans*, 274.
71. "Speech Anniversary of the Opening of Methodist Hospital," September 25, 1969, Mayor Victor Hugo Schiro Collection, CANOPL.
72. "Victor Schiro Fundraising Letter," June 4, 1968, Victor Hugo Schiro Collection 1957–1970, CANOPL; "John B. Koelmay to D. Canella Sept. 18," 1969, Mayor Victor Hugo Schiro Collection, CANOPL.
73. Starr, *The Social Transformation of American Medicine*, 290.
74. Starr, *The Social Transformation of American Medicine*, 291.
75. Department of Defense, "Assessment of Post-Attack Health Resources," July 1, 1970.

Chapter Seven

1. "Tenant Unit Prepares Fight," *Times Picayune*, December 15, 1970.
2. "Flint Goodridge Board of Management Minutes," September 23, 1963, Flint Goodridge Hospital Collection, Dillard University Archives, FGHC.
3. "Flint Goodridge Board of Management Minutes," September 27, 1965, FGHC.
4. "Flint Goodridge Board of Management Minutes," November 29, 1965, FGHC.
5. "Charles Kohlmeyer Jr. to J. Hilbert Schieb," February 2, 1966, FGHC.
6. "Charles Kohlmeyer Jr. to Al Fluery," April 19, 1967, FGHC.
7. "Flint Goodridge Board of Management Minutes," March 24, 1966, FGHC.
8. "Flint Goodridge Board of Management Minutes," December 12, 1966, FGHC.
9. "Letter Jesse Bankston to C. C. Weil," February 2, 1967, FGHC.
10. "Letter Jesse Bankston to C. C. Weil," March 1, 1967, FGHC.
11. "Letter Jesse Bankston to C. C. Weil," February 2, 1967, FGHC.
12. "Letter Jesse Bankston to C. C. Weil," February 2, 1967, FGHC.
13. "Flint Goodridge Board of Management Minutes," May 18, 1967, FGHC.
14. "Flint Goodridge Board of Management Minutes," March 14, 1967, FGHC.
15. "Flint Goodridge Board of Management Minutes," January 29, 1968, FGHC.
16. "Flint Goodridge Board of Management Minutes," May 18, 1967, FGHC.
17. Joseph W. Thomas, "Expansion Report Flint-Goodridge Hospital," May 12, 1969, FGHC.
18. "Letter Charles Kohlemeyer Jr. to Broadus Butler," December 4, 1969, FGHC.
19. "Tulane Annual Report 1969–1970," LRCTU.
20. "Tulane Annual Report 1969–1970," LRCTU.
21. "H.E.A.L. Pamphlet," Charles Cassidy Bass Papers, LRCTU.
22. "Health Complex Is Need," *Times Picayune*, January 25, 1970.
23. "Proposed Medical Center is Attacked, Defended," *Times Picayune*, December 19, 1970.

24. "Application for block grant from Neighborhood Development Program 1972," H. EA.L. Collection, CANOPL.

25. "Board of Governors Meeting Minutes," January 13, 1971, Ernest "Dutch" E. Morial Collection, ARC.

26. "Tulane University Hospital Board of Management Meeting Minutes," March 28, 1973, TUHC.

27. "Tulane University Hospital Board of Management Meeting Minutes," March 23, 1973, TUHC.

28. "Tulane University Hospital Board of Management Meeting Minutes," March 20, 1975, TUHC.

29. Starr, *The Social Transformation of Medicine*.

30. "Tulane University Hospital Board of Management Meeting minutes," November 17, 1971, TUHC.

31. "Tulane University Hospital Board of Management Meeting minutes," March 28, 1972, TUHC.

32. "Tulane University Hospital Board of Management Meeting Minutes," July 7, 1971, TUHC.

33. "Report on Financial Feasibility Study for Proposed Tulane Medical Center Hospital, Clinical Facilities and Parking Garage," August 5, 1972, TUHC.

34. Government Accountability Office, "Report to the Congress 6412," (1978) https://www.gao.gov/assets/130/122753.pdf.

35. "Tulane Medical Center Newsline #20," December 1977, TUHC.

36. "Annual Report of the Office of Medical Admissions," September 1, 1971; Tulane University Hospital Board of Management Meeting March 21, 1974, TUHC.

37. "Board of Management Meeting Minutes," September 27, 1977, TUHC.

38. Salvaggio, *New Orleans' Charity Hospital*, 202.

39. "Crisis at Charity," Human Relations Council, July 1970, NAACP Collection, ARC; "Charity Hospital Crisis Agenda," June 4, 1970, NAACP Collection, LCUNO.

40. Human Relations Council, "Monthly Reports June and September 1969," NAACP Collection, ARC.

41. This refusal of Medicaid patients led to an inundation at Flint Goodridge and Charity, resulting in Charity being forced to turn away as many as fifty patients a day. Institute of Medicine, *Health Care in a Context of Civil Rights*, 175.

42. *Cook v. Ochsner Foundation Hospital*, 61 F.R.D. 354 (E.D.La.1972).

43. Institute of Medicine, *Health Care in a Context of Civil Rights*, 182.

44. NAACP Legal Defense Fund 1981/82 Pamphlet, NAACP Collection, ARC; Hoffman, *Health Care for Some*, 146; "Hospital Oks terms of consent decree," *Times Picayune*, August 29, 1989.

45. Human Relations Council Newsletter, May–June 1971, ARC.

46. NOHD Annual Report 1973, NOHD.

47. Gould, "Childhood Lead Poisoning."

48. "Letter Doris H. Thompson, Director of Health to Charles Herndon, U.S. Dept. of Agriculture," August 10, 1973, NOHD.

49. See, Nelson, *Body and Soul*; Fernández, *The Young Lords*; Hoffman, "¡Viva La Clinica!"; Lloyd, *Health Rights Are Civil Rights*.

50. Nelson, *Body and Soul*, 6.

51. "Letter Rodney C. Jung to J. Gilbert Schaub," August 26, 1970, Housing Authority of New Orleans Collection, CANOPL.

52. Germany, *New Orleans After the Promises*, 64.

53. "Letter Evonne Lacy, Gertrude Johnson, and Margaret Tillie to Rodney Jung," April 10, 1969, New Orleans Health Department Collection, CANOPL.

54. Germany, *New Orleans After the Promises*, 198–201.

55. Germany, *New Orleans After the Promises*, 203.

56. "Pamphlet 1968–1973, Your Economic Opportunity Committee," Economic Opportunity Corporation Records, ARC; "June 16, 1970 Health and Medical Service Committee Report," Economic Opportunity Corporation Records, ARC.

57. "Memo," April 2, 1973, NOHD.

58. "Final Report on Title XIX Special Demonstration Project under Section 1115 New Orleans Model Cities Neighborhood Health Program FY 1973," NOHD.

59. "Model Cities Report 1973," NOHD.

60. "Resolution of the Neighborhood Health Council Concerning Health Services" 1973, Housing Authority of New Orleans Records, CANOPL.

61. "A Study: An Integrated Approach to Human Services Planning," The Public Development Assistance Foundation, November 1973, NOHD.

62. "Model Cities 1973 Report," NOHD.

63. Germany, *New Orleans After the Promises*, 205–207.

64. "Letter Terrance H. Duvernay to Doris Thompson," April 3, 1973, NOHD.

65. "Letter Allie Mae Williams to Doris H. Thompson," May 19, 1972, Housing Authority of New Orleans Collection, CANOPL.

66. Nelson, *Body and Soul*, 6

67. Arend, *Showdown in Desire*, 11.

68. Arend, *Showdown in Desire*, 27.

Chapter Eight

1. "Testimony of Dr. William Adams," House Committee on Interstate and Foreign Commerce Hearing on the Hospital Construction Act Amendments, May 5–8, 1958, *Hearings Volume 4* (Washington: Government Printing Office, 1958), 73.

2. "Flint Goodridge Hospital," *FOLKS*, February 6, 1983.

3. "Pamphlet," 1978, FGHC.

4. "Minutes of the Board of Management," March 12, 1981, FGHC.

5. "Minutes of the Board of Management." March 12, 1981, FGHC.

6. "Expansion Report," 1969, FGHC.

7. Institute of Medicine, *Health Care in a Context of Civil Rights*, 176.

8. "Report," November 22, 1975, FGHC.

9. "George Thomas Jr. Interview," 1986, George Thomas Jr. Papers, ARC.

10. "Board of Management Minutes," March 24, 1969, and September 4, 1979, FGHC.

11. "Report," November 22, 1975, FGHC.

12. "Position Memorandum," July 21, 1972, FGHC.

13. "Letter Quillie Parker to Henry Whyte," June 16, 1981, FGHC.

14. "Hospital's Fate Hinges on Bid by Black Doctors," *Times Picayune*, July 4, 1982.
15. "Flint Goodridge Hospital Sold," *Louisiana Weekly*, April 17, 1982.
16. "Black-Owned Hospital Sold in New Orleans," *New York Times*, March 7, 1983.
17. "Board Letter to All Physicians," November 21, 1984, FGHC.
18. "Letter David Golden to Sidney Barthelemey," May 1, 1985, Councilman Sidney J. Barthelemy Subject Files, CANOPL.
19. "Dillard Agrees to Sell Flint-Goodridge to Chain," *Times Picayune*, January 5, 1983.
20. "Black-Owned Hospital Sold in New Orleans," *New York Times*, March 7, 1983.
21. Rice and Jones, *Public Policy and the Black Hospital*, 101.
22. Starr, *The Social Transformation of American Medicine*, 428; Stevens, *In Sickness and in Wealth*, 334.
23. Starr, *The Social Transformation of American Medicine*, 430.
24. Starr, *The Social Transformation of American Medicine*, 434.
25. Starr, *The Social Transformation of American Medicine*, 464.
26. Starr, *The Social Transformation of American Medicine*, 464.
27. In 1972, Lifemark Corporation bought St. Claude General Hospital; in 1973, American Health Services Inc. bought DePaul Sanitarium; in 1977, HCA opened the Lakeview Regional Medical Center in Covington; in 1982, Tenet Healthcare opened Doctors Hospital of Jefferson; in 1984, Tenet opened Meadowcrest Hospital in Gretna; in 1985, Tenet opened St. Jude Hospital in Kenner; in 1995, Tulane merged with HCA; in 1996, Tenet purchased the Ear, Eye, Nose and Throat Hospital, and Mercy and Baptist Hospitals—Mercy became the Lindy Boggs Medical Center and Baptist the Memorial Medical Center; in 1997, Tulane/HCA acquired DePaul Hospital; in 2003, United Medical Corporation purchased Bywater Hospital; in 2003, Universal Health Services acquired Pendleton Memorial Hospital; in 2004, Universal Health Services bought Lakeland Medical Center; in 2004, Tenet sold Doctors Hospital of Jefferson to East Jefferson General Hospital; and in 2005, Lakeside Hospital for Women in Metairie and Lakeview Regional Medical Center in Covington merged with Tulane/HCA.
28. LCMC Health, "Historical Timeline of Touro Infirmary Hospital in New Orleans."
29. Department of Health and Hospitals, "Health Education Authority of Louisiana Projects," (2012).
30. Franklin, "A New Kind of Medical Disaster in the United States," 186.
31. "The Community Development Plan," February 13, 1975, NOHD.
32. "The Community Development Plan," February 13, 1975, NOHD.
33. "Transition Team Task Force on Health Progress Report," February 13, 1978, Ernest "Dutch" E. Morial Papers, ARC.
34. "NOHD Cost Report Summary," July 1, 1983 through June 30, 1984, NOHD.
35. "1985 Budget Statement," New Orleans Health Department Collection, CANOPL.
36. "NOHD Budget Message 1986," NOHD.
37. "NOHD Budget Narrative 1987," NOHD.
38. "NOHD Budget Statement 1991," NOHD.
39. "An Assessment of Need for Primary Health Care Services," May 1991, Mayor Marc H. Morial Papers, CANOPL.
40. New Orleans Sickle Cell Anemia Foundation Collection, ARC.
41. Sisco, "St. Thomas Clinic Celebrates Major Expansion."

42. Kilpatrick and Beasley, "Urban Public Hospitals," 148.

43. Dr. Frederick P. Cerise, "Letter to Governor Blanco and Members of the Governor's Health Care Reform Panel," June 24, 2004, State of Louisiana Department of Health and Hospitals Records, Louisiana State Archives, 2–6.

44. "NOHD 1991 Assessment," New Orleans Health Department Collection, CANOPL.

45. Rudowitz et al., "Health Care in New Orleans," 9.

46. "NOHD 1991 Assessment," NOHD.

47. "NOHD 1991 Assessment," NOHD.

48. "NOHD 1991 Assessment," NOHD.

49. "OPMS Charity Hospital Study Committee Report," December 1983, OPMS.

50. Salvaggio, *New Orleans' Charity Hospital*, 241–242.

51. Laborde, "A Year of Change and Turmoil"; Pope, "Charity Avoids Repairs"; Roberts and Durant, *A History of the Charity Hospitals of Louisiana*, 50.

52. Roberts and Durant, *A History of the Charity Hospitals of Louisiana*, 44–54.

53. Ott, "The Closure of New Orleans' Charity Hospital After Hurricane Katrina," 56–60.

54. Franklin, "A New Kind of Medical Disaster in the United States," 186.

55. Barrouquere, "Senate Approves Plan to Give LSU More Control of Hospitals."

56. Stephens *Governor's Health Care Reform*, 4.

57. Shuler, "Majority Favor Keeping State Charity Hospitals."

58. Moller, "Senators Blast Care at Charity Hospitals."

59. Ott, "The Closure of New Orleans' Charity Hospital After Hurricane Katrina," 69.

60. Lincoln, "The History of Tulane University's School of Medicine's Involvement with Charity Hospital"; Rudowitz et al., "Health Care in New Orleans."

61. Evans et al., *Social Determinants of Health*, 16.

62. Allen, *Uneasy Alchemy*, 1.

63. Cohen, "Development Atop a City Dump."

64. Newkirk, "The Poisoned Generation."

65. Evans et al., *Social Determinants of Health*, 16.

Conclusion

1. "Interview with Malik Rahim," August 6, 2015, Joel Buchanan Archive of Black History, University of Florida.

2. "Interview with Malik Rahim," May 23, 2006, Oral Histories of the American South Collection, University of North Carolina at Chapel Hill.

3. Morris, "Latino Health Outreach Project at Common Ground Health Clinic."

4. Assistant Secretary for Planning and Evaluation, *Role of Faith-Based and Community Organizations*.

5. "Interview with Malik Rahim," May 23, 2006, Oral Histories of the American South Collection, University of North Carolina at Chapel Hill.

6. "Study Shows Hurricane Katrina Affected 20,000 Physicians."

7. Freemantle, "Trapped Hospital Workers Kept Most Patients Alive."

8. Ott, "The Closure of New Orleans' Charity Hospital," 77–81.

9. Zigmond and Robeznieks, "Still in Recovery."

10. Franzel, *Hurricane Katrina*.
11. Pope, "LSU Hospital Wins Level 1 Designation for Emergency Room."
12. Clark, "Rebuilding the Past," 753.
13. *Framework for a Healthier Greater New Orleans* Executive Summary, November 10, 2005.
14. Clark, "Rebuilding the Past," 755.
15. *Thurman et. al v. Nagin*, Civil District Court for the Parish of Orleans 09-7244 (2009).
16. Gratz, "Why Was New Orleans's Charity Hospital Allowed to Die."
17. Clark, "Rebuilding the Past," 755.
18. Gratz, "Why Was New Orleans's Charity Hospital Allowed to Die."
19. Ott, "The Closing of New Orleans' Charity Hospital," 91–104.
20. Joseph, "STAT List."
21. RMJ M. Hillier, "Medical Center of New Orleans Charity Hospital: Feasibility Study," (2008).
22. Gratz, "Why Was New Orleans' Charity Hospital Allowed to Die."
23. Buchanan, "Hospital Building Accelerates."
24. van Holm and Wyczalkowski, "Gentrification in the Wake of Hurricane."
25. Moller, "LRA Agrees to $74 Million Down Payment on Hospital."
26. Urban League of Greater New Orleans, *State of Black New Orleans*, 129.
27. Worthy, "St. Thomas Opens New State of the Art Health Center in Gentilly."
28. New Orleans Musicians' Clinic & Assistance Foundation, "About Us."
29. Adelson, "Programs that Provide Health Care."
30. New Orleans Health Department, "Community Health Improvement plan, 2nd Revision" (2016).
31. Urban League of Greater New Orleans, *State of Black New Orleans*, 129.
32. Urban League of Greater New Orleans, *State of Black New Orleans*, 27.
33. Adelson, "Programs that Provide Health Care."
34. Barnes et al., *Louisiana Health Insurance Survey 2017*.
35. Urban League of Greater New Orleans, *State of Black New Orleans*, 126.
36. Urban League of Greater New Orleans, *State of Black New Orleans*, 128.
37. Broussard et al., *Advancing Health Equity in New Orleans*.
38. Urban League of Greater New Orleans, *State of Black New Orleans*, 126.
39. Robeznieks, "Miles to Go."
40. Van Holm and Wyczalkowski, "Gentrification in the Wake of a Hurricane."
41. Corporation for Enterprise Development, *The Racial Wealth Divide in New Orleans*.
42. Corporation for Enterprise Development, *The Racial Wealth Divide in New Orleans*. The Asian American and Latino American populations both grew in the period, from 2 and 3 percent, respectively, in 2000 to 4 and 6 percent by 2015. While beyond the scope of this work, the Latino population in New Orleans has also faced inequality in access to health care and racial health disparity.
43. In 2015, African Americans had an unemployment rate of 15.3 percent compared to 5.1 percent for whites. Corporation for Enterprise Development, *The Racial Wealth Divide in New Orleans*. In 2016, the median Black household income was $25,324, compared to $67,884 for whites. Plyer and Gardere, *The New Orleans Prosperity Index*.

44. Over 71 percent of Black households earned less than what MIT estimated was a living wage of $47,200 in New Orleans in 2016, compared to 31 percent of white households. Henrici et al., *Get to the Bricks*, viii.

45. Corporation for Enterprise Development, *The Racial Wealth Divide in New Orleans*.

46. Evans et al., *Social Determinants of Health and Crime in Post-Katrina Orleans Parish*, 16; Broussard et al., *Advancing Health Equity in New Orleans*, 8.

47. Broussard et al., *Advancing Health Equity in New Orleans*, 8.

48. Curth, "New Orleans Facing HIV Epidemic."

49. Broussard et al., *Advancing Health Equity in New Orleans*.

50. New Orleans Health Department, *Health Disparities in New Orleans*, 3.

51. Louisiana Budget Project, *Location and Life Expectancy in New Orleans*; Arias et al., *U.S. Small-Area Life Expectancy Estimate Project*.

52. See, for example, Pardies et al., "A Systematic Review of the Extent and Measurement of Healthcare Provider Racism."

53. Adkins-Jackson et al., "How to Measure Racism in Academic Health Centers."

54. Kiefer, "Tulane School of Medicine Placed on Probation."

55. Broussard et al., *Advancing Health Equity in New Orleans*, 10.

56. Alsan et al., *Does Diversity Matter for Health?*

57. Joseph, "STAT List."

58. U.S. Bureau of Labor Statistics, "Table 1."

59. Massachusetts Institute of Technology, "Living Wage Calculation for New Orleans-Metairie, LA."

60. McAuley, "Seeking Public Money."

Bibliography

Archives and Collections Used

Amistad Research Center, New Orleans (ARC)
    Albert and Jessie Dent Family Papers
    American Missionary Association Collection
    A. P. Tureaud Papers
    Daniel Ellis Byrd Papers
    Economic Opportunity Corporation Records
    Ernest "Dutch" E. Morial Papers
    George Thomas Jr. Papers
    Henry E. Braden III Papers
    Joseph Hardin Papers
    Kim Lacy Rogers Collection
    Marc H. Morial Papers
    National Association for the Advancement of Colored People,
        Office of Field Director of Louisiana Records (NAACP)
    New Orleans Sickle Cell Anemia Foundation Collection
    Rivers Frederick Papers
    Robert Elijah Jones Papers
    Rosa Freeman Keller Papers
    Small Collection
City Archives, New Orleans Public Library, New Orleans (CANOPL)
    City Directories
    City Planning and Zoning Commission Records
    Commission Council Series
    Councilman Sidney J. Barthelemy Subject Files
    H.E.A.L. Collection
    Hospitals Collection
    Hospital & Insanity Records
    Housing Authority of New Orleans Collection
    Mayor Andrew McShane Papers
    Mayor Arthur J. O'Keefe Records
    Mayor Chep Morrison Records
    Mayor Ernest N. Morial Records
    Mayor Marc H. Morial Papers
    Mayor Martin Behrman Records
    Mayor Robert S. Maestri Records
    Mayor Sidney J. Barthelemey Records

Mayor Victor Hugo Schiro Collection
New Orleans Health Department Collection (NOHD)
New Orleans Planning Records
Records of the City Councils
Rosa Keller Papers
Sanborn Fire Insurance Maps
Woods Directory
WPA Photograph Collection
Dillard University Archives, New Orleans (FGHC)
    Flint Goodridge Hospital Collection
Ethel and Herman Midlo Center for New Orleans Studies,
      University of New Orleans, New Orleans
    Oral History Project Collection
Historic New Orleans Collection, New Orleans
    Franck-Bertacci Photographers Collection
Howard University Archives, Washington, D.C.
    Peter Marshall Murray Papers
Joel Buchanan Archive of Black History, University of Florida, Gainesville
    African American History Project Oral Histories
Louisiana Collection, University of New Orleans (LCUNO)
    A. P. Tureaud Collection
    Charity Hospital School of Nursing Collection
    Community Services Council of New Orleans, Inc. Collection
    Department of Health & Hospitals Vertical Files
    Edgar Hull Papers
    Marcus Christian Collection
    National Association for the Advancement of Colored People,
        New Orleans Branch Collection (NAACP)
    Patricia Williams Collection
    Sidney J. Barthelemy Collection
Library of Congress, Washington, D.C.
    African American Pamphlet Collection
    Archives du Ministère de la Guerre
    Maps Collection
Louisiana Research Center, Tulane University, New Orleans (LRCTU)
    Charles Cassidy Bass Papers
    Charles Rouseve Papers
    Council of Social Agencies of New Orleans Records
    Edgar B. Stern Collection
    Edmond Souchon Papers
    Henry Dickson Bruns Papers
    John Minor Wisdom Collection
    Joseph Jones Papers
    Medical Documents Collection
    New Orleans Social Council Collection

Orleans Parish Medical Society Collection (OPMS)
Rosemonde E. & Emile Kuntz Collection
Rudolph Matas Papers
Société Française Records
Stanford E. Chaille Papers
Tulane University Hospital Collection (TUHC)
United States Marine Hospital Records
Louisiana State Archives, Baton Rouge
   State of Louisiana Department of Health and Hospitals Records
Louisiana State Museum Historical Center, New Orleans
   Antebellum Period Collection
   Charity Hospital Papers
   Master Calendar Collection
Notarial Archives, Washington, D.C.
Records of the French Superior Council in New Orleans
   National Archives and Records Administration, College Park (NARA)
   Records of the Bureau of Refugees, Freedmen, and Abandoned Lands
Rudolph Matas Library of the Health Sciences, Tulane University, New Orleans (RMTU)
   Charity Hospital Records (CHC)
   Medical College of Louisiana Records
Southeastern Architectural Archive, Tulane University, New Orleans
   James R. Lamantia Jr. Office Records and Collection
   Leon Francis Dufrechou Office Records
   Miscellaneous Photographs Collection
   Rathbone DeBuys Office Records
   Robert Mills Papers
   Sanborn Fire Insurance Maps Collection
   Theodore Lilenthal New Orleans Photographs Collection
State Library of Louisiana, Baton Rouge
   Louisiana Works Progress Administration Collection
University of North Carolina at Chapel Hill Library, Chapel Hill
   Oral Histories of the American South Collection

Primary Source Periodicals

Chicago Defender
Congress Reports
The Crisis
DeBow's Journal
FOLKS
Journal of the American Medical Association
Journal of the National Medical Association
Louisiana Board of Health Annual Report
Louisiana Historic Quarterly
Louisiana Weekly
New Orleans Medical and Surgical Journal
New Orleans Medical News and Hospital Gazette
New Orleans States-Item
New York Times
Pittsburgh Courier
Public Health Bulletin
Public Health Reports
The Saturday Evening Post
Southwestern Christian Advocate

Times Picayune
Transactions of the American
   Medical Association
Transactions of the American
   Surgical Association
Who's Who of the Colored Race

Government Documents

Bureau of the Census, Mortality Statistics 1905, 1910
Department of Defense, "Assessment of Post-Attack Health Resources," July 1, 1970
Department of Health and Hospitals, "Health Education Authority of Louisiana Projects," (2012)
Government Accountability Office, "Report to the Congress 6412," (1978)
Louisiana Board of Health Annual Report, 1883–1884, 1906–1907
Louisiana Code Noir (1724)
New Orleans Health Department, "Community Health Improvement Plan, 2nd Revision" (2016).
New Orleans Sewerage and Water Board, Twenty-Sixth Semi-Annual Report (1912)
"Testimony of Dr. William Adams," House Committee on Interstate and Foreign Commerce Hearing on the Hospital Construction Act Amendments, May 5-8, 1958, Hearings Volume 4 (Washington: Government Printing Office, 1958)

Court Cases

Cook v. Ochsner Foundation Hospital, 61 F.R.D. 354 (E.D.La.1972)
Harmon v. Tyler, 273 U.S. 668 (1927)
The Josefa Segunda, 18 U.S. 5 Wheat. 338 338 (1820)
Thurman et al. v. Nagin, Civil District Court for the Parish of Orleans 09-7244 (2009)

Miscellaneous Primary Sources

Abraham Flexner, "Medical Education in the United States and Canada: A Report to the Carnegie Foundation for the Advancement of Teaching" (New York: Carnegie Foundation, 1910)
A. W. Dent, "The Role of a Negro Clinic in the Control of Tuberculosis in a Large Southern City," *Transactions of the Thirty-Seventh Annual Meeting of the National Tuberculosis Association* (1941)
RMJ M. Hillier, "Medical Center of New Orleans Charity Hospital: Feasibility Study," (2008)

Works Cited

Adams, Thomas Jessen, and Matt Sakakeeny, eds. *Remaking New Orleans: Beyond Exceptionalism and Authenticity*. Durham, NC: Duke University Press, 2019.
Adelson, Jeff. "Programs that Provide Health Care to Thousands on Verge of Going Broke." *Times Picayune*, April 29, 2014.
Adler, Jeffrey. *Murder in New Orleans: The Creation of Jim Crow Policing*. Chicago: University of Chicago Press, 2019.

Allen, Barbara L. *Uneasy Alchemy: Citizens and Experts in Louisiana's Chemical Corridor Disputes.* Cambridge, MA: MIT Press, 2003.

Alsan, Marcella, Owen Garrick, and Grant C. Graziani. *Does Diversity Matter for Health?* Cambridge, MA: National Bureau of Economic Research, 2018.

Arend, Orissa. *Showdown in Desire: The Black Panthers Take a Stand in New Orleans.* Fayetteville: University of Arkansas Press, 2009.

Arias, E., L. A. Escobedo, J. Kennedy, C. Fu, and K. Cisewski. *U.S. Small-Area Life Expectancy Estimate Project.* Atlanta: Centers for Disease Control, 2018.

Artiga, Samantha, and Kendal Ortega. "Key Facts on Health and Health Care by Race and Ethnicity." *Kaiser Family Foundation*, November 12, 2019.

Assistant Secretary for Planning and Evaluation. *Role of Faith-Based and Community Organizations in Providing Relief and Recovery Services after Hurricane Katrina and Rita.* Washington, DC: U.S. Department of Health and Human Services, 2008.

Bankole-Medina, Katherine. *Slavery and Medicine: Enslavement and Medical Practices in Antebellum Louisiana.* Oxfordshire, UK: Routledge, 1998.

Barnes, Stephen, Mike Henderson, Dek Terrell, and Stephanie Virgets. *Louisiana Health Insurance Survey 2017.* Accessed August 12, 2022. http://ldh.la.gov/assets/media/2017-Louisiana-Health-Insurance-Survey-Report.pdf.

Barrouquere, Brett. "Senate Approves Plan to Give LSU More Control of Hospitals." *The Advocate*, June 23, 2003.

Blassingame, John H. *Black New Orleans, 1860–1880.* Chicago: University of Chicago Press, 1973.

Bonilla-Silva, Eduardo. "More than Prejudice: Restatement, Reflections, and New Directions in Race Theory." *Sociology of Race and Ethnicity* 1, no. 1 (2015): 75–89.

Broussard, Danielle, Lisa Richardson, Maeve Wallace, and Katherine Theall. *Advancing Health Equity in New Orleans: Building on Positive Change in Health.* New Orleans: The Data Center, 2018.

Buchanan, Susan. "Hospital Building Accelerates in New Orleans After Homes Were Moved." *Huffington Post*, August 8, 2012.

Byrd, William, and Linda A. Clayton. *An American Health Dilemma: A Medical History of African Americans and the Problem of Race.* New York: Routledge, 2000.

Campanella, Richard. *Cityscapes of New Orleans.* Baton Rouge: Louisiana State University Press, 2017.

———. "An Ethnic Geography of New Orleans." *Journal of American History* 94, no. 3 (December 2007): 704–715.

———. *Geographies of New Orleans: Urban Fabrics Before the Storm.* Lafayette: University of Louisiana, 2006.

Carpenter, Arthur Eldred. "Gateway to the Americas: New Orleans's for Latin American Trade, 1900–1970." PhD diss., Tulane University, 1987.

———. "Social Origins of Anti-Communism: The Information Council of the Americas." *Louisiana History: The Journal of the Louisiana Historical Association* 30, no. 2 (Spring 1989): 117–143.

Carrier, Jim. *Charity: The Heroic and Heartbreaking Story of Charity Hospital in Hurricane Katrina.* Ranger Media, 2015.

Centers for Disease Control and Prevention. "CDC Research on SDOH." Accessed May 7, 2019. www.cdc.gov/socialdeterminants/index.htm.

Cherrie, Lolita V. "A Black Physician in the Jim Crow South: Dr. Raleigh J. Coker." November 6, 2014. www.creolegen.org/2014/11/06/a-black-physician-in-the-jim-crow-south-dr-raleigh-j-coker-1885-1953/.

Clark, Mary A. "Rebuilding the Past: Health Care Reform in Post-Katrina Louisiana." *Journal of Health Politics, Policy, and Law* 35, no. 5 (October 2010): 743–769.

Cohen, Ariella. "Development Atop a City Dump." *The Lens*, January 11, 2012.

Colten, Craig E. "Basin Street Blues: Drainage and Environmental Equity in New Orleans, 1890–1930." *Journal of Historical Geography* 28, no. 2 (2002): 237–257.

Connor, Catherine A. "The University That Ate Birmingham: The Healthcare Industry, Urban Development, and Neoliberalism." *Journal of Urban History* 42, no. 2 (March 2006): 284–305.

Cornley, Paul B. "Segregation and Discrimination in Medical Care in the United States." *Journal of the American Medical Association* 46 (1956): 1074–1081.

Corporation for Enterprise Development. *The Racial Wealth Divide in New Orleans*. Washington, DC: Corporation for Enterprise Development, 2016.

Covey, Herbert C. *African American Slave Medicine: Herbal and Non-Herbal Treatments*. Lanham, MD: Lexington Books, 2007.

Cruzat, Heloise Hulse. "The Ursulines of Louisiana." *Louisiana Historical Quarterly* 2, no. 1 (1919): 5–23.

Curth, Kimberly. "New Orleans Facing HIV Epidemic." *Fox 8*, November 18, 2016.

Decuir, Sharlene Sinegal. "Attacking Jim Crow: Black Activism in New Orleans 1925–1941." PhD diss., Louisiana State University, 2009.

de Grummon, Jane Lucas. *Renato Beluche: Smuggler, Privateer, and Patriot, 1780—1860*. Baton Rouge: Louisiana State University Press, 1983.

Devore, Donald E. *Defying Jim Crow: African American Community Development and the Struggle for Racial Equality in New Orleans, 1900–1960*. Baton Rouge: Louisiana State University Press, 2015.

Downs, Jim. *Sick from Freedom: African-American Illness and Suffering during the Civil War and Reconstruction*. Oxford: Oxford University Press, 2012.

Duffy, John. *The Samaritans: A History of American Public Health*. Urbana: University of Illinois Press, 1990.

Emanuel, Rachel L., and Alexander P. Tureaud Jr. *A More Noble Cause: A. P. Tureaud and the Struggle for Civil Rights in Louisiana*. Baton Rouge: Louisiana State University Press, 2011.

Evans, Benjamin F., Emily Zimmerman, Steven H. Woolf, and Amber D. Haley. *Social Determinants of Health and Crime in Post-Katrina Orleans Parish*. Richmond, VA: Center on Human Needs, 2012.

Fairclough, Adam. *Race & Democracy: The Civil Rights Struggle in Louisiana, 1915–1972*. Athens: University of Georgia Press, 1995.

Fernández, Johann. *The Young Lords: A Radical History*. Chapel Hill: University of North Carolina Press, 2020.

Fett, Sharla M. *Working Cures: Healing, Health, and Power on Southern Slave Plantations*. Chapel Hill: University of North Carolina Press, 2002.

Finley, Keith. "Lynching." Accessed April 12, 2019. https://64parishes.org/entry/lynching.

Florida, Richard. "Where Eds and Meds Industries Could Become a Liability." CityLab, November 26, 2013.

Fogel, Robert William. *Without Consent or Contract: The Rise and Fall of American Slavery.* New York: W. W. Norton, 1989.

Fortier, Alcee, ed. *Louisiana: Comprising Sketches of Parishes, Towns, Events, Institutions, and Persons, Arranged in Cyclopedic Form*, Vol. 3. New Orleans: Century Historical Association, 1914.

Fossier, A. E. "The Charity Hospital of New Orleans." *New Orleans Medical and Surgical Journal* 39 (1923): 728–730.

Franklin, Evangeline. "A New Kind of Medical Disaster in the United States." In *There is No Such Thing as a Natural Disaster*, edited by Gregory Squires and Chester Hartman, 185–195. New York: Routledge, 2006.

Franzel, Jeanette M. *Hurricane Katrina Trends in the Operating Results of Five Hospitals in New Orleans Before and After Hurricane Katrina.* Washington, DC: U.S. Government Accountability Office, 2008.

Freemantle, Tony. "Trapped Hospital Workers Kept Most Patients Alive." *Houston Chronicle*, September 18, 2005.

French, B. F. *Collections of Louisiana.* New York: D. Appleton, 1851.

Gaines, Kevin. *Uplifting the Race: Black Leadership Politics and Culture in the Twentieth Century.* Chapel Hill: University of North Carolina Press, 1996.

Gamble, Vanessa Northington. *Making a Place for Ourselves: The Black Hospital Movement, 1920–1945.* Oxford: Oxford University Press, 1995.

Germany, Kent. *New Orleans After the Promises: Poverty, Citizenship and the Great Society.* Athens: University of Georgia Press, 2007.

Gotham, Kevin Fox. *Authentic New Orleans: Tourism, Race, and Culture in the Big Easy.* New York: New York University Press, 2007.

Gould, Elise. "Childhood Lead Poisoning: Conservative Estimates of the Social and Economic Benefits of Lead Hazard Control." *Environmental Health Perspectives* 117, no. 7 (2009): 1162–1167.

Gratz, Roberta Brandes. "Why Was New Orleans's Charity Hospital Allowed to Die." *The Nation*, May 16, 2011.

Haas, Edward F. *DeLesseps S. Morrison and the Image of Reform.* Baton Rouge: Louisiana State University Press, 1974.

Hall, Gwendolyn Midlo Hall. *Africans in Colonial Louisiana: The Development of Afro-Creole Culture in the Eighteenth Century.* Baton Rouge: Louisiana State University Press, 1995.

Hayes, Phoebe. "Emma Wakefield-Paillet, MD." Accessed January 11, 2020. https://64parishes.org/emma-wakefield-paillet-md.

Haynes, Stephen R. *Noah's Curse: The Biblical Justification of American Slavery.* New York: Oxford University Press, 2002.

Henrici, Jane, Chandra Childers, and Elyse Shaw. *Get to the Bricks: The Experience of Black Women from Public Housing after Hurricane Katrina.* Washington, DC: Institute for Women's Policy Research, 2015.

Hine, Darlene Clark. *Black Women in White: Racial Conflict and Cooperation in the Nursing Profession, 1890–1950.* Bloomington: Indiana University Press, 1989.

Hirsch, Arnold R. *Making the Second Ghetto: Race and Housing in Chicago, 1940–1960.* Chicago: University of Chicago Press, 1983.

Hoffman, Beatrix. *Health Care for Some: Rights and Rationing in the United States Since 1930*. Chicago: University of Chicago Press, 2012.

———. "¡Viva La Clinica!": The United Farm Workers' Fight for Medical Care," *Bulletin of the History of Medicine* 93, no. 4 (2019): 518–549.

Hogarth, Rana A. *Medicalizing Blackness: Making Racial Difference in the Atlantic World, 1780–1840*. Chapel Hill: University of North Carolina Press, 2017.

Horowitz, Andy. *Katrina: A History, 1915–2015*. Cambridge, MA: Harvard University Press, 2020.

"How to Measure Racism in Academic Health Centers." *AMA Journal of Ethics* 23, no. 2 (February 2021): 140–145.

Institute of Medicine. *Health Care in a Context of Civil Rights*. Washington, DC: The National Academies Press, 1981.

Johnson, Rashauna. *Slavery's Metropolis: Unfree Labor in New Orleans During the Age of Revolutions*. Cambridge: Cambridge University Press, 2016.

Johnson, Walter. *Soul by Soul: Life Inside the Antebellum Slave Market*. Cambridge, MA: Harvard University Press, 2001.

Joseph, Andrew. "STAT List: These 10 Cities Had the Biggest Jumps in Hospital Jobs." STAT News, October 11, 2017.

Keller, Rosa. *Memoirs*. New Orleans: 1977.

Kemp, Kathryn W. "Jean and Kate Gordon: New Orleans Social Reformers, 1898–1933." *Louisiana History: The Journal of the Louisiana Historical Association* 24, no. 4 (Autumn 1983): 389–401.

Kenny, Stephen C. "A Dictate of Both Interest and Mercy? Slave Hospitals in the Antebellum South." *Journal of the History of Medicine and Allied Sciences* 65, no. 1 (2010): 1–47.

———. "Specimens Calculated to Shock the Soundest Sleeper: Deep Layers of Anatomical Racism Circulated On-Board the Louisiana Health Exhibit Train." In *Bodies Beyond Borders: Moving Anatomies, 1750–1950*, edited by Kaat Wils, Raf de Bont, and Sokhieng Au. Leuven, Belgium: Leuven University Press, 2017.

Kiefer, Philip. "Tulane School of Medicine Placed on Probation," *The Lens*, July 6, 2021.

Kilpatrick, Anne Osborne, and Lynn W. Beasley. "Urban Public Hospitals: Evolutions, Challenges, and Opportunities in an Era of Health Reform." *Journal of Health and Human Services Administration* 18, no. 2 (1995): 143–162.

Klein, Herbert S., Stanley L. Engerman, Robin Haines, and Ralph Shlomowitz. "Transoceanic Mortality: The Slave Trade in Comparative Perspective." *William & Mary Quarterly* 58, no. 1 (January 2001): 93–188.

Klein, Russell C. *A History of LSU School of Medicine New Orleans*. New Orleans: Louisiana State University Medical Alumni Association, 2010.

Laborde, Karen. "A Year of Change and Turmoil." *New Orleans City Business*, May 31, 1993.

Lahut, Jake. "Fauci Says the Coronavirus Is 'Shining a Bright Light' on 'Unacceptable' Health Disparities for African Americans." *Business Insider*, April 7, 2020.

Larson, Edward. *Sex, Race, and Science: Eugenics in the Deep South*. Baltimore, MD: Johns Hopkins University Press, 1995.

LCMC Health. "Historical Timeline of Touro Infirmary Hospital in New Orleans." Accessed January 11, 202. https://www.lcmchealth.org/touro/about-us/touro-timeline/.

Lincoln, Douglas R. "The History of Tulane University's School of Medicine's Involvement with Charity Hospital." Accessed February 20, 2020. http://www2.tulane.edu/~matas/historical/charity/.

Lloyd, Jenna. *Health Rights Are Civil Rights: Peace and Justice Activism in Los Angeles, 1963–1978.* Minneapolis: University of Minnesota Press, 2014.

Long, Carolyn Morrow. *A New Orleans Voudou Priestess: The Legend and Reality of Marie Laveau.* Gainesville: University of Florida Press, 2006.

Long, Gretchen. *Doctoring Freedom: The Politics of African American Medical Care in Slavery and Emancipation.* Chapel Hill: University of North Carolina Press, 2016.

Louisiana Budget Project. *Location and Life Expectancy in New Orleans.* Baton Rouge: Louisiana Budge Project, 2018.

Louisiana Department of Health. "Louisiana Coronavirus Information." Accessed June 1, 2021. https://ldh.la.gov/Coronavirus/.

Marler, Scott P. *The Merchants' Capital: New Orleans and the Political Economy of the Nineteenth-Century South.* New York: Cambridge University Press, 2013.

Massachusetts Institute of Technology. "Living Wage Calculation for New Orleans-Metairie, LA." Accessed August 15, 2022. https://livingwage.mit.edu/metros/35380.

Matas, Rudolph. *History of Medicine in Louisiana.* Baton Rouge: Louisiana State University Press, 1962

McAuley, Anthony. "Seeking Public Money, New Orleans BioDistrict Paints Picture of a Vibrant New Sector." *Times Picayune,* August 14, 2021.

McBride, David. *Integrating the City of Medicine: Blacks in Philadelphia Health Care, 1910–1965.* Philadelphia: Temple University Press, 1989.

McKee, Guian. "The Hospital City in an Ethnic Enclave: Tufts-New England Medical Center, Boston's Chinatown, and the Urban Political Economy of Health Care." *Journal of Urban History* 42, no. 2 (March 2016): 259–283.

Miller, Z. L. "Urban Blacks in the South, 1865–1920: The Richmond, Savannah, New Orleans, Louisville, and Birmingham Experience." In *The New Urban History,* edited by L. F. Schnore, 184–227. Princeton, NJ: Princeton University Press, 1975.

Mintz, Steven. "Childhood and Transatlantic Slavery." Accessed January 1, 2018. http://chnm.gmu.edu/cyh/items/show/57.

Mohr, Clarence L. *Tulane: The Emergence of a Modern University, 1945–1980.* Baton Rouge: Louisiana State University Press, 2001.

Moller, Jan. "LRA Agrees to $74 Million Down Payment on Hospital." *Times Picayune,* December 15, 2006.

———. "Senators Blast Care at Charity Hospitals." *Times Picayune,* June 3, 2005.

Monroe Work Today. "Map of White Supremacy White Violence." Accessed April 12, 2019. www.monroeworktoday.org/explore/.

Moore, Leonard L. *Black Rage in New Orleans: Police Brutality and African American Activism from World War II to Hurricane Katrina.* Baton Rouge: Louisiana State University Press, 2010.

Morris, Benjamin. "Latino Health Outreach Project at Common Ground Health Clinic." *Uptown Messenger,* April 30, 2011.

National Institute on Minority Health and Health Disparities. "Death Rates Table 5 Year Average." https://hdpulse.nimhd.nih.gov/data/recenttrend/data.php?0&11&0&9599&001&999&00&1&0&0&2&1.

Nelson, Alondra. *Body and Soul: The Black Panther Party and the Fight against Medical Discrimination*. Minneapolis: University of Minnesota Press, 2013.

Newkirk, Vann R., II. "The Poisoned Generation." *The Atlantic*, May 21, 2017.

New Orleans Health Department. *Heath Disparities in New Orleans*. New Orleans: New Orleans Health Department, 2013.

New Orleans Musicians' Clinic & Assistance Foundation. "About Us." Accessed August 15, 2022. https://neworleansmusiciansclinic.org/about/about-nomc/history-of-the-nomc/.

Northup, Solomon. *Twelve Years a Slave*. 1853.

Nystrom, Justin A. *New Orleans After the Civil War: Race, Politics, and the New Birth of Freedom*. Baltimore, MD: John Hopkins Press, 2010.

Olivarius, Kathryn Meyer. *Necropolis: Disease, Power, and Capitalism in the Cotton Kingdom*. Cambridge, MA: Harvard University Press, 2022.

Ott, Kenneth Brad. "The Closure of New Orleans' Charity Hospital After Hurricane Katrina." Master's thesis, University of New Orleans, 2012.

Oviedo, Brian H. *National Register of Historic Places Inventory/Nomination Form: The Houmas*. Washington, DC: National Park Service, 1979.

Owens, Deirdre Cooper. *Medical Bondage: Race, Gender, and the Origins of American Gynecology*. Athens: University of Georgia Press, 2017.

Pardies, Yin, Mandy Truong, and Naomi Priest. "A Systematic Review of the Extent and Measurement of Healthcare Provider Racism." *Journal of General Internal Medicine* 29, no. 2 (February 2014): 364–387.

Plyer, Allison, and Lamar Gardere. *The New Orleans Prosperity Index*. New Orleans: The Data Center, 2018.

Pope, John. "Charity Avoids Repairs." *Times Picayune*, March 23, 1995.

———. "LSU Hospital Wins Level 1 Designation for Emergency Room." *Times Picayune*, December 16, 2008.

Prince, K. Stephen. *The Ballad of Robert Charles: Searching for the New Orleans Riot of 1900*. Chapel Hill: University of North Carolina Press, 2021.

Pritchett, Jonathan, and Myeong-Su Yun. *The In-Hospital Mortality Rates of Slaves and Freemen: Evidence from Touro Infirmary, New Orleans, Louisiana, 1855–1860*. Bonn, Germany: Institute for the Study of Labor, 2008.

Radford, Gail. *Modern Housing for America: Policy Struggles in the New Deal Era*. Chicago: University of Chicago Press, 1996.

Rao, S.L.N. "On Long-term Mortality Trends in the United States, 1850–1968." *Demography* 10, no. 3 (August 1973): 405–419.

Rice, Mitchell F., and Woodrow Jones. *Public Policy and the Black Hospital: From Slavery to Segregation to Integration*. Westport, CT: Greenwood, 1994.

Richardson, Joe M. "Albert W. Dent: A Black New Orleans Hospital and University Administrator." *Louisiana History: The Journal of the Louisiana Historical Association* 37, no. 3 (Summer 1996): 309–323.

Roberts, Jonathan, and Thomas J. Durant Jr. *A History of the Charity Hospitals of Louisiana: A Study of Poverty, Politics, Public Health and the Public Interest.* Lewiston, NY: Mellen Press, 2009.

Roberts, Samuel K., Jr. *Infectious Fear: Politics, Disease, and the Health Effects of Segregation.* Chapel Hill: University of North Carolina Press, 2009.

Robeznieks, Andis. "Miles to Go: New Orleans's Mental Health Services Still on the Mend." *Modern Health Care*, August 29, 2016.

Rogers, Kim Lacy. *Righteous Lives: Narratives of the New Orleans Civil Rights Movement.* New York: New York University Press, 1994.

Rosenberg, Charles E. *The Care of Strangers: The Rise of America's Hospital System.* New York: Basic Books, 1987.

Rosenberg, Charles E. "Martinet, Louis Andre." Oxford African American Studies Center. May 31, 2013. https://oxfordaasc.com/view/10.1093/acref/9780195301731.001.0001/acref-9780195301731-e-38685.

Rothman, Joshua. "Before the Civil War, New Orleans Was the Center of the U.S. Slave Trade." *Smithsonian Magazine*, April 19, 2021.

Roudanez, Mark Charles. "Grappling with the Memory of New Orleans." *The Atlantic*, October 25, 2015.

Rudowitz, Robin, Diane Rowland, and Adele Shartzer. "Health Care in New Orleans Before and After Katrina." Supplement, *Health Affairs* 25, no. S1 (2006): 393–406.

Russell, William Howard. *My Diary North and South.* Boston: T. O. H. P. Burnham, 1863.

Salvaggio, John E. *New Orleans' Charity Hospital.* Baton Rouge: Louisiana State University Press, 1992.

Savitt, Todd L. "Entering a White Profession: Black Physicians in the New South 1880–1920." *Bulletin of the History of Medicine* 61, no. 4 (Winter 1987): 507–540.

———. "Straight University Medical Department: The Short Life of a Black Medical School in Reconstruction New Orleans." *Louisiana History* 41 (2000): 175–201.

Schwartz, Marie Jenkins. *Birthing a Slave: Motherhood and Medicine in the Antebellum South.* Cambridge, MA: Harvard University Press, 2010.

Shah, Nyan. *Contagious Divides: Epidemics and Race in San Francisco's Chinatown.* Berkeley: University of California Press, 2001.

Shuler, Marsha. "Majority Favor Keeping State Charity Hospitals." *The Advocate*, January 12, 2005.

Simpson, Andrew T. *The Medical Metropolis: Health Care and Economic Transformation in Pittsburgh and Houston.* Philadelphia: University of Pennsylvania Press, 2019.

Sisco, Annette. "St. Thomas Clinic Celebrates Major Expansion." *Times Picayune*, March 28, 2012.

Smith, Douglas L. "Black Communities Mobilize." In *The African American Experience in Louisiana: From Jim Crow to Civil Rights*, edited by Charles Vincent. Lafayette: University of Louisiana at Lafayette, 2002.

Smith, Susan L. *Sick and Tired of Being Sick and Tired: Black Women's Health Activism in America, 1890–1950.* Philadelphia: University of Pennsylvania Press, 1995.

Souther, J. Mark. *New Orleans on Parade: Tourism and the Transformation of the Crescent City.* Baton Rouge: Louisiana State University Press, 2006.

Stange, Marion. *Vital Negotiations: Protecting Settlers' Health in Colonial Louisiana and South Carolina, 1720–1763*. Göttingen, Germany: Vandenhoeck & Ruprecht, 2012.

Starr, Paul. *The Social Transformation of American Medicine: The Rise of a Sovereign Profession and the Making of a Vast Industry*. New York: Basic Books, 1982.

Stephens, Kevin U. *Governor's Health Care Reform: Region 1 Consortium Update*. Louisiana Regional Health Care Consortium Region One, March 17, 2005.

Stevens, Rosemary. *In Sickness and in Wealth: American Hospitals in the Twentieth Century*. New York: Basic Books, 1989.

"Study Shows Hurricane Katrina Affected 20,000 Physicians, Up To 6,000 May Have Been Displaced." *Science News*, September 28, 2005.

Sumpter, Amy R. "Segregation of the Free People of Color and the Construction of Race in Antebellum New Orleans." *Southeastern Geographer* 48, no. 1 (May 2008): 19–37.

Tadman, Michael. "The Demographic Cost of Sugar: Debates on Slave Societies and Natural Increase in the Americas." *American Historical Review* 105, no. 5 (December 2000): 1534–1575.

Tansey, R. "Bernard Kendig and the New Orleans Slave Trade." *Louisiana History* 23, no. 2 (1982): 159–178.

Thomas, Karen Kruse. *Deluxe Jim Crow: Civil Rights and American Health Policy, 1935–1954*. Athens: University of Georgia Press, 2011.

University of Richmond. "Mapping Inequality: Redlining in New Deal America." Accessed August 12, 2022. https://dsl.richmond.edu/panorama/redlining/#loc=15/29.9420/-90.0910&opacity=0.8&city=new-orleans-la&area=D34.

Urban League of Greater New Orleans. *State of Black New Orleans 10 Years Post-Katrina*. New Orleans: Urban League of Greater New Orleans, 2015.

U.S. Bureau of Labor Statistics. "Table 1. Employment and Wage Data for Food Preparation and Serving Related Occupations, New Orleans Metropolitan Area, May 2021." Accessed August 15, 2022. www.bls.gov/regions/southwest/news-release/occupationalemploymentandwages_neworleans.htm#table1.

"U.S. Hospitals and the Civil Rights Act of 1964." *Hospitals and Health Networks Magazine*, June 3, 2014.

van Holm, Eric Joseph, and Christopher K. Wyczalkowski. "Gentrification in the Wake of Hurricane: New Orleans After Katrina." *Urban Studies* 56, no. 13 (2018): 2763–2778.

Vidal, Cecile, ed. *Louisiana: Crossroads of the Atlantic World*. Philadelphia: University of Pennsylvania Press, 2014.

Vincent, Charles. "Aspects of the Family and Public Life of Antoine Dubuclet: Louisiana's Black State Treasurer." *Journal of Negro History* 66, no. 1 (Spring 1981): 26–36.

Wailoo, Keith. *Dying in the City of the Blues: Sickle Cell Anemia and the Politics of Race and Health*. Chapel Hill: University of North Carolina Press, 2001.

Waldman, Anna, and Joshua Kaplan. "Sent Home to Die." *ProPublica*, September 2, 2020.

The War Department. *Reports of the Extent and Nature of the Materials Available for the Preparation of a Medical and Surgical History of the Rebellion*. Philadelphia: J.B. Lippincott & Co., 1865.

Ward, Thomas J., Jr. *Black Physicians in the Jim Crow South*. Fayetteville: University of Arkansas Press, 2010.

Washington, Harriet A. *Medical Apartheid: The Dark History of Medical Experimentation on Black Americans from Colonial Times to the Present.* New York: Doubleday, 2007.
Washington, Harriet A., Robert B. Baker, Ololade Olakanmi, Todd L. Savitt, Elizabeth A. Jacobs, Eddie Hoover, and Matthew K. Wynia. "Segregation, Civil Rights, and Health Disparities: The Legacy of African American Physicians and Organized Medicine, 1910–1968." *Journal of the National Medical Association* 101, no. 6 (June 2009): 513–527.
Williams, Robert W., Jr. "Martin Behrman and New Orleans Civic Development, 1904–1920." *Louisiana History: The Journal of the Louisiana Historical Association* 2, no. 4 (Autumn 1961): 373–400.
Willoughby, Christopher D. E. *Masters of Health: Racial Science and Slavery in U.S. Medical Schools.* Chapel Hill: University of North Carolina Press, 2022.
Willoughby, Urmi Engineer. *Yellow Fever, Race, and Ecology in Nineteenth-Century New Orleans.* Baton Rouge: Louisiana State University Press, 2017.
Winant, Gabriel. *The Next Shift: The Fall of Industry and the Rise of Health Care in Rust Belt America.* Cambridge, MA: Harvard University Press, 2021.
Woodruff, Emily. "High Lead Levels at Old Incinerator Site in Central City Trigger Residents' Fears." *Times Picayune*, August 9, 2019.
Worthy, Tyree. "St. Thomas Opens New State of the Art Health Center in Gentilly." *Gentilly Messenger*, September 4, 2017.
Wynes, Charles E. "Dr. James Durham, Mysterious Eighteenth-Century Black Physician: Man or Myth." *Pennsylvania Magazine of History and Biography* 103, no. 3 (July 1979): 325–333.
Zigmond, J., and A. Robeznieks. "Still in Recovery." *Modern Health Care* 36, no. 33 (August 2006): 6–7.

Index

Note: Page numbers in italics refer to figures.

Accreditation Council for Graduate Medical Education, 213
Adams, William, 119, 121, 131–132, 133, 135–136, 175–176
Adkins-Jackson, Paris, 213
Affordable Care Act (2010), 3, 206–207
African Communities League, 193
Aid to Families with Dependent Children (AFDC), 184
Alexander, W. W., 106, 108
Algiers-Fischer (neighborhood), 170, 172
Algiers Point, 208
Almonaster y Roxas, Don Andres de, 20, 24
Alvin, Hubert, 138–139
American College of Surgeons, 109, 119
American Federation of Musicians (AFM), 185
American Medical Association, 88–89, 109, 112, 113, 119, 132, 136
American Missionary Association, 54, 61, 65, 66, 105
Andres (child), 24
anemia, 168, 171; sickle cell, 169, 173, 178, 179, 184, 185
anesthesia, 43
Aram, Marie, 24
Aron, Jack, 155
Aron Charitable Foundation, 163
Ashley, Samuel S., 66
asthma, 2; racial disparities and, 3, 192, 209
Atomic Energy Commission, 95
Augusta, Ga., 12

B. W. Cooper (neighborhood), 87, 115, 116
Baltimore, 11, 86, 184
bananas, 82
Banks, William, 63–64
Bankston, Jesse, 152
Barbara Ann (enslaved woman), 28–29
Bartholomew, Harland, 86
Bass, C. C., 92–94, 109, 156
Baton Rouge General Hospital, 133
Battle of Liberty Place (1874), 70, 71, 72
Beard, Cornelius, 40–42, 49, 63, 69, 70, 72
Beard, J. A., 27, 28
Beasley, Joseph, 171
Behrman, Martin, 90
Bellevue Hospital, 20
Beluche, Renato, 38
Bennett, J. Jefferson, 155, 157
Bensadon, Joseph, 36
BioDistrict, 11, 16, 195, 203, 204, 212, 215, 216
Biomedical Research and Development Park, 198
Birmingham, Ala., 155
Black Codes, 13, 19, 31, 60, 71
Black Panther Party (BPP), 15, 150, 169, 173–174, 193, 194
Blanco, Kathleen, 191, 200, 202
bleeding, 43, 44
Bloomenthal, Dan, 139, 140
Blue Cross Blue Shield, 199
Boggs, Hale, 152
Bonilla-Silva, Eduardo, 6
Bonin, Garland, 136–137
Boston Club, 71
Bowles, Ferris, 193
Bozeman, Nathan, 43–44, 63
Braden, Henry, 162
Brazile-Brown, Elsie, 139
Brent House Hotel, 145

Brickell, D. Warren, 40, 49, 63, 64, 66–67; Africans disparaged by, 27; Battle of Liberty Place viewed by, 70, 72; racist experiments by, 41–42, 43–45
Broadmoor (neighborhood), 82
bronchitis, 28
Brown, John, 29
Brown, Marguerite, 131
Brown v. Board of Education (1954), 125, 130, 156
Bruns, J, Dickson, 63, 69–72
Buchanan v. Warley (1917), 86
Burnside, John, 38
Business Council of New Orleans, 199
Butler, Keith, 180
Butler, Vera, 204
Butts, John, 41
Bywater (neighborhood), 182, 208
Bywater Hospital, 182, 190

Calliope Projects, 115, 116, 169
Campbell, G. W., 35
Cao, Anh, 203
Cabell, Walter, 36
Camp Parapet, 53
cancer, 2, 110, 191–192; racial disparities and, 3, 209
Caricabura, Arrieta, and Company, 38
Carl Mackley Houses, 114
Carnegie Foundation, 89
Carrollton (neighborhood), 172, 208
Cartwright, Samuel D., 26–27, 29, 41, 56, 97, 129
Castle, Callie, 134
cataracts, 42
catarrh, 28
Cely (enslaved person), 28
Cenas, August, 39
Centers for Disease Control and Prevention, 2–3
Central Business District, 34, 35, 53, 63, 82, 88, 211
Central City (neighborhood), 14, 68, 170, 208; Black medical district in, 98–104, 105; exclusionary zoning in, 87; hospital proposed for, 79, 80; poverty and health problems in, 168, 169; slum clearance in, 114–116, 157, 158
Chaille, Stanford, 35
Chalmette General Hospital, 144
Charity Hospital, 156, 215, 218, 219; Black and indigent patients at, 3–5, 12, 15, 16, 62–63, 69, 72, 75, 94, 97, 112, 131, 150, 151, 153, 161–167, 177, 182, 185–189, 210, 212; decline and closure of, 15–16, 150, 162–163, 173, 176, 180, 185–186, 188–191, 195–196, 203, 212; dental care at, 171; emergency room overused at, 187, 190; growth of, 84, 85, 92, 114, 116, 149; HEAL funds received by, 157, 159; immigrants as patients at, 12, 35, 37, 39, 69; after Katrina, 196–198, 202, 208; inaccessibility of, 182; LHCA takeover of, 188; LSU vs., 16, 155, 191, 195–200, 202, 205, 212; maximum income restrictions at, 39, 75, 111; medical school of, 64, 67; medical schools linked to, 40–42, 45, 85, 144; nursing program of, 93, 131; under occupation, 59–61; opening of, 19–20; poor reputation of, 34; racism and desegregation at, 4, 13, 15, 51, 56–57, 59–61, 63, 70, 72–73, 90–91, 95, 97, 101, 123–124, 130, 131, 134–135, 137–141, 145, 159, 174, 210; relocation of, 82; slave trade linked to, 13, 18–25, 27, 30, 33, 37–39, 43; staffing of, 108, 122; training at, 35, 66
Charity Hospital Medical College, 64, 67
Charles, Robert, 73
Charleston, S.C., 12, 34
Chataubaudaux, Thimoleon de, 24
Chaumette, Joseph, 47, 48, 76, 120
Chicago Defender, 109
Children's Hospital, 125
cholera, 28, 31, 39, 53, 55–56, 57
Choppin, Samuel, 40, 42, 63, 69–72
Circus Street Infirmary, 35, 63, 82
Citizens' Committee of New Orleans, 133
Citizens' Council, 9, 128–130
City Hospital for Mental Diseases, 82
civic improvement leagues, 8

Civil Rights Act (1964), 14, 123, 142, 143, 148, 164–166, 211; hospitals covered by, 1, 9, 134; Medicare and Medicaid linked to, 136; resistance to, 137, 140, 149
Civil Rights cases (1883), 73
civil rights movement, 123–148
Clark, Joseph, 99–100
Clark, Mary, 202
Clark, S. D. M., 96
Coca-Cola Company, 147
Code Noir, 13, 19, 22, 23
coffee, 82
Cohen, Walter L., 79, 80
Coker, Raleigh, 104, 120
Cole, D. R., 33
Colored Hospital, 14, 100–103
Colored Hospital Association, 80, 102–103, 109
Comiskey, James, 158
Common Ground (health clinic), 193–195, 206
Community Chest, 105, 112, 118
Community Improvement Agency (CIA), 157
Company of the Indies, 19, 21, 22; during slave trade, 23
La Concorde (fraternal organization), 68
Confederate Memorial Hospital (Shreveport), 134–135
"contraband camps," 53
Cook, Rosezella, 164
Cook, Samuel, 179–180
Cook v. Ochsner (1970), 165–166
Cooper, Deirdre Owens, 42–43
Corps d'Afrique Hospital, 52, 54, 55, 59
cotton, 30
Council on Medical Education, 89
Covey, Herbert, 28
COVID-19 pandemic, 1–2, 16, 212
Cozey, Henry, 28
Creoles, 47, 49, 67–68, 120
Crescent City Regiment, 71
Crisis (periodical), 105, 106, 109
critical race theory, 6

Crow, Scott, 193
The Crusader (newspaper), 76–77
Cuyamel Fruit, 84

Daughters of Charity, 185, 188
Davis (hospital supervisor), 142
Davis, A. L., 131
Davis, Viola, 132
deBoisblanc, Ben, 196
de Boré, Jean Etienne, 37–38
Delgado Hospital, 85, 184, 199
dementia, 31
Dennar, Princess, 213
Dent, Edgar, 108, 109, 110, 112–114, 117, 118
dental care, 111, 171
DePaul Hospital, 63, 208
depression of 1873, 62
Desire (neighborhood), 15, 150, 169, 170, 173–174, 192, 193, 208
diabetes, 2, 3, 178, 179, 192, 209
diarrhea, 28, 53, 55, 57
Dillard, James Hardy, 106
Dillard University, 104–106, 118, 150, 153, 154; Flint Goodridge sold by, 175–176, 178–180; nursing program at, 99, 117, 178; origins of, 103
diphtheria, 111, 168
Disproportionate Share Hospital (DSH) funding, 189
dissection, 42
Doctor Hospitals Group Inc. (DHGI), 178–180
Domingo (hospital worker), 24
Dove, Robert, 46
Dowling, John, 149, 158
Dubuclet, Antoine, 67
Dubuclet, Eugene, 67
Duc de Noaille (ship), 21
"dumping" of patients, 162, 163, 186, 189
Durham, James, 24, 46–47, 120
dysentery, 21, 28, 30, 35, 53, 55, 57

Eagle Life Insurance Company, 104
Ear, Eye, Nose, and Throat Hospital, 79, 82, 93, 143, 157, 198

East Jefferson General Hospital, 144, 166, 196, 197
Economic Opportunity Corporation (EOC), 170–171
Edna Pilsbury Health Center, 170
Edwards, John Bel, 207
Ellender, Allen, 130
Emancipation Proclamation (1863), 52
Embree, Edwin, 105, 107, 109
emergency medical services (EMS), 184
Emergency Medical Treatment and Active Labor Act (1986), 186
environmental racism, 167, 191
Epps, Edwin, 18
Ezekiel (enslaved man), 29

Family Health Inc., 171, 172
Fauci, Anthony, 2
Federal Emergency Management Agency (FEMA), 196, 201, 202–203
federally qualified health centers (FQHCs), 195, 206–207
Federation of Civic Leagues, 91, 102
Fenner, Darwin S., 156
Fenner, Erasmus Darwin, 33, 40, 42, 65, 73, 156; death of, 64; racist experiments by, 41, 44, 45
Fett, Sharla, 28
First District Baptist Association, 78, 79
Fishbein, Morris, 91–92, 95
Flexner, Abraham, 89
Flexner Report (1910), 78, 89
Flint, John, 75, 90
Flint Goodridge Hospital, 74–75, 77, 79–81, 88, 89, 94, 111, 112, 116, 122, 167; Black physicians employed by, 126, 133, 136, 165, 175; decline of, 15, 113, 118–119, 149, 150–154, 176–180, 185–186; desegregation and, 124–127; Dillard linked to, 104; expansion plans of, 100, 101, 103, 114, 115, 117, 121, 123, 124, 125, 151–154; Hill-Burton and HEAL funds denied to, 124, 125, 145, 157, 162, 211–212; initial challenges to, 105–109; opening of, 3, 14, 52, 76, 82, 90, 99, 107; public health advances of, 121, 126; "racial uplift" movement embraced by, 109–110; relocation of, 104; white physicians' exodus from, 152–153
Flint Medical College, 74–77, 80, 211; closure of, 88–89, 104, 108, 114, 117, 120, 161; nursing program of, 93; opening of, 14, 82
Flood, William, 38–39
flooding, 50, 53, 73, 86, 88
Florida (neighborhood), 170
folk medicine, 46, 48, 49
Fort Jackson, 53
Foster, Dayle, 132
Foster, Mike, 189, 198
Foster, Thomas, 36
Foundation for Historical Louisiana, 204
Fourteenth Amendment, 60
Francisco (child), 24
Franklin Infirmary, 34–35
Frederick, T. Rivers, 102, 108, 119, 120
Frederick Douglass Memorial Hospital, Philadelphia, 107, 108
Freedmen's Bureau, 54–59, 65
Freedmen's Hospital, 13, 55, 57, 59, 60–61, 69, 210
Freedmen's Savings and Trust Company, 53
French Hospital, 63, 93
French Quarter, 34
Freret (neighborhood), 81
Frohm, Jessie, 123, 131

Galathe, M. A., 1
Gamble, Vanessa Northington, 10
Gayllard (hospital worker), 24
Geddes, Joseph, 99
Gentilly (neighborhood), 84, 104, 106, 145, 208
gentrification, 204–205, 206, 215, 216
German Coast uprising (1811), 31
Gert Town (neighborhood), 203
G.I. Bill (1944), 144
glaucoma, 171
Goldstein, Moises, 106
Gordon, Jean, 96
Gordon, Jeff, 139

Gordon, Kate, 84, 95–97
Gordon Plaza, 192
Great Depression, 91, 111–113, 119, 153
Greater New Orleans Biosciences Economic Development District, 198
Greater New Orleans Community Health Connection (GNOCHC), 206, 207
Greater New Orleans Health Planning Group, 199
Great Migration, 121
Great Society, 156, 159, 172, 182
"the Group," 131, 133
Guimbilotte, Oscar, 47, 48

Haiti, 25, 31
Haley, Oretha Castle, 134, 185
Hall, Gwendolyn Midlo, 22
Hardin, Joseph, 90, 120, 131
Harmon v. Tyler (1927), 86
Harris, E. H., 56
Harrison, John, 39
Hathaway Home for the Poor and Friendless, 61
Health Education Authority of Louisiana (HEAL), 154–160, 182, 203, 220; biosciences district likened to, 198, 199; Black residents and businesses displaced by, 15, 149, 158, 159, 215; LSU's and Tulane's support for, 155; Tulane aided by, 160, 176, 181, 211
Health Insurance Connector, 201
health maintenance organizations (HMOs), 181
Healthy Start Initiative, 207
heart disease, 2; racial disparities and, 3, 110, 192, 209
Heath, T. Restin, 101–102
Henderson, Stephen, 38
Hibernia National Bank, 147
Higgins Industries, 146
Hill-Burton Act (Hospital Survey and Construction Act, 1946), 8, 12, 14, 123, 131–134, 144, 165, 175; bed quota of, 162; conditions attached to, 166; Flint Goodridge denied funds under, 124, 125, 145, 154, 211–212; Methodist Hospital funds from, 145, 147; NAACP litigation over, 9
Hine, Darlene Clark, 10
Hines, Dr., 18
Hirsch, Arnold, 8
HIV/AIDS, 2, 3, 184, 191, 192, 209
Hoffman Triangle (neighborhood), 2, 209
Hollier, Larry, 205
Home for the Incurables, 142
Home Owners' Loan Corporation, 92
Horowitz, Andy, 5
Hospital Affiliates International (HAI), 161, 181
Hotel Dieu (University Hospital), 63, 93, 157, 191, 197–198, 200; desegregation resisted by, 159, 165; enslaved patients at, 36, 37, 45, 51, 52, 61, 62; free Blacks barred from, 52, 54; LHCA purchase and renaming of, 188–189; opening of, 34–35, 82
Housing Act (1937), 114
Housing Authority of New Orleans (HANO), 151, 154, 167, 169, 192
Howard, Oliver O., 55
Howard University, 65, 89, 113, 120, 122
Hull, Ellis, Jr., 142–143
Humana Inc., 179
Human Relations Council, 139, 164
Hunt, Thomas, 39
Hurricane Betsy (1965), 146, 150
Hurricane Katrina (2005), 5, 15, 160, 176, 187, 192–208
hypertension, 171, 178, 184, 209

Illinois Central Railroad, 82, 182
Industrial Canal, 145
infant mortality, 2, 30, 62, 121, 154; racial disparities and, 3, 74, 110, 168, 192, 209
Ingalls, T. R., 39
Intercoastal Waterway, 145
Intracoastal Mississippi River–Gulf Outlet Canal, 145
Irish Channel (neighborhood), 170, 208
Irwin, Emmet Lee, 94, 128–129, 132, 213
Isolation Hospital, 82

J. Aron Charitable Foundation, 163
Jamaica, 24
Jefferson, Thomas, 129
Jeunes Amis (fraternal organization), 68, 69
Jindal, Bobby, 189, 207, 208
Jinks (enslaved person), 28
John (enslaved man), 29
John Dibert Tuberculosis Hospital, 84, 85, 97
Johns Hopkins University, 107
Johnson, Andrew, 58
Johnson, Lyndon, 134, 136, 154, 156
Johnson, Rashauna, 37
Johnson, Sharon, 193
Johnson, Walter, 28
Joint Commission of Hospital Accreditation, 119
Joly, Joseph, 48
Joly, Nicola, 48
Jones, A. P., 42
Jones, Kyle, 213
Jones, Lois, 138
Jones, R. E., 99
Jones, Virginia, 140–141
Josefa Segunda (slave ship), 38, 39
Joseph (carpenter), 24
Josephine (patient), 61
Juana (hospital worker), 24
Jung, Rodney C., 135, 170

Karenga, Maulana, 193
Kearsley, John, Jr., 46
Keeler, Mystis, 139
Keller, Rosa, 125, 127
Kellogg, William Pitt, 69–70
Kendig, Bernard, 27, 36
Kennedy, John A., 133
Kiblinger, Ada, 96
kidney disease, 209
King, Martin Luther, Jr., 142
Kitty (enslaved woman), 28
Knight, H. W., 105
Knights of Pythias, 88, 94–95
Koelemay, John, 146, 147
Kolhmeyer, Charles, Jr., 151

LaBranche, Emile, 99
Lafitte (neighborhood), 115, 169
Lakeview (neighborhood), 209
Lakeside Hospital for Women, 144
Lakeview Regional Medical Center, 144
Landrieu, Mary, 203
Landrieu, Moon, 158, 170, 173
Landry, Eldridge, 232–233n8
Landry, L. B., 80, 120
Landry, Oliver, 232–233n8
Landry, Pierre, 232–233n8
Latin America, 82, 84, 93, 156, 210
Latino Outreach Project, 194
Laveau, Marie, 48
LCMC Health, 203, 205–206
lead poisoning, 2, 167–169, 184, 192
Leavitt, Mike, 200, 201
Legha, Rupinder, 213
Leland University, 65
life expectancy, 2, 49–50, 192, 209, 210
Lifemark Company, 182, 190
Lincoln, Abraham, 60
Lizzy (enslaved woman), 28
Logan, Samuel, 70
London, Katherine, 131
Long, Earl, 125
Long, Gretchen, 10, 120
Long, Huey, 85, 91, 92
Louis, Jean, 19–20
Louisiana Anti-Tuberculosis League, 84
Louisiana Board of Health, 97
Louisiana Board of Nurse Examiners, 114
Louisiana Dental Association, 156
Louisiana Health Care Authority (LHCA), 188–189
Louisiana Health Care Redesign Collective, 200, 201
Louisiana Life Insurance Company, 119
Louisiana Native Guard, 52
Louisiana State College, 65
Louisiana State Medical Society, 156
Louisiana State University (LSU), 113, 119, 155–157, 185, 189, 199–205; Charity Hospital closure sought by, 16, 155, 191, 195–200, 202, 205, 212; desegregation

resisted by, 159; growth of, 92, 215; medical school of, 85, 116–117, 122, 127, 131, 132, 149, 198
Lower Ninth Ward, 153, 154, 170, 177, 182
Loyola University, 185
Lucas, George, 80, 90, 120, 131
Luis (child), 24
Luzenberg, Charles A., 34, 39
Luzenberg Hospital, 63
Lying-in Hospital, 82
lynching, 73

Mackie, J. Monroe, 35, 39
MacLean, Basil, 118, 119
Macy Foundation, 163
Magdalena (hospital worker), 24
Magnolia Projects, 114–115, 116, 169, 177
Maison de Santé, 34
Making the Second Ghetto (Hirsch), 8
malaria, 25, 26, 62, 83, 84
Mallalieu, Willard Francis, 75, 76
Mallow, James, 79
malnutrition, 30, 50, 54, 168, 171
Maria (child), 24
Marigny (neighborhood), 68, 208
Marine Hospital, 55, 60, 72, 93, 182
Marr, Robert, 70
Martinet, Louis, 76
Mary, Charles, 141
Matas, Rudolph, 97
maternal mortality, 2, 119, 168, 192
Mattingly, C. Walter, 127
Mayo, Sara, 96
McBride, David, 10
McEnery, John, 70, 72
McKenna, Dwight, 180
measles, 28
Mechanics' Institute Massacre (1866), 56–57
Medicaid, 4, 5, 9, 123, 136, 150–151, 162–167, 171, 187, 201, 206; Black institutions hurt by, 8; discrimination and, 7; expansion of, 16, 186, 195, 207, 212; racial integration mandated by, 14–15; reimbursements from, 15, 153, 176, 177, 180, 186, 189; state cuts in, 184

Medical College of Louisiana, 39–40
Medicare, 4, 5, 9, 123, 136, 150–151, 155, 161–167, 171, 187; Black institutions hurt by, 8; discrimination and, 7; racial integration mandated by, 14–15; reimbursements from, 15, 153, 176, 177, 180, 186, 189
Medicare for All, 3
Meharry College, 89, 113, 120, 122, 178
mental health, 154, 161, 172, 183, 207–208
Mercier, Alfred, 35
Mercy Hospital, 81, 165
Merrill Lynch, 147
Metairie Hospital, 144
Methodist Episcopal Church (MEC), 67, 75, 90, 101–102, 105
Methodist Hospital, 144–148, 150, 164, 187, 205
Michoud Assembly Facility, 145–146, 147, 148
Mid-City (neighborhood), 172, 203, 204, 208
midwifery, 48, 49, 110–111
Milan (neighborhood), 208
Militia (enslaved person), 28
Milliken Memorial Children's Hospital, 85
Milne Home for Destitute Girls, 96
Mobile, Ala., 12, 34
Model Cities program, 12, 15, 150, 153–154, 170–173, 185, 211
Modesty (enslaved woman), 29
Montane, John, 48–49
Moore, John, 29
Moore, Queen Mother, 193
Moore, Sarah, 28
Morial, Ernest, 133, 162, 183
Morrison, deLesseps, 125, 126
Mudge, Caroline, 76, 90
Murphy, Ellen, 79–80

Nagin, Ray, 201
Napoleon Bonaparte, emperor of the French, 25
Natchez revolt (1729), 24
National Aeronautics and Space Administration (NAS), 145–146

National Association for the Advancement of Colored People (NAACP), 15, 86, 102, 123, 126, 131, 134, 135, 138–143, 149, 164–166, 175; attacks on, 129, 132; Hill-Burton litigation by, 9; physicians in, 80, 90, 91, 120, 133; separate Black hospitals opposed by, 109
National Industrial Recovery Act (1933), 91, 114
National Institutes of Health, 160, 163
National League of Nursing Education, 114
National Legal Program on Health Programs of the Poor, 164
National Medical Association, 132, 136
National Medical Enterprises (NME), 175–176, 179
National Negro Health Week, 100
National Organization for Public Health Nursing, 114
National Recovery Administration, 111
National Tenants Organization, 164
Neighborhood Development Program (NDP), 158
Neighborhood Health Council Concerning Health Services, 171–172
Nelson, Alondra, 169
Newman, James T., 61, 66–67, 72, 75, 78–80, 102, 103, 120
Newman, Philip, 79
New Orleans Adolescent Hospital, 208
New Orleans Dispensary, 79
New Orleans East (neighborhood), 16, 145–148, 187, 205, 208
New Orleans Health Corporation, 172
New Orleans Health Department (NOHD), 167–170, 172–173, 182–185, 186–187, 199, 207, 211
New Orleans Hospital and Dispensary for Women, 93
New Orleans Improvement Association (NOIA), 132, 175
New Orleans Medical College, 75–76
New Orleans Medical News and Hospital Gazette, 42, 43, 44–45, 49
New Orleans Musicians' Clinic, 185, 206

New Orleans Regional Medical Center, 198
New Orleans School of Medicine, 33, 40, 41, 44, 64–65, 71
New Orleans School of Tropical Medicine and Hygiene, 84
New Orleans Sickle Cell Anemia Foundation, 185
New Orleans Tribune, 47, 67
New Orleans Tuberculosis League, 84, 97
New Orleans University, 65, 75, 78, 103–104, 109, 211
Nicholls, Francis, 72
Nickerson, F. S., 53
Ninth Ward, 88, 153, 154, 169, 170, 177, 182
Nixon, Richard, 159, 172, 181, 183
Northup, Solomon, 17–18
nursing, 48, 93, 101, 107, 114, 117–118, 178, 214
nursing homes, 181

obstetrics and gynecology, 43
Ochsner, Alton, 127, 129, 144
Ochsner Foundation Hospital, 4, 185, 187, 199, 200, 201; construction of, 125; growth of, 5, 15, 144, 150, 163, 176, 181–182, 198, 211; after Katrina, 196, 197; origins of, 144–145; racial discrimination by, 1, 2, 212
Odom, Charles, 137
Ogden, Fred, 69, 72
O'Keefe, Arthur J., 103
Olivarius, Kathryn Meyer McAllister, 49
Orleans Anti-Tuberculosis Hospital, 84, 97
Orleans Infirmary, 63
Orleans Parish Medical Society (OPMS): Blacks barred from, 51, 94, 108, 119, 127, 129, 135, 136, 210; Charity Hospital expansion and, 91, 187–188; desegregation opposed by, 128, 135; Methodist Hospital and, 146; origins of, 72; race-specific data collection opposed by, 137
Osetors, Ben, 61
Our Lady of the Lake Hospital, 133
Owners and Tenants Association of Greater New Orleans (OTAGNO), 149, 158, 159

Page, Charles, 48
Panama-Pacific Exposition (1915), 83
patent medicines, 32
Paugi (hospital worker), 24
Peck, David, 47, 48
Pedro (carpenter), 24
People's Action Center, 164
People's Free Clinic, 15, 150, 173
People's Institute for Survival and Beyond, 211
Peniston, Anthony, 26, 40, 41
Perez, Leander, 130
Performing Arts Medicine Association, 185
Perier, Étienne, 22
Perron, Myrtle, 138
Phillip (carpenter), 24
Phyllis Wheatley clubs, 75
Phyllis Wheatley Sanitarium and Training Hospital for Nurses, 75
Pilsbury Health Center, 170
Plessy v. Ferguson (1896), 73, 77
pneumonia, 28, 43, 44, 55, 57, 69, 110
Potens, Aimee, 47, 48
Poydras, Julien de Lallande, 38
preferred provider organizations (PPOs), 181
prenatal care, 110, 171
Presbyterian Hospital, 81, 82, 93, 96
Press Park, 192
PricewaterhouseCoopers, 200
Pritchett, Jonathan, 35–36
Provident Hospital, Baltimore, 107–108, 109
Provident Hospital, Chicago, 107, 109
Provident Sanitarium and Nurse Training School, 78, 80–81, 104
Public Works Administration (PWA), 8, 9, 91–92, 94, 108, 114–117
Pythian Temple, 88, 94, 95

Rahim, Malik, 193–195
Rand Corporation, 199
Reagan, Ronald, 182, 183–184
Reconstruction, 6, 51, 60, 69, 71, 72
Redeemers, 72
redhibition, 22, 28–29, 30, 210
Reynolds, Eliza, 141

Reynolds, Joseph, 141
Richard, H. J., 42
Richard Milliken Memorial Children's Hospital, 85
Richardson, Tobias, 64
rickets, 29, 30
RMJM Hiller, 204
Road Home program, 204
Robert (free Black man), 17
Roberts, Samuel, Jr., 10
Rockefeller Foundation, 101, 105, 108
Roman, Andre, 32
Roosevelt, Franklin, 91
Rosenwald, Julius, 106–107, 112
Rosenwald Fund, 105, 108–110, 112, 113, 117–118, 161
Rosette (hospital worker), 24
Roudanez, Charles Louis, 47, 48, 67, 68, 76, 120
Royal Hospital, 12, 18–19, 20, 22–23
Rush, Benjamin, 46
Russell, William Howard, 32

St. Bernard (neighborhood), 169, 170
St. Bernard General Hospital, 144
St. Claude (neighborhood), 182
St. Phillip (refugee camp), 53
St. Roch (neighborhood), 208
St. Tammany Parish Hospital, 144
St. Thomas (neighborhood), 169
St. Thomas Health Services Clinic, 185
St. Thomas Housing Redevelopment Council, 185
Salvaggio, John, 95
Sanders, James, 141–142
San Francisco, 11
Sarah Goodridge Hospital, 76
Sara Mayo Hospital, 135, 136
Savannah, Ga., 34
Savitt, Todd, 10
Schiro, Victor, 133, 135, 139, 145, 146–147, 148, 170
Schor, Kenneth, 146
scientific racism, 9, 13, 19, 44, 45, 63, 65, 128–130, 213

scurvy, 21, 54
Seventh Ward, 208
Seventh Ward Civic League, 100
Sibley, A. O., 36
sickle cell anemia, 169, 173, 178, 179, 184, 185
Simkins v. Moses H. Cone Memorial Hospital (1963), 132, 134
Sims, J. Marion, 43
Sisters of Charity, 34, 37, 63, 185
"slave hospitals," 7, 12, 13, 32–35, 45, 63, 209
Slidell Memorial Hospital, 144
Sloan Foundation, 163
"slum clearance," 14, 92, 100, 114–116, 157, 158, 203–204, 218
smallpox, 17, 18, 39, 42; deaths from, 25, 53, 55, 57; hospitalization for, 21, 54, 57, 63; inoculation against, 32, 46
Smith, E. Bathurst, 39
Smith, Howard, 70
Smith, James McCune, 47, 48
Smith, Susan, 10
Smyth, Andrew, 63–64
Soublet, Brenda, 139
Soublet, Louis, 139
Souchon, Edmond, 63–64, 65, 73
Southern Baptist Hospital, 81, 165
Southern Bell Telephone, 147
Southern Historical Society, 71
Southern University, 131
Spelman College, 114
Spirit of Charity (clinic), 196–197
Stafford, Ethelred, 79
Stallings, Olive, 79
sterilization, 96
Stern, Edgar, 99, 108, 112, 119, 125
Stevens, Gerald, 179
Stone, Warren, 34, 71
Stone's Infirmary, 63, 82
Straight University, 61, 65–67, 78, 103–104, 211
stroke, 2, 192
sugarcane, 25, 30
Surgical and Women's Hospital, 63
syphilis, 110

Tebault, Charles, 70
Tenet Healthcare Corporation, 181, 196
Thomas, George, Jr., 127, 177
Thomas, Samuel, 54
Times Picayune, 97–98
Tiocou, François, 23–24
Toledano, Christopher, 51
Total Community Action (TCA), 169–170, 172
tourism, 7, 9, 11, 82, 210
Touro, Judah, 36
Touro Infirmary, 45, 63, 79, 125, 203; Blacks barred from, 61; HMO formed by, 181; after Katrina, 197; opening of, 35, 93; slave trade linked to, 27, 29, 30, 35–36, 62
Tremé (neighborhood), 34, 68, 115, 157, 172
transfusions, 42
tuberculosis, 50, 73, 83, 95, 154, 168–169, 184; deaths from, 55, 62, 69, 74, 84, 97, 110; hospitalization for, 57; public health campaigns against, 9, 84, 96–97; racial disparities and, 130; treatment for, 110
Tuberculosis and Public Health Association of Louisiana, 110
Tuberculosis Committee of New Orleans, 110
Tulane Gravier (neighborhood), 157, 159, 201, 204; housing discrimination in, 92; medical district in, 15, 37, 82, 88, 104, 116, 149, 211
Tulane/HCA, 181
Tulane University (University of Louisiana), 16, 40, 66, 70–71, 116, 122, 185, 190, 199; anatomical museum of, 65; Blacks barred from, 13, 73, 51–52, 78, 119, 132, 145; Civil War occupation of, 64; hospital of, 4, 15, 85, 149, 155–156, 157, 159, 160–163, 176, 187, 189, 196–198; opening of, 39, 82, 67; public health at, 84, 178; tropical medicine at, 94
Tureaud, A. P., 14, 123, 131, 132
Turner, Jack, 28
Tuskegee Institute, 100
Twelve Years a Slave (Northup), 17, 18
typhoid, 31, 83, 84
typhoid pneumonia, 43, 44

Unified New Orleans Plan, 201
L'Union (newspaper), 47
Union Cotton Press, 38
Union of New Orleans Musicians, 185
United Confederate Veterans, 71
United Farm Workers, 169
U.S. Life Insurance, Annuity and Trust Company, 36
U.S. Marine Hospital, 55, 60, 72, 93, 182
US Organization, 193
U.S. Public Health Service, 117, 160, 199
Unity Industrial Life, 104
Universal Health Services, 181
Universal Negro Improvement Association, 193
University of Alabama, 155
University Medical Center New Orleans (UMCNO), 11, 204–205, 212, 215
University of Chicago, 107
University of Maryland, 107–108
University of New Orleans, 198
University of Pennsylvania, 108
Upper Ninth Ward, 182
Uptown (neighborhood), 208

VA Hospital, 11, 143, 157, 200, 201–202, 203
Valsin (enslaved man), 51
Van Holm, Eric Joseph, 205
La Venus (ship), 22
vesicovaginal fistula, 43
Vining, Ruby, 120
voodoo, 48

wages, for health care professionals, 214–215
Wagner Act (1935), 115
Wailoo, Keith, 10
Wakefield-Paillet, Emma, 76
Walden R. B., 134–135
Walmsley, T. Semmes, 106

Walsh, John, 155
Ward, E. H., 99
Ward, Thomas, Jr., 10
Warehouse District, 88
Warmoth, Henry Clay, 60, 66, 69
Warren, Charles, 57–59
Washington, Booker T., 91, 100
Weil, C. C., 118, 121, 125
Wellman, Creighton, 84
West, George, 46
West, Gordon, 134
West Jefferson General Hospital, 144, 166, 196, 197
White Citizens' Council, 9, 128–130
"white flight" hospitals, 5, 15, 124, 143–148, 150, 187
White League, 9, 52, 65, 69–72, 129
whooping cough, 28, 111, 168
Williams, Marie, 131
women's rights, 96
Woodside Dairy, 104
Works Progress Administration (WPA), 14, 116, 203–204, 218
worms, 31
WWOZ (radio station), 185
Wyczalkowski, Christopher, 205

Xavier University, 178, 198

yellow fever, 26, 35, 41, 47, 73, 84; deaths from, 25, 36, 39, 49, 57, 62, 74; sanitation problems linked to, 83
Young Female Benevolent Association, 68
Young Lords, 169
Yun, Myeong-Su, 35–36

Zemurray, Samuel, 84
zoning, 86–88, 167

www.ingramcontent.com/pod-product-compliance
Lightning Source LLC
Chambersburg PA
CBHW020257140125
20345CB00002B/62